Peripheral Nerve Disorders 2

Blue Books of Practical Neurology
(*Volumes 1–14 published as BIMR Neurology*)

Peripheral Nerve Disorders 2

Edited by

Arthur K. Asbury MD
University of Pennsylvania School of Medicine,
Philadelphia, Pennsylvania, USA

and

P. K. Thomas CBE, MD, DSc
Royal Free Hospital School of Medicine and Institute of Neurology,
University of London, UK

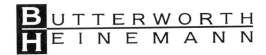

Butterworth-Heinemann Ltd
Linacre House, Jordan Hill, Oxford OX2 8DP

ℛ A member of the Reed Elsevier plc group

OXFORD   LONDON   BOSTON
MUNICH   NEW DELHI   SINGAPORE   SYDNEY
TOKYO   TORONTO   WELLINGTON

First published 1995

© Butterworth-Heinemann Ltd 1995

British Library Cataloguing in Publication Data
A catalogue record for this book is available from the British Library

ISBN 0 7506 1765 9

Library of Congress Cataloging in Publication Data
A catalogue record for this book is available from the Library of Congress

Typeset by Keyword Typesetting Services Ltd, Wallington, Surrey
Printed in Great Britain at the University Press, Cambridge

Contents

Contributors

A. K. Asbury MD
University of Pennsylvania School of Medicine, 290 John Morgan Building, Philadelphia, PA 19104-6055, USA

C. F. Bolton MD, FRCP(C)
Clinical Neurological Sciences, Victoria Hospital, London, Ontario N6A 4G5 Canada

P. F. Chance MD
Division of Neurology, The Children's Hospital of Philadelphia, and Department of Neurology and Pediatrics, University of Pennsylvania School of Medicine, Philadelphia, PA 19104-6055, USA

D. R. Cornblath MD
Department of Neurology, Pathology 627b, The Johns Hopkins University School of Medicine, Baltimore, MD 21287, USA

J. W. Griffin MD
Department of Neurology, Meyer 6-109, Johns Hopkins Hospital, 600 N Wolfe Street, Baltimore, MD 21287, USA
(alternative address: Johns Hopkins University School of Medicine, Baltimore)

A. E. Harding MD, FRCP
University Department of Clinical Neurology, Institute of Neurology, Queen Square, London WC1N 3BG, UK

R. A. C. Hughes MD, FRCP
Department of Neurology, UMDS, Guy's Hospital, London SE1 9RT, UK

J. R. Kaplan MD
Montefiore Medical Park, Department of Neurology, 1575 Blondell Avenue, Bronx, NY 10461, USA

N. Latov MD, PhD
Department of Neurology, Neurological Institute, 630 W 168th Street, New York, NY 10032, USA

C. J. Mathias DPhil, FRCP
Autonomic Unit, University Department of Clinical Neurology, National Hospital for Neurology and Neurosurgery and Institute of Neurology, Queen Square and Cardiovascular Medicine Unit, Department of Medicine, St Mary's Hospital Medical School/Imperial College of Science, Technology and Medicine, University of London, UK

J. C. McArthur MBBS, MPH
Department of Neurology, Meyer 6-109, The Johns Hopkins University School of Medicine, Baltimore, MD 21287, USA

J. L. Ochoa DSc, MD, PhD
Neuromuscular Disease Unit, Good Samaritan Hospital and Medical Centre, and Oregon Health Sciences Centre, 1040 NW 22nd Avenue Suite NSC-460, Portland, OR 97210, USA

D. E. Pleasure
Departments of Neurology and Pediatrics, University of Pennsylvania School of Medicine, Philadelphia, PA 19104-6055, USA

J. R. Pleasure MD
Department of Pediatrics, University of Pennsylvania School of Medicine, Philadelphia, PA 19104-6055, USA

M. M. Reilly MRCPI
University Department of Clinical Neurology, Institute of Neurology, The National Hospital, Queen Square, London WC1N 3BG, UK

G. Said
Department de Neurologie, Hôpital de Bicêtre (Université Paris-Sud), 78 rue du Général Leclerc, Le Kremlin Bicêtre 94270, France

H. H. Schaumburg MD
Department of Neurology, Forchheimer Room G-9, Albert Einstein College of Medicine, 1300 Morris Park Avenue, Bronx, NY 10461, USA

A. J. Steck
Kantonspital Basel, Neurologische Universitäts-Klinik, Petersgraben 4, CH-4035 Basel, Switzerland

P. K. Thomas CBE, MD, DSc
Department of Clinical Neurosciences, The Royal Free Hospital School of Medicine, Rowland Hill Street, London NW3 2PF, and University Department of Clinical Neurology, Institute of Neurology, Queen Square, London WC1N 3BG, UK

P. D. Thompson MB, PhD, FRACP
University Department of Medicine and Department of Neurology, Royal Adelaide
Hospital, Adelaide, South Australia

Series Preface

The *Blue Books of Practical Neurology* series is the new name for the *BIMR Neurology* series which was itself the successor to the *Modern Trends in Neurology* series. As before, the volumes are intended for use by physicians who grapple with the problems of neurological disorders on a daily basis, be they neurologists, neurologists in training, or those in related fields such as neurosurgery, internal medicine, psychiatry, and rehabilitation medicine.

Our purpose is to produce monographs on topics in clinical neurology in which progress through research has brought about new concepts of patient management. The subject of each monograph is selected by the Series Editors using two criteria: first, that there has been significant advance in knowledge in that area and, second, that such advances have been incorporated into new ways of managing patients with the disorders in question. This has been the guiding spirit behind each volume, and we expect it to continue. In effect we emphasize research, both in the clinic and in the experimental laboratory, but principally to the extent that it changes our collective attitudes and practices in caring for those who are neurologically afflicted.

C. D. Marsden
A. K. Asbury
Series Editors

Preface

In the 12 years since the publication of the first volume of *Peripheral Nerve Disorders*, the flow of new information on peripheral neuropathies has grown to a torrent. A few examples suffice to make the point. A number of neuropathies have been newly recognized, such as multifocal motor neuropathy, neuropathies associated with acquired immunodeficiency syndrome (AIDS), neuropathies associated with Borreliosis, and neuropathies due to previously uncharacterized neurotoxins (taxol and suramin, for example). The revolution in molecular genetics brought about by spectacular advances in recombinant DNA technology has resulted in the precise identification of many molecular genetic defects responsible for hereditary neuropathies. These powerful techniques have also generated a wave of new information concerning the role of neurotrophic factors and their receptors in the biology of peripheral nerve and insights into the cell biology of Wallerian degeneration.

Some neuropathies have essentially disappeared, such as those secondary to exposure to γ-diketone solvents, and those secondary to other neurotoxic substances no longer in current use, such as monomeric acrylamide, thalidomide, perhexilene and dimethylaminopropionitrile. Implementation of appropriate public health measures has been primarily responsible. A particular disorder, the axonal neuropathy associated with eosinophilia–myalgia syndrome, came and then disappeared when its basis was recognized as being due to ingestion of L-tryptophan, which was probably adulterated. Another transient epidemic in which peripheral nerve was affected, along with other tissues, was the Spanish oil syndrome.

Antibody-associated neuropathies and their pathogenesis in terms of immune mediation of peripheral nerve dysfunction have attracted intense interest, and also controversy. The role of circulating antibodies that bind to glycoconjugates continues to be the subject of major debate. Likewise, the neuromuscular disorders encountered in the setting of critical illnesses, sepsis and organ failure requiring intensive care have also attracted a great deal of attention.

From a therapeutic standpoint, the role of plasmapheresis has been firmly established in the management of Guillain–Barré syndrome. More recently, high-dose immunoglobulin therapy also has been demonstrated to be effective in the course of Guillain–Barré syndrome and further trials are nearing completion. Another important advance has come through the Diabetes Control and Complications Trial in the United States, which has established convincingly that strict glycaemic control produces a substantial reduction in the occurrence of diabetic neuropathy, although at the cost of an increased number of hypoglycaemic events. Indeed, one of the major advances of the recent decade has been the growing skill and experience in mounting successful, large scale, well-organized and properly designed clinical trials for the study of peripheral neuropathies and their treatment.

In this new volume, emphasis is placed on the advances of the past decade, and no attempt is made to rehash those subjects that were well covered in the first volume and for which relatively little progress has been made since. For instance, the chapter on compression and entrapment neuropathies by Harrison and Gilliatt in the first volume remains as cogent now as when it was first written in 1983.

Finally, it is with deep sadness and sense of loss that we acknowledge the untimely death in August, 1991 of Roger W. Gilliatt, co-editor of the first volume.

A. K. Asbury
P. K. Thomas

1
The clinical approach to neuropathy

A. K. Asbury and P. K. Thomas

INTRODUCTION

In this chapter we summarize our clinical approach to peripheral neuropathies. Particular emphasis is placed on the underlying logic and the sequence of thought used in evaluating the patient with neuropathy. Sets of principles do exist that guide the seasoned examiner of patients with peripheral neuropathies, but these are frequency unstated and simply chalked up to experience. It is our intent to state explicitly the principles and the logic sequence.

A second and related purpose is to place into context the more specialized chapters that follow, and to provide a framework through which they may be more readily understood and applied.

Third, some aspects of peripheral neuropathies have not changed much in the decade since the first volume was published. These areas are reviewed and brought up to date briefly as part of this chapter; they include focal neuropathies, nerve ischaemia, vasculitis and neuropathy, acquired amyloidosis and neuropathy, and the treatment of diabetic neuropathy. Those aspects of peripheral nerve disorders that are either new or in which our understanding has become rapidly enhanced through research are covered in more detail in succeeding chapters.

PATHOLOGICAL PROCESSES

Peripheral nerve is limited in the ways it can react to injury. When dealing with a particular patient with a neuropathy, it is helpful to ask which of the few known reactions of nerve is taking place. The major processes are:

(1) Wallerian degeneration (the response to transection);
(2) segmental demyelination;
(3) axonal atrophy and degeneration;
(4) primary disorders of nerve cell bodies.

The occurrence of paranodal or segmental demyelination is often referred to as myelinopathy. Conditions that cause axonal degeneration with preservation of the cell bodies are referred to as axonopathies; these include both Wallerian degeneration and axonal atrophy and degeneration. Primary disorders affecting the cell bodies that lead to death of the whole neuron are termed neuronopathies.

Wallerian degeneration

For Wallerian degeneration to occur, it must be preceded by physical interruption of an otherwise healthy axon or a group of axons, as in a nerve trunk. If a nerve trunk is severed, the most obvious changes occur distal to the transection site. Paralysis and anaesthesia in the distribution of the nerve trunk are immediate. Axons and myelin sheaths degenerate distal to the site of transection, and conduction fails in myelinated fibres within days, or longer for some unmyelinated axons. Regeneration from the proximal stump begins early but proceeds slowly, and recovery is variable, but may be both incomplete and dysfunctional.

Quality of recovery depends upon the extent of Schwann tube, nerve sheath and surrounding soft tissue destruction. Other factors include the proximodistal site of injury and the age of the individual. Although direct trauma to a nerve trunk is the usual cause of Wallerian degeneration, there are others. Nerve trunk ischaemia, whether focal or multifocal, may produce extensive distal degeneration if blood flow is critically reduced. As a general rule, nerve trunk ischaemia severe enough to produce focal axonal damage and distal Wallerian degeneration results from widespread pathological processes affecting small vessels and capillaries of the size of the vasa nervorum. Multifocal nerve trunk ischaemia, as occurs with systemic vasculitis, is a frequent basis for multiple mononeuropathy (mononeuropathy multiplex) encountered clinically.

Demyelination

Segmental demyelination means damage to myelin sheaths with sparing of axons. Conduction block is the functionally important expression of demyelination. An axon that is blocked displays a functional deficit as severe as if the axon were transected. Although nerve transection and conduction block may show similar degrees of paralysis or sensory deficit acutely, they differ in terms of outlook, degree of muscle wasting, tempo of recovery and electrophysiological properties. For instance, in demyelinating neuropathies, conduction block is often transient and remyelination may be rapid, measured in days or weeks, and is frequently complete. This is much more favorable and rapid than the course of recovery expected with Wallerian degeneration.

In the past, often-studied models of segmental demyelination in peripheral nerve were those produced by diphtheria toxin and lead salts. The lesion resulting from these intoxications was thought to be prototypical. Changes observed were widening of nodal gaps, paranodal retraction and breakdown of myelin, and eventual disintegration of whole internodes of myelin. But other ways have been described in which myelin sheath may be damaged as a primary event. For instance, with acute nerve compression, telescoping (intussusception) of myelin occurs at the nodes of Ranvier, representing a type of mechanical injury to myelin (Ochoa, 1980). With certain myelinotoxic agents such as hexachlorophene or triethyltin, striking oedema occurs with the myelin sheath. In other demyelinating neuropathies such as the Guillain–Barré syndrome, peeling and engulfment of myelin by activated macrophages at the nodes of Ranvier and at other sites along the internode are the pathological hallmarks. In sum, a variety of recognizable morphological patterns may converge with a common result – demyelination. The electrophysiological counterpart of all of these is qualitatively the same.

Secondary segmental demyelination also occurs. Here primary axonal changes, usually chronic shrinkage and atrophy, are attended by recurrent myelin breakdown and reconstitution. Along atrophic axons, uniform demyelinative–remyelinative changes occur over many consecutive internodes, in contrast to primary demyelinating processes which tend to show a random hit-or-miss distribution. Protracted axonal atrophy eventually leads to progressive breakdown and resorption of the axon, back to and including the parent nerve cell body. Axonal atrophy and secondary demyelination occur in some chronic polyneuropathies such as that associated with uraemia (Dyck *et al.*, 1971), in distal nerve fibres in chronic iminodiproprionitrile (IDPN) intoxication (Long *et al.*, 1980), in permanent axotomy (Dyck *et al.*, 1981) and in nerve fibres distal to chronic constriction (Baba *et al.*, 1982).

Axonal degeneration

Axonal degeneration implies a metabolic derangement within neurons which manifests as distal axonal breakdown. The clinical effect is that of a distal symmetric stocking–glove polyneuropathy with characteristic electrodiagnostic features which allow it to be distinguished from a demyelinating process. Although it has long been said that the longest and largest fibres are at risk, this rule is often breached when the details of polyneuropathies are examined. Exogenous toxins, systemic metabolic disorders and some inherited neuropathies are the usual cause of axonal degeneration of peripheral nerve, but the exact sequence of events in nerve tissue which culminates in axonal degeneration remains obscure.

Neuronopathy

Neuronopathy signifies primary destruction of the nerve cell body. Either the lower motor neuron or the primary sensory neuron may be affected. When the anterior horn cell is the target of disease, as in poliomyelitis or motor neuron disease, motor neuronopathy is the result. Sensory neuronopathy means damage to dorsal root ganglion cells, often resulting in striking sensory syndromes. Examples include acute sensory neuronopathy (Sterman *et al.*, 1980) and inflammatory disorders of dorsal root ganglia and cranial ganglia, such as carcinomatous sensory neuropathy (Dalmau *et al.*, 1992), herpes zoster and Sjögren's syndrome (Griffin *et al.*, 1990). Once sensory neuronopathies run their course and the pathologic processes are no longer active, the sensory deficit becomes fixed and little or no recovery takes place. The subject of predominantly motor or sensory neuropathic (or neuronopathic) disorders is considered at more length in Chapter 4.

Axonopathy versus neuronopathy

It has been known for some years that pyridoxine (vitamin B_6) ingested chronically in doses of 250–1000 mg per day may result in a sensory neuropathy, mainly of the large fibre type (Schaumburg *et al.*, 1983). If the condition is diagnosed and the vitamin ingestion discontinued, recovery takes place, but the completeness of recovery depends on the duration and severity of the neuropathy. The same is true of the sensory neuropathy induced by the chemotherapeutic agent, cisplatin. Returning to pyridoxine, the inadvertent single administration of massive amounts of pyridoxine to two young adults resulted in a profound sensory ablation in these individuals which left them permanently deafferented and unable to sit or stand (Albin *et al.*, 1987). These observations suggest that modest sensory neuropathy caused by pyridoxine is reversible but that more severe neuropathy is not.

An experimental study in rats by Xu *et al.* (1989) provides further insight. When they administered pyridoxine to rats in large single doses (1200 mg/kg) the rats rapidly became severely ataxic and could be shown to have degeneration of the large dorsal root ganglion cells by 7 days. Intermediate doses produced less damage with a longer latency, and small doses of pyridoxine produced only some shrinkage of the nerve cell bodies of the large dorsal root ganglion cells and distal axonal breakdown. The latter appeared to be a fully reversible lesion. Whether pyridoxine produces an axonopathy or a neuronopathy is therefore dose related. Although these observations provide considerable insight into the relationship between axonopathy and neuronopathy in pyridoxine intoxication, they provide no information as to what pyridoxine is doing at the tissue and subcellular levels. It is equally uncertain how generalizable these dose–response observations might be.

MANIFESTATIONS OF NEUROPATHY

Typical polyneuropathy

The prototypical polyneuropathy is a distal symmetrical motor–sensory axonal process that has a stocking–glove disturbance of sensation and a similar pattern of weakness. Typically this type of neuropathy is associated with exogenous intoxications, such as by medications, alcohol abuse, heavy metal exposure and industrial organic chemicals; or by endogenous metabolic disturbances such as nutritional disorders, chronic renal failure or malignancies. Clinical manifestations of such a polyneuropathy will be familiar to many readers, but are summarized in the following paragraphs to emphasize the full range of manifestations. It should be noted that an acquired demyelinating polyneuropathy, given a similar temporal evolution, could also fit the same clinical description.

The first symptoms are commonly distal dysaesthesias. Frequently these are described as tingling, prickling, burning or band-like sensations in the balls of the feet, tips of the toes or in a more generalized fashion over the soles of the feet. Symmetry of symptoms and findings in a distal graded fashion are the rule, but occasionally dysaesthesias may appear on the sole of one foot earlier than the other, or be more pronounced unilaterally. When this occurs, the examiner must take care to distinguish between polyneuropathy, which is a graded nerve length-dependent process, and multiple mononeuropathy (mononeuropathy multiplex) in which individual distal cutaneous nerves may be damaged in a fashion giving rise to multifocal symptoms and signs. If the polyneuropathy remains mild, that is, confined to dysaesthesias of the soles of the feet, careful examination may fail to disclose detectable motor or sensory signs.

As the polyneuropathy worsens, sensory deficit for cutaneous modalities will appear on the soles of the feet and begin to creep over the dorsa of both feet. Ankle jerks disappear and weakness of dorsiflexion of the toes, best demonstrated in the great toe, is likely to appear. The only functional sign of weakness at this point may be inability to walk on the heels, due to mild weakness of ankle dorsiflexion. With continued worsening, the sensory disturbance can be expected to move centripetally in a graded stocking-like pattern. Dysaesthesias often will become more intense by this time, and perhaps are experienced as pain. Patient complaints may include such phrases as 'my feet are numb', 'my feet feel like wood', 'I feel as though I am walking on stumps', or 'I feel as though there is a coating or a layer of something over my skin'. Heel walking may be impossible by this time, and the feet may slap while walking. Later, the knee jerks disappear and foot drop worsens, resulting in a steppage gait.

By the time sensory disturbance has ascended to the upper shin, dysaesthesias are usually noticed in the finger tips. The degree of painfulness varies widely from one patient to the next, but pain may be a major complaint. Frequently, minimal stimuli delivered to hyperaesthetic areas of skin, once perceived, may be experienced as a deep, searing, burning pain. This phenomenon is frequently referred to as hyperpathia, or more precisely, allodynia. More discussion of neuropathic pain is presented below and in Chapter 3.

When the polyneuropathy involves the large afferent fibres subserving muscle spindle stretch and tendon organs, not only do reflexes disappear, but also unsteadiness of gait, called sensory ataxia, may occur due to the proprioceptive loss. This unsteadiness is out of proportion to the degree of muscle weakness.

Progression proceeds symmetrically in a graded manner, spreading proximally up the thighs and towards the elbows. Concurrent spread of motor weakness occurs, and is usually greater in the extensor muscles than in the corresponding flexors. Weakened muscles atrophy as denervation proceeds and this is usually accompanied by pan–sensory loss and areflexia. When the sensory disturbance reaches mid-thigh, a small tent-shaped area of cutaneous hyperaesthesia may be demonstrated on the lower abdomen. The patient is usually unaware of this finding. As the neuropathy progresses, the tent-shaped area of hyperaesthesia widens and extends rostrally toward the sternum. The explanation is that this represents dying back according to nerve length of the intercostal and lumbar segmental nerves. In polyneuropathies of such severity, the patient generally cannot stand or walk or hold objects in the hands. Sensory loss may also develop over the vertex of the head and centrally in the face.

In the most extreme cases, ventilatory capacity may be reduced due to weakness of intercostal muscles or diaphragm or both. Respiratory assistance is then necessary. Such patients are bed-ridden.

The tempo of progression is highly variable, ranging from a couple of days in the most fulminant cases of Guillain–Barré syndrome or porphyric neuropathy to many months or indeed years. Most acquired axonal polyneuropathies are either subacute or chronic and progress over many weeks to months or perhaps even years.

Preceding and concurrent events

Key features to the diagnosis of peripheral neuropathies are frequently not described or even noticed by patients. Easily forgotten events occurring in the period before the onset of symptoms are generally not reported; therefore inquiry must be made. It is important to ask about recent viral illnesses, symptoms of systemic illness or of constitutional dysfunction, the initiation of new medications, possible exposure to solvents, pesticides, heavy metals, or other potential toxins; similar symptoms in others either at home or at work; abuse of alcohol; and the presence of pre-existing medical illness such as polycythaemia, chronic renal failure, or intestinal malabsorption. The examiner should always ask if the patient would otherwise feel well if free of the neuropathic symptoms. In this way one obtains a sense of whether systemic illness co-exists.

Progression

One should always inquire carefully as to how progression occurred. It is not enough to know that symptoms began 4 months ago and progressed to the present state of dysfunction. Worsening may be steady and uniform, or accelerating, or minimally changing or even static after initial rapid progression, or relapsing and remitting. Examples of differing types of progression are illustrated in Figure 1.1. Although the

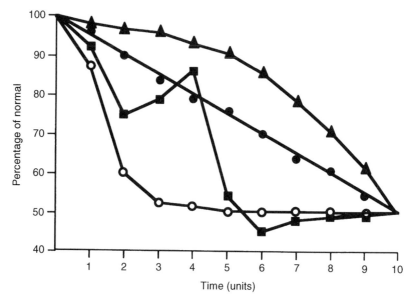

Figure 1.1 Examples of different clinical evolution of neuropathy in four patients. Each patient was affected from the same interval (10 units of time) and has the same degree of dysfunction now (50% of normal), but each has come to this point by a different route: (▲) represents an ominously accelerating course; (○) represents a course with rapid onset and then plateauing, and is thus much less ominous; (●) represents an inexorably progressive course, cause for concern; (■) describes a fluctuating course, now improving. It is important to identify and characterize these differences in evolution by history, because of the differing implications for diagnosis and outlook.

duration of symptoms is similar in the four examples given, the evolution is widely divergent, and the prognostic implication of each of the four examples is different from the others.

NATURE OF SYMPTOMS

The symptoms of neuropathic disorder, although varied and diverse, fall under the general headings of motor, sensory (including pain) and autonomic.

Motor

The predominant motor symptom is muscular weakness. Degree and distribution depends upon the severity and basis of the neuropathy. If weakness is not accompanied by major sensory loss, dexterity and fine movements are not disproportionately affected; this is different from what occurs with an upper motor neuron lesion. In polyneuropathies, the early motor symptoms tend to be distal in distribution. Distal weakness may cause tripping on rugs, door sills and stair risers because of minor degrees of foot drop. If the fingers are weak, patients may also complain of difficulty in winding an alarm clock, removing the lid from a jar or turning a key in a lock. These particular tasks require adequate strength of intrinsic hand muscles (see Chapter 2 for more on the pathophysiology of motor weakness).

Sensory

The wide spectrum of sensory symptoms is impressive, and subsumes both positive and negative phenomena. Positive symptoms include tingling, pins and needles, and other dysaesthesias, some of which may be described as unpleasant or even painful experiences. Neuropathic pain, the extreme example of a positive symptom, is dealt with in more detail below. Negative symptoms refer to numbness and other loss or absence of feeling. This includes the loss of proprioception and thus imbalance and difficulty with stance and gait, generally referred to as sensory ataxia. On examination, a principal feature of sensory ataxia is a positive Romberg sign, meaning disproportionate loss of balance with eyes closed compared with eyes open. Another feature of sensory ataxia is involuntary movement of fingers and hands (pseudoathetosis) when the arms are outstretched and the eyes closed. This is suppressed through visual feedback when the eyes are open.

Neuropathic pain

Pain due to damage peripheral nerves is a complex subject. Neuropathic pain may be divided into two major types, namely dysaesthetic pain and nerve trunk pain. Although painfulness in peripheral neuropathies is often a combination of these two types of pain, it is useful to think of the characteristics of each type as it occurs in relatively pure form. Dysaethetic pain and nerve pain are compared and contrasted in Table 1.1, along with a hypothesis as to their separate bases. In addition to these two major types of neuropathic pain, patients with rapidly evolving

Table 1.1 Characteristics of two major forms of neuropathic pain

	Dysaesthetic pain	*Nerve trunk pain*
Descriptors	Burning, tingling, raw, searing, crawling, drawing	Aching, occasionally knife-like
Recognition	Unfamiliar; never experienced before	Familiar; 'like a toothache'
Distribution	(1) Cutaneous or subcutaneous usually (2) Distal	(1) Deep (2) Relatively proximal
Constancy	Variable, may be intermittent, jabbing, lancinating, shooting	Usually continuous, but waxes and wanes
Better/worse	Little makes it better; worse following activity	Better with rest or optimal position; worse with movement, nerve stretch or palpation
Basis of pain (hypothetical)	Increased firing of damaged or abnormally excitable nociceptive fibres, particularly sprouting, regenerating fibres	Increased firing due to physiological stimulation of endings of undamaged afferents from nerve sheaths themselves (nervi nervorum)
Examples	(1) Causalgia (2) Small-fibre polyneuropathy	(1) Root compression (2) Brachial neuritis

denervation of muscle, as with Guillain–Barré syndrome or acute poliomyelitis, may complain of muscle pain and tenderness which they describe as like having over-exercised on the previous day.

Autonomic

Symptoms of sympathetic and parasympathetic dysfunction have an even wider diversity than sensory symptoms and are discussed in detail in Chapter 5.

PATTERNS OF NEUROPATHY

Symmetry

In polyneuropathies, the findings are symmetrical on both sides of the body. The anticipated pattern of symmetry for most polyneuropathies is one in which the motor and sensory deficits and attenuation of reflexes are distal and graded in severity. From a sensory standpoint, the stocking–glove pattern described above under the section Typical polyneuropathy is the expectation. If sensory hyperaesthesia to cutaneous modalities fades just above the ankle in one leg but extends almost to the knee in the other, the findings are asymmetrical and should alert the examiner to processes other than pure polyneuropathy. Similarly, if one foot slaps when the patient walks but the other does not, the process is not symmetrical. Further, muscles of extension and abduction tend to be weakened to a greater extent in acquired symmetrical neuropathies than do muscles of flexion and adduction. For example the dorsiflexors of the toes and ankles tend to be weaker than the plantar flexors in most polyneuropathies. Occasionally this dictum is violated, as in some cases of long-standing hereditary neuropathies, where the plantar flexors may be as weak as the dorsiflexors of the ankles (Harding and Thomas, 1980).

Legs versus arms

Legs are more severely affected than the arms in most polyneuropathies. There are exceptions, as in lead neuropathy in which manifestations of bilateral wrist drop may predominate, and occasionally as in porphyric neuropathy, in which arms may be more affected than legs and proximal muscles more than distal ones, even though symmetry is generally preserved.

Proximal versus distal

In some instances, even when the neuropathy is symmetrical and affects the legs more than the arms, the proximal limb muscles are either more involved or just as involved as the distal ones. A demyelinating basis for the neuropathy can be suspected and looked for on electrodiagnostic examination. Sensory neuropathies are rarely proximally accentuated but this can occur in Tangier disease (Kocen *et al.*, 1967) and porphyric neuropathy.

Nerve trunk or root versus graded findings

Exception to the distal, graded and symmetrical pattern of neuropathies raises the likelihood of a multifocal process affecting individual nerve trunks and roots. Such processes include focal ischaemia of nerve trunks and roots as in vasculitis, multifocal demyelination of nerve, other widespread processes affecting nerve such as hyperlipidaemic deposits in perineurium, amyloid accumulation in nerve, sarcoid involvement of peripheral nerves, and infectious processes affecting nerve trunk such as leprosy or Lyme disease. A common manifestation of a multifocal process is exemplified by sensory disturbances extending as high as the head of the fibula on the lateral aspect of the leg but only extending above the malleolus on the medial aspect, thus suggesting focal lesions of the L5 and S1 roots or the sciatic nerve trunks rather than a polyneuropathy.

Plexopathy

Both brachial and lumbosacral plexuses are subject to focal or multifocal lesions which produce either unilateral or bilateral signs and symptoms. Lesions affecting the brachial plexus are relatively common, and display characteristic signs quite different from those expected either in mononeuropathies of the upper limb or polyneuropathies. The usual causes are direct trauma to the brachial plexus, brachial neuritis (neuralgic amyotrophy), cervical ribs or cervical bands, infiltration of the plexus by malignancy, and radiation therapy. When the upper portion of the plexus, which originates from the C5, C6 and C7 roots, is damaged, weakness and atrophy of the shoulder and proximal arm muscles ensues. Damage to the lower brachial plexus, which arises from the C8 and T1 roots, produces more distal weakness, atrophy and sensory deficit in the forearm and hand. As a generalization, brachial neuritis, or damage from localized radiation more than 6000 rads, or certain types of trauma (arm jerked downward) result in upper plexus findings; in contrast, malignant infiltration, cervical rib and cervical bands, and other types of trauma (arm jerked upwards) induce lower plexus signs.

Lesions of lumbosacral plexus generally result in asymmetrical mixtures of partial femoral, obturator and sciatic neuropathies. Examples of causes are trauma, including surgical and obstetric trauma, retroperitoneal haemorrhage, infiltration of plexus by malignant tumour, irradiation and lumbosacral plexitis, a controversial disorder which is postulated to be the lower-extremity counterpart of brachial neuritis. Further details may be found in Donaghy (1993).

OTHER CONSIDERATIONS IN ASSESSING NEUROPATHY

Motor versus sensory deficits

In every neuropathy judgment should be reached as to the relative balance of motor and sensory findings. In many polyneuropathies, the severity of the motor findings is roughly equal to the severity of sensory disturbance, but this general principle is frequently violated. In Guillain–Barré syndrome, findings may be predominantly or virtually exclusively motor, and in some neuropathies associated with dysproteinaemia, the manifestations are almost exclusively sensory. This can be true in processes that are either predominantly axonal or predominantly demyelinating. A major reason for weighing motor versus sensory is to consider the possibility of disorder that is almost purely one or the other, and therefore possibly a neuronopathy. Examples of primary motor neuronopathies include acute anterior poliomyelitis, hereditary spinal muscular atrophies and the lower motor neuron form of motor neuron disease; primary sensory neuronopathies with destruction of dorsal root ganglion cells may occur with small cell lung carcinoma or breast carcinoma, or intoxications due to pyridoxine, taxol or cisplatin (see previous discussion on Pathologic processes). Although our capacity to diagnose neuronopathies, either motor or sensory, is still indirect and sometimes based on observing that no recovery takes place long term, it is still an important category of disorders to keep in mind because the prognostic implications are so much worse than for axonopathic or demyelinating processes in nerve (also see Chapter 4).

Large-fibre versus small-fibre neuropathies

All motor axons, except the gamma efferents to intrafusal muscle fibres, are large myelinated fibres, whereas peripheral sensory fibres are represented by the full range in size of myelinated and unmyelinated axons. As a clinical generalization, temperature and pain sensation are mediated by unmyelinated and small myelinated fibres, but proprioception, vibratory sense and the afferent limb of the muscle stretch reflex are subserved by large myelinated fibres. Touch sensibility is mediated by both large and small fibres, and autonomic functions are effected mainly by unmyelinated fibres.

These anatomical facts are of clinical utility. In neuropathies affecting mainly small fibres, diminished cutaneous sensation, as measured by pain and temperature testing, is the dominant finding. It is often accompanied by burning painful dysaesthesias and autonomic dysfunction. Touch is generally spared, along with motor power, balance and tendon jerks. Examples of small-fibre neuropathy include some instances of amyloid neuropathy and distal diabetic polyneuropathy. In contrast, large-fibre neuropathies are characterized by areflexia, imbalance from sensory ataxia, variable degress of motor weakness and minimal distal numbness. Although tingling and machinery-like dysaesthesias may be prominent in large-fibre neuropathies, they are generally not described as painful.

Axonal versus demyelinating neuropathies

This distinction is usually made electrodiagnostically, and is not generally possible to predict reliably by the clinical history and examination alone, athough the preservation of muscle bulk in chronically weak muscles favours a demyelinating process. The distinction of neuropathies that are primarily demyelinating from those that are primarily axonal is important, because of the differences in approach to diagnosis and management and also because of the likelihood of recovery and its anticipated rate. Once a demyelinating process abates and remyelination commences unimpeded, recovery may take place rapidly, proceeding from paralysis to recovery in just a few weeks. In contrast, in most axonal neuropathies in which denervation of muscles and sensory deficits are widespread, recovery is measured in months to a few years because of the requirement for successful regeneration.

Alteration of reflexes

Diminution or disappearance of reflexes is the rule in neuropathies. A key factor in reflex loss is involvement of the afferent limb of the reflex arc emanating from muscle spindles. As such, areflexia may be an early and prominent finding in polyneuropathies affecting large fibres, regardless of whether the neuropathy is axonal or demyelinating in nature. In predominantly motor neuropathies, such as the acute motor axonal subtype of Guillain–Barré syndrome (McKhann *et al.*, 1993), reflexes become reduced concurrently with and proportional to motor weakness, and reflexes do not completely disappear until the limbs are almost flaccid.

Enlargement of nerve trunks

Palpation of the nerve trunk to detect focal or diffuse enlargement or other abnormalities is a frequently forgotten part of the neurological examination. If peripheral neuropathy is the clinical question, it is both logical and practical to examine directly the organ in question. In mononeuropathies, the entire palpable course of the nerve trunk in question should be explored manually for focal thickening, the presence of a neurofibroma, point tenderness, nerve trunk pain from putting the nerve on stretch, and Tinel's phenomenon (elicitation of a tingling sensation in the sensory distribution of the nerve by tapping along the course of the nerve). In more generalized neuropathies, the examiner should assess the size of the common peroneal trunk in the popliteal fossa and near the fibular head and the ulnar nerve at the elbow, following it proximally into the medial upper arm. Care must be taken not to over-interpret findings on palpation of the ulnar nerve at the elbow, because the epineurial sheaths of the ulnar nerve where it lies in the bicipital groove may normally be quite thick. If generalized nerve trunk enlargement is suspected, smaller cutaneous nerve trunks can also be readily palpated, including the sensory branch of the superficial peroneal nerve in the lower leg and dorsum of the foot, the great auricular nerve as it passes cephalad over the sternocleidomastoid muscle, and the two branches of the radial cutaneous nerve as they pass superficially over the extensor tendons of the thumb. These two latter cutaneous twigs are more readily felt if the thumb is extended. Either beaded, fusiform enlargement of nerve trunks or uniform thickening may be encountered. In some genetically determined neuropathies of the hypertrophic variety, uniform thickening of nerve trunks, often of the calibre of a clothes line or larger, may be found.

ASSOCIATED MANIFESTATIONS

Constitutional features

These are malaise, weight loss, anorexia and fever. Although the presence of any of these constitutional symptoms is not specific for particular underlying medical illnesses, it does strongly suggest that general possibility.

Systemic disease

In addition to inquiring about constitutional symptoms, the examiner should also be alert to the possibility of associated systemic illness. The presence of diabetes, liver disease, abdominal pain or gastrointestinal disturbance, hyperlipidaemia, malignancies including lymphomas, nutritional disorders and dietary extremes, chronic renal failure, a wide range of medications, alcoholism, HIV seropositivity, and a story consistent with Lyme disease are all important clues to diagnosis. Also exogenous intoxications which result in neuropathy often have associated systemic effects.

COURSE OF NEUROPATHY

Tempo

The rate at which neuropathy evolves varies from a fulminant course of hours to a day or so to an indolent process extending over a life-time. Neuropathies termed acute generally evolve over days to weeks, subacute over weeks to months and chronic from months to years. Generally speaking, a polyneuropathy with a slowly progressive course extending more than 5 years is quite likely to be determined genetically, particularly if the major manifestations are atrophy and motor weakness with few positive sensory symptoms. Acquired neuropathies having a chronic course over many years are diabetic distal sensory neuropathy and paraproteinaemic neuropathies in which progression may be quite slow.

If major fluctuations occur in the course of neuropathy it brings to mind two possibilities: (1) relapsing forms of demyelinating polyneuropathy, or (2) repeated toxic exposure. Other factors may also be responsible for fluctuation of symptoms; for instance, in catamenial sciatica endometrial implants on the sciatic nerve trunk in the pelvis produce symptoms only in relation to the menses. Slow fluctuation in symptoms taking place over weeks or months (reflecting changes in the activity of the neuropathy) should not be confused with day-to-day variation or diurnal undulations of symptoms. The latter are common to all neuropathic disorders. An example is carpal tunnel syndrome in which dysaesthesias may be prominent at night but absent during the day.

Severity

As mentioned, severity of neuropathy ranges from subclinical involvement demonstrable only by electrodiagnostic examination or quantitative sensory testing to profound sensory loss and flaccid paralysis requiring respiratory support. The issue facing the examiner is always one of predicting severity. For instance, in a patient with mild symptoms the question becomes whether this will be only a minimal neuropathy, a nuisance at worst, or whether this represents the early stages of a much more severe disorder. For neuropathies expected to be monophasic, such as Guillain–Barré syndrome, reassurance can be taken from plateauing of the clinical course. Once worsening ceases in Guillain–Barré syndrome, it usually does not commence again, and the beginnings of recovery are not far off. In indolent, exceptionally chronic neuropathies, the distinction between insidious progression and a static state is often difficult or impossible to judge. Even so, predicting eventual severity is often possible by projecting minimal or no worsening. Observing the course over time is the best predictor.

Recovery

A number of mechanisms can be cited by which recovery of function occurs in peripheral neuropathies. Repair of nerve itself through either remyelination or regeneration is the most important (see the previous section on Pathologic processes). Peripheral nerve retains the capacity for recovery of function as long as the nerve cell body remains viable. A striking example concerns recovery from long-standing uraemic polyneuropathy, particularly in younger patients. Some individuals with chronic renal failure maintained on periodic haemodiaylsis for several years may exhibit what appears to be a static motor–sensory polyneuropathy. If such patients undergo successful renal transplantation, full recovery from the long-standing polyneuropathy may ensue over the succeeding 6–12 months.

Motor recovery may take place even when anterior horn cells are destroyed. This process, collateral re-innervation, occurs through distal sprouting of intramuscular motor nerve twigs of surviving motor units which can re-innervate adjacent denervated muscle fibres. This enlarges remaining motor units, and may restore full power and bulk of muscle, although usually at the expense of fine control. Collateral re-innervation is readily demonstrated by needle electromyography or through fibre type grouping using histochemical methods on muscle biopsy. It is uncertain whether a similar phenomenon occurs on the afferent side through collateral re-innervation of sensory endings.

ELECTRODIAGNOSIS

The range of electrodiagnostic studies that can be applied for the diagnosis and elucidation of peripheral neuropathies continues to expand. Here we give only a brief overview of the more important techniques that are currently available. Detailed accounts are given in texts such as Kimura (1989) and Brown and Bolton (1993). It must be emphasized very firmly that electrodiagnostic studies should be considered as an extension of the clinical evaluation and not merely as a laboratory test. Such studies may be undertaken by the neurologist at the time of his or her initial examination or by a clinical neurophysiologist. If the latter, it is vital that the particular question or questions requiring solution should be clearly formulated.

Electrodiagnostic examination

Needle electromyography (EMG)

The electrical activity of muscle fibres can be examined by an intramuscular recording, usually with a coaxial needle electrode. This records from a restricted region of the muscle. For specialized purposes, needles that record the activity of single muscle fibres (single fibre EMG, SFEMG) or single motor unit potentials (macro EMG) can be employed.

For routine needle EMG, recordings from multiple sites are usually required to obtain adequate sampling. When a normal muscle is at rest it is electrically silent. On voluntary contraction, potentials appear that are derived from the summated activity of the muscle fibres innervated by single motor axons. With increased force of contraction, the number of such motor unit potentials increases, as does their firing rate, producing an overlapping 'interference' recruitment pattern. In denervating disorders, the number of motor unit potentials is decreased but their firing rate is maintained. After chronic partial denervation with collateral re-innervation, the motor unit potentials may be of increased amplitude and duration and are often polyphasic. The motor unit recruitment pattern is reduced with upper motor neuron lesions and psychogenic weakness but the firing rate of individual motor unit potentials is reduced and their parameters are normal. In primary muscle disease, the number of motor unit potentials tends to be preserved despite muscle weakness but they are brief, their amplitude is reduced and they are polyphasic.

The occurrence of spontaneous electrical activity or potentials produced by needle movement can be diagnostically helpful. For example, fasciculations are spontaneous sporadic motor unit potentials. Although often considered to indicate anterior horn cell disease, such potentials can be a conspicuous finding in some demyelinating neuropathies. Other types of spontaneous or evoked motor unit activity are seen in myokymia and neuromyotonia. These are discussed in Chapter 2. Fibrillation potentials, which are brief and of low amplitude, are derived from the spontaneous discharge of single muscle fibres or may be evoked by needle movement. They are a frequent finding in denervated muscle. Fibrillations are also encountered in some myopathies, particularly polymyositis, where they are probably related to segmental muscle fibre necrosis leading to isolation of portions of the fibres from their innervation. Crescendo – decrescendo bursts of high frequency discharges are characteristic of myotonic disorders and are related to instability of the muscle fibre membrane.

They must be distinguished from brief pseudomyotonic runs provoked by needle movement in denervated muscles.

In muscle cramps, profuse motor unit activity is recorded. This contrasts with the contractures that can be encountered in some metabolic myopathies where the muscle is electrically silent: the contractile apparatus is activated distal to the sarcolemma.

Nerve conduction studies

The examination of motor and sensory conduction, including evoked muscle and nerve action potential amplitude, is essential in the investigation of peripheral nerve disorders. Motor nerve conduction velocity is measured by recording with surface electrodes over the relevant muscle with stimulation of its motor nerve at two or more sites. Conduction velocity is obtained from the latency of onset of the evoked muscle action potential and measurement of the distance between stimulation points (Figure 1.2). The latency on stimulation at the point closest to the muscle is referred to as the distal motor latency. For some nerves such as the facial or femoral, only this single value can be recorded. Conduction in the proximal portions of motor nerve fibres can be examined by recording F wave latencies (see below) or by stimulation of motor roots paraspinally using high voltage electrical stimulation (Figure 1.3).

The amplitude of the compound muscle action potential (CMAP) gives valuable information. It will be reduced in denervating processes or if there is conduction

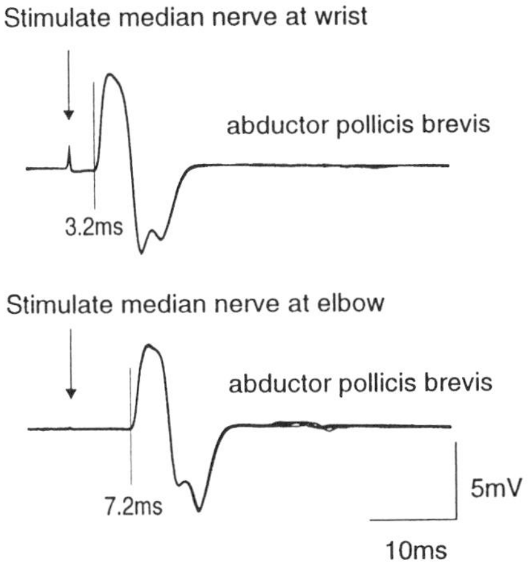

Stimulate median nerve at wrist

abductor pollicis brevis

3.2ms

Stimulate median nerve at elbow

abductor pollicis brevis

7.2ms

5mV

10ms

Distal motor latency = 3.2ms
Latency from stimulation at elbow = 7.2ms
Distance = 250mm
Nerve conduction velocity = 62.5 metres/ sec
CMAP amplitude (negative component):
6mV (wrist stimulation), 5.2mV (elbow stimulation)

Figure 1.2 Motor conduction in the median nerve on recording from abductor pollicis brevis with stimulation at the wrist and elbow. Figure kindly provided by Dr. P. Thompson.

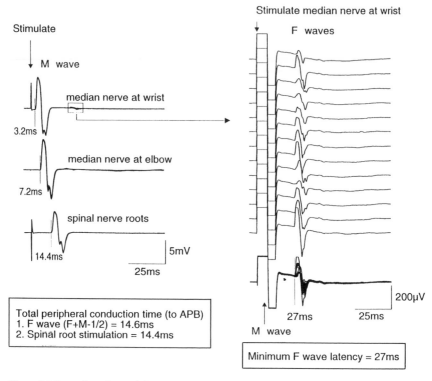

Figure 1.3 Recordings from abductor pollicis brevis with stimulation, in the three traces to the left of the figure, at the wrist and elbow and over the spinal nerve roots. Calculation of total conduction time from the spinal roots to the muscle using F wave latency gives a value (14.6 ms) that is closely similar to that obtained with stimulation paraspinally over the spinal roots (14.4 ms). Recordings of F wave responses are seen in the traces shown on the right of the figure which are at higher amplification and with stimulation at the wrist. The superimposed traces in the lowermost part of the figure indicate that, in the normal subject, F wave latency varies little, although the amplitude in successive sweeps differs. Figure kindly provided by Dr. P. Thompson.

block, causing an abrupt reduction on the size of the potential between a more distal and a more proximal stimulation site. Considerable care must be taken before deciding that conduction block is present as spurious reductions in CMAP can be produced by phase cancellations in dispersed compound action potentials (Kimura *et al.*, 1986). The criteria for the recognition of conduction block have been discussed by Cornblath *et al.* (1991).

The recording of F waves (Figure 1.3) is helpful for the examination of conduction in the proximal regions of motor nerve fibres. Motor nerve stimulation, in addition to giving rise to an orthodromic volley and a direct muscle response (M wave), an antidromic volley ascends to the spinal cord where the anterior horn cells are activated, causing a reflected volley that descends to activate the muscle, the F wave (Figure 1.3). This response may be delayed or absent with selective proximal demyelination as may occur in the Guillain–Barré syndrome.

Sensory nerve conduction is examined by stimulating a sensory nerve trunk and recording from the nerve at one or more points proximally (Figure 1.4). At times it is more convenient to employ antidromic rather than orthodromic recording. Both the velocity of the potential and its amplitude are informative. Potentials may also be recorded from mixed nerve trunks. Cutaneous electrical stimulation and the recording of dermatomal somatosensory evoked potentials (Katifi and Sedgwick, 1987) may be helpful.

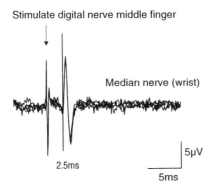

Stimulate digital nerve middle finger

Median nerve (wrist)

5μV

2.5ms

5ms

Onset nerve action potential = 2.5ms
Distance = 150mm
Nerve conduction velocity = 60 metres/ sec
Nerve potential amplitude (peak to peak = 15μV)

Figure 1.4 Median sensory nerve action potential with stimulation of the digital nerves of the middle finger on recording with surface electrodes at the wrist; five traces have been superimposed. Figure kindly provided by Dr. P. Thompson.

These techniques, both motor and sensory, only examine the larger and faster conducting fibres comprising the Aα group. It is possible to record small-calibre fibres with near-nerve needle electrode recording and averaging a large number of responses, but this is an exacting experience for the patient and not generally employed. A technique that appeared to offer promise for the assessment of conduction in small-calibre sensory fibres in neuropathies was the recording of cerebral somatosensory evoked potentials evoked by CO_2 laser stimulation (Kakigi *et al.*, 1989). These were found to be selectively lost in syringomyelia (Kakigi *et al.*, 1991). The technique unfortunately proved not to be helpful as it is difficult to record these potentials from persons who are in mid-life or older (Purves, 1994).

The intraneural recording of nerve fibre activity, including that of unmyelinated C fibres, has provided interesting information (Fagius and Wallin, 1980) but this is purely a research procedure.

Uses of electrodiagnosis

Electrophysiological studies are helpful in the investigation and management of most patients with peripheral nerve disorders (Figure 1.5). At the outset, the suspicion of peripheral neuropathy can be confirmed by nerve conduction studies, although in selective small-fibre sensory neuropathies this may not be possible. Quantitative thermal sensory testing can provide suggestive evidence but the confidence limits for the results of this psychophysical test are wide. Moreover, an abnormal result does not distinguish between peripheral nerve and CNS disease. This is not a frequent problem but nerve biopsy may be required to establish the diagnosis (see Chapter 14). In unusual patients with a central distal axonopathy (Thomas *et al.*, 1984), there is a selective degeneration of the centrally directed axons of the primary sensory neurons. The clinical picture may mimic that of a peripheral neuropathy very closely, but sensory nerve action potentials are normal. Diagnostic help may be obtained by the recording of somatosensory evoked responses.

EMG studies are usually decisive in distinguishing between a denervating process and a myopathy, and from simulated weakness, although neuropathy and myopathy can co-exist at times, for example in paraneoplastic syndromes or vitamin E deficiency. Disturbances of neuromuscular transmission can be investigated by the examination of the response to repetitive stimulation and by measuring 'jitter' in an SFEMG recording (Stålberg and Trontelj, 1979).

A common clinical problem in assessing a patient is in establishing the level of involvement by the disease process, e.g. spinal cord, spinal roots, limb girdle plexuses or peripheral nerve trunks. In a motor syndrome a distinction can often be achieved by EMG sampling at multiple sites from the paraspinal muscles to the periphery. In cases of suspected anterior horn cell diseases the finding of subclinical abnormalities of sensory conduction will question the diagnosis. The recording of dermatomal evoked potentials may be helpful in assessing lower-limb spinal root compression (Katifi and Sedgwick, 1987).

Both in diffuse and focal neuropathies a distinction can usually be made between axonopathies and demyelinating neuropathies (Figure 1.5). In axonopathies conduction velocity is either within normal limits or only mildly reduced, particularly if there is selective loss of the larger and faster-conducting fibres. More severe reductions are observed in demyelinating neuropathies, either diffuse or focal, with reductions in conduction velocity to 60 per cent of normal or less. Sensory nerve action potentials are of reduced amplitude or absent, partly because of loss of nerve fibres but also because of temporal dispersion from unequal degrees of slowing in the constituent fibres. Severely reduced nerve conduction velocity is also encountered in the early stages of regeneration after axonal degeneration.

In demyelinating neuropathies, unequal degrees of slowing between different nerves or segments of nerves, or the presence of conduction block, may suggest that the patient has chronic inflammatory demyelinating polyneuropathy rather than an inherited or other type of acquired demyelinating neuropathy.

Nerve conduction studies can be informative for following the progress of a neuropathy, for example in monitoring treatment, although alterations in nerve conduction velocity tend to be slow. EMG sampling is particularly valuable in following recovery after focal nerve injury and it may be decisive in deciding whether surgical intervention is merited if there is doubt as to whether or not nerve transection has occurred.

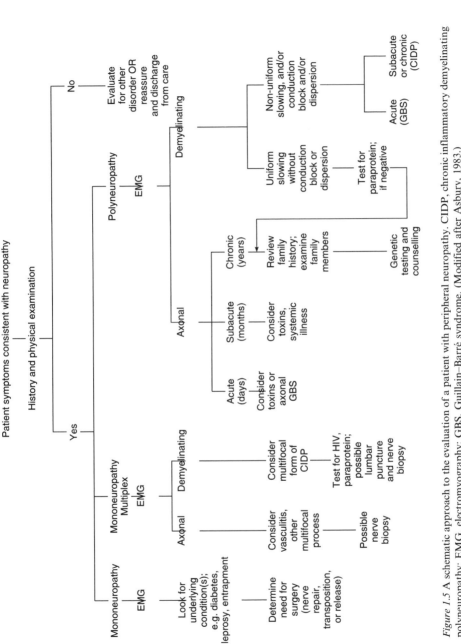

Figure 1.5 A schematic approach to the evaluation of a patient with peripheral neuropathy. CIDP, chronic inflammatory demyelinating polyneuropathy; EMG, electromyography; GBS, Guillain–Barré syndrome. (Modified after Asbury, 1983.)

Nerve biopsy

The indications for nerve biopsy or biopsy of other tissues containing peripheral nerve are discussed in Chapter 14.

CLINICAL DIAGNOSIS OF NEUROPATHIES

The logic used to analyse and diagnose peripheral neuropathies, particularly poly-neuropathies, is exceedingly cumbersome. The sequence, in simplified form, goes as follows. First, a diagnosis of polyneuropathy is rendered, and second, a known association is sought. The association process requires sifting through more than 100 known associations (drugs, other toxins, metabolic disorders, dysimmune states, genetically determined disorders, infectious disorders), pinpointing one, and ruling out all of the others. Too often, no association or causative condition is discovered. Sometimes, the examiner is too successful and identifies two or three known associations (for example, diabetes, alcoholism and paraproteinaemia). Next, one must decide how much, if any, an associated condition or disorder contributes to the neuropathy. For instance, is the diabetes too mild to be respon-sible for the neuropathy? Or, is the use of alcohol substantial enough to explain the neuropathy?

A better method of approaching clinical diagnosis of neuropathies is to categorize each case into a general subtype using the clinical history, findings on neurological examination and the electrodiagnostic information in order to arrive at the initial synthesis. In each instance a judgment should be made as to whether the process is acute, subacute or chronic; whether it is a polyneuropathy or a multiple mononeuro-pathy (ordinarily single mononeuropathies are easily distinguished); whether axonal or demyelinating or mixed; whether motor–sensory or predominantly one or the other; if sensory, whether large-fibre or small-fibre in type.

Once one arrives at this general formulation, the possibilities in the differential diagnosis of specific causes and associations are greatly reduced. For example, a chronic demyelinating motor–sensory polyneuropathy present for a decade or more is probably hereditary, and most likely Charcot–Marie–Tooth neuropathy, type 1, although other considerations include monoclonal gammopathy such as that related to anti-myelin-associated glycoprotein or perhaps chronic inflammatory demyelinat-ing polyneuropathy (CIDP). Diabetic polyneuropathy may be this chronic, but usually presents an axonal or mixed pattern electrodiagnostically.

Certain categories of neuropathy occur much more frequently than others of the more than 100 combinations possible with this scheme. For instance, subacute or chronic axonal motor–sensory polyneuropathies are relatively common, and suggest metabolic disorders or toxins. Acute predominantly motor demyelinating polyneuro-pathy is very likely to be Guillain–Barré syndrome, although the concurrence of systemic illness or constitutional symptoms should arouse suspicion of associated conditions. Rarely, neuropathy due to buckthorn berry intoxication or diphtheritic polyneuritis, which are other causes of acute predominantly motor demyelinating polyneuropathy can be mistaken for Guillain–Barré syndrome. The overall approach is shown in Figure 1.5.

SPECIAL ASPECTS OF PERIPHERAL NEUROPATHIES

Ischaemia of nerve

Compared with other tissues, peripheral nerve is relatively resistant to ischaemia, because of the abundance of its circulation. In addition to a rich intraneural network of vasa nervorum, there are extensive anastomotic connections with the nutrient arterial supply to nerve. Experimentally, major arteries must be extensively ligated in order to produce nerve ischaemia in a limb. From a clinical standpoint, several situations of arterial compromise can bring about neuropathic symptoms and signs due to ischaemia. The most common basis is widespread small vessel disease, such as vasculitis, affecting vasa nervorum in numerous sites. The resulting multifocal neuropathy is the hallmark of nerve ischaemia. In addition, acute occlusion of a major artery to a limb, especially if transient as with a large embolus, can result in an ischaemic monomelic neuropathy (Wilbourn *et al.*, 1983; Levin, 1989). Major arteriovenous shunting in a limb can also produce an ischaemic monomelic neuropathy, both clinically (Bolton *et al.*, 1979; Wytrzes *et al.*, 1987) and experimentally (Sladky *et al.*, 1991). Another basis for ischaemia of peripheral nerve includes disorders altering the rheological properties of the blood itself such as in polycythaemia vera (Yiannikas *et al.*, 1983), and rarely in cryoglobulinaemia or Waldenström's macroglobulinaemia. On occasion, showers of embolic material may cause neuropathy (Bendixen *et al.*, 1992).

The role of ischaemia in diabetic neuropathies has long been argued but has not been settled. (For a review, see Thomas and Tomlinson 1993.) The evidence for nerve ischaemia is stronger in the focal and multifocal neuropathies of diabetes than for the more common polyneuropathy.

Vasculitis and neuropathy

Necrotizing vasculitis has a predilection for small arteries and arterioles, the size range of vasa nervorum. As a consequence, peripheral nerve damage is a frequent occurrence in many of the vasculitic syndromes encountered clinically. In polyarteritis nodosa, it is estimated that about 50 per cent of patients with this multisystem disorder exhibit peripheral neuropathy. Neuropathic manifestations are also common in the vasculitides associated with connective tissue disorders, such as rheumatoid arthritis, systemic lupus erythematosus, Churg–Strauss syndrome, Sjögren syndrome, Wegener granulomatosis and others. Rarely, a non-systemic vasculitis affecting only peripheral nerve can be an obscure cause of peripheral neuropathy (Kissel *et al.*, 1985; Dyck *et al.*, 1987). Vasculitic damage of vasa nervorum usually presents clinically as a multiple mononeuropathy because of the multifocal nature of the process. In severe cases, this feature may become difficult to demonstrate because of confluence of clinical deficits giving a relatively distal symmetrical graded pattern. The history will usually reveal the multifocal nature of the neuropathy. The electrodiagnostic and pathological features of nerve ischaemia indicate a primarily axonal disorder (Fujimura *et al.*, 1991).

Neuropathy and vasculitis are discussed by Lisak and Levinson in Chapter 7 of the first volume (1984). More recent publications on the subject include Moore (1989), Panegyres *et al.* (1990), Said *et al.* (1988), Kissel *et al.* (1985, 1989) and a major review by Chalk *et al.* (1993).

Focal neuropathies

Isolated peripheral nerve lesions are related to processes that produce localized damage. These include mechanical injury (external pressure, entrapment, traction, direct blows, penetrating wounds); thermal, electrical and radiation injury; vascular lesions; focal inflammatory demyelination; granulomatous, neoplastic and other infiltrative processes; and primary peripheral nerve tumours. Recent comprehensive reviews have been provided by Stewart (1993) and Dawson *et al.* (1990).

As emphasized by Wilbourn (1993), there has been growing skepticism concerning the attribution of vague upper-limb symptoms to the thoracic outlet syndrome. The same is true for a number of other syndromes considered to be due to peripheral nerve damage from so-called 'repetitive strain injury'. Clear confirmation by electrophysiological or other studies is often lacking. Such questions frequently arise in medicolegal practice, often in an occupational context.

The localization of focal nerve lesions can be problematic. For example, selective atrophy of the lateral part of the thenar eminence due to a T1 root lesion can masquerade as a median nerve lesion, or malignant infiltration of the lower brachial plexus can mimic an ulnar nerve lesion. A possible explanation is provided by new information concerning the fascicular anatomy of peripheral nerve. Older studies by Sunderland (1978) suggested that repeated interchange of fibres between fascicles in nerve trunks takes place along their length. This view has been increasingly challenged, based on dissection (Jabalay *et al.*, 1980) and microneurography (Schady *et al.*, 1983; Hallin, 1990) of human nerve and experimental tracer studies in monkeys (Brushart, 1991). These studies suggest that segregation of fibres in terms of their destination takes place proximally and is maintained throughout their course.

Entrapment and compression neuropathies comprise a large proportion of focal neuropathies. The statement has been made that patients with diffuse neuropathies show increased susceptibility to compression injury (Gilliatt and Harrison, 1984). It is true that an individual with a diffuse neuropathy, and consequently a reduced complement of nerve fibres, is less able to afford loss of fibres from superimposed entrapment or compression injury. This might provide the explanation for the so-called double crush syndrome (Upton and McComas, 1973), although other interpretations based on interference with axonal transport have also been advanced.

It is general clinical experience that patients with diabetes are more liable to develop compression and entrapment neuropathies but community-based surveys are lacking. Focal nerve injury caused by external compression or entrapment is related both to axoplasmic displacement and secondary myelin damage (Ochoa, 1980). Increased vulnerability in diabetes could possibly result from reduced compliance of the Schwann cell basal laminal ensheathment which is abnormally rigid in diabetes (King *et al.*, 1989). Apart from hereditary neuropathy with liability to pressure palsies (HNPP), and probably for diabetic neuropathy, firm evidence that there is an increased susceptibility to compression injury is lacking in other polyneuropathies, such as uraemic neuropathy or the Guillain–Barré syndrome.

Patients with HNPP consistently show electrophysiological if not clinical evidence of a generalized neuropathy. DNA studies to look for a chromosome 17p11.2 deletion (see Chapter 6) are unrewarding in patients with unexplained focal neuropathies unless there is evidence of a generalized neuropathy (A. E. Harding and P. K. Thomas, unpublished observations).

There is increasing interest in focal demyelinating inflammatory neuropathy, originally recognized in the brachial plexus (Adams *et al.*, 1965; Cusimano *et al.*, 1988), particularly because it may respond to immunosuppressive therapy (see Chapter 4). This condition can also pick out individual limb nerves such as the median or ulnar in the upper limbs or the tibial in the lower. An instructive case who presented with unilateral leg pain and myokymia in muscles innervated by the tibial nerve was reported by Mitsumoto *et al.* (1990). Electrophysiological studies revealed a mononeuropathy of the tibial nerve. Prominent localized enlargement of this nerve in the lower thigh and popliteal region was demonstrated on magnetic resonance imaging (MRI). On the reasonable assumption that this was a nerve tumour, the affected segment was excised surgically. Histological examination showed it to be an example of focal inflammatory demyelinating neuropathy. Such cases on electrophysiological studies may exhibit a marked focal reduction in nerve conduction velocity, this not being displayed by tumours. If focal slowing is found in a patient with localized nerve enlargement, exploration and intraoperative fascicular biopsy would be merited.

Other focal neuropathies associated with nerve enlargement include localized amyloidoma (Birch, 1993) and focal hypertrophic neurofibrosis (Simpson and Fowler, 1966). This latter condition continues to be a puzzle. These patients present with a mononeuropathy. Histologically the nerve shows compartmentation into multiple onion bulb-like structures resembling a chronic hypertrophic demyelinating neuropathy. The whorls, however, are composed of cells with the ultrastructural and immunocytochemical features of perineurial cells (Bilboa *et al.*, 1984). The minifascicles may or may not contain axons. Focal hypertrophic neurofibrosis has been attributed either to recurrent trauma (Ochoa and Neary, 1975) or to neoplasia, leading to the use of the term perineurioma (Bilboa *et al.*, 1984). Recently the suggestion has been made that this condition arises as a result of breaching of the perineurial diffusion barrier, the compartmentation being a secondary response (Johnson and Kline, 1989). The issue is not yet resolved although the condition is distinct from focal inflammatory demyelinating polyneuropathy.

New medical and surgical procedures may give rise to unexpected focal neuropathies as a side effect. Devastating combined median, ulnar and radial nerve lesions, caused by high arteriovenous fistulas in the arm established for renal dialysis, have already been mentioned. Antebrachial Cimino–Brescia fistulas can lead to the carpal tunnel syndrome, presumably as a result of a vascular steal phenomenon (Harding and LeFanu, 1977). Prolonged renal dialysis may also give rise to the carpal tunnel syndrome from the deposition of amyloid in the transverse carpal ligament, as mentioned in the section on Amyloid and neuropathy. The amyloid is derived from β_2 microglobulin which is retained in the circulation (Shirahama *et al.*, 1985). It is normally eliminated by the kidneys but is inadequately removed by dialysis (Chanard *et al.*, 1986). Complications from amyloid deposition develop more rapidly in patients who commence dialysis at an older age (Kurer *et al.*, 1991).

Paralysis of the diaphragm from phrenic nerve damage may develop when the internal thoracic (internal mammary) artery is harvested for use in coronary artery bypass graft operations (Landymore and Howell, 1990; O'Brien *et al.*, 1991) and is considered to be caused by compromise to the vascular supply to the nerve (Setina *et al.*, 1993). Sensory impairment and hyperaesthesia of the skin over the anterior chest wall may also develop. Right phrenic nerve injury may occur during orthotopic liver transplantation (McAlister *et al.*, 1993). Other examples of nerve injury related to newly devised invasive procedures could be given.

Diabetic neuropathies

Several clinical patterns of neuropathy, focal, multifocal and generalized, occur in the setting of diabetes mellitus, and often more than one type co-exists in the same patient. Approximately 50% of diabetic patients have evidence, either clinical or subclinical, of neuropathy, and in 13% neuropathy is symptomatic (Dyck *et al.*, 1993). Some of the peripheral motor and sensory syndromes encountered in the setting of diabetes are detailed elsewhere (see Chapter 4); a practical classification of the diabetic neuropathies appears in Table 1.2.

The strongest risk factor for the development of a diabetic neuropathy is the duration of hyperglycaemia (Pirart, 1978), although there are clearly other factors at play (Said *et al.*, 1992). Mechanisms by which hyperglycaemia eventually results in damage to peripheral nerves are still unsettled. The relative roles of tissue glycation (Brownlee *et al.*, 1988), of damage to vasa nervorum and consequent hypoxia–ischaemia of nerve (Giannini and Dyck, 1994), or of other metabolic dysfunction in nerve are undetermined.

These uncertainties notwithstanding, a number of recent clinical trials have proved valuable. Principal among these was the Diabetes Control and Complications Trial (DCCT Research Group, 1993). This decade-long trial of intensive glycaemic management in two cohorts with a total of over 1400 patients with insulin-dependent diabetes produced robust data showing a reduction by 60% of the occurrence of peripheral neuropathy in those patients managed intensively. An important adverse event seen with intensive treatment was two to three times more frequent severe hypoglycaemia episodes than in those receiving conventional therapy.

Another major effort to control the complication of neuropathy in diabetes involves aldose reductase inhibitors, but so far these have not been shown to be effective. Trials of ponalrestat (Statil) showed no effect (Florkowski *et al.*, 1991; Ziegler *et al.*, 1991; Faes *et al.*, 1993). Large trials of sorbinil, a once promising agent, disclosed no evidence of beneficial effect on peripheral nerve (Sorbinil Retinopathy Trial Research Group, 1993), and a discouraging number of hyper-

---

Table 1.2 Classification of diabetic neuropathies

Rapidly reversible phenomena
  Reduced nerve conduction velocity
  Increased resistance to ischaemic conduction failure
  'Hyperglycaemic neuropathy'

Symmetric polyneuropathies
  Sensory and sensorimotor polyneuropathy
  Autonomic neuropathy
  Acute painful neuropathy
  Proximal lower-limb motor neuropathy

Focal and multifocal neuropathies
  Cranial nerve lesions
  Thoracoabdominal neuropathy
  Focal limb neuropathies
  Diabetic amyotrophy

Mixed forms

---

sensitivity reactions occurred in patients receiving sorbinil. Tolrestat, another promising aldose reductase inhibitor, appears not to have unacceptable adverse effects, but efficacy is yet to be demonstrated. A large trial involving sural nerve biopsy studies is in progress. Other agents under study for the prevention of the complication of neuropathy in diabetes include γ-linolenic acid, said to show modest effect (Keen *et al.*, 1993) and acetyl-L-carnitine, for which results are not yet available.

Dysaesthetic pain in the extremities of diabetic patients with neuropathy remains a refractory problem. Recent controlled trials show that both amitripytyline and desipramine, both of which are tricyclic antidepressants, have equal efficacy in blunting this virulent pain, but fluoxetine was no different from placebo (Max *et al.*, 1992).

Amyloid and neuropathy

Amyloid is the poorly degradable, tissue-deposited end-product of abnormal β-pleating of a variety of proteins including transthyretin, gelsolin, apoprotein A1, immunoglobulin light chains, protein A and β_2-microglobulin. For all practical purposes, the only important amyloid disorders that are associated with generalized neuropathies are the dominantly inherited point-mutations of transthyretin (see Chapter 7) and the immunoglobulin light chain alterations responsible for primary systemic amyloidosis. At a general medical centre, primary systemic amyloidosis is much more frequent than other types of amyloidosis. Neuropathy is the presenting symptom in a fraction of all cases, perhaps 20%, and is often manifested as carpal tunnel syndrome (CTS) (Kyle and Dyck, 1993). However, CTS, while usually not associated with systemic disorders, is linked with several amyloid diseases. In some of these, CTS is the only neuropathic manifestation. For example, β_2-microglobulin-derived amyloid deposition may result in CTS in chronic dialysis patients (Shirahama *et al.*, 1985), and amyloid deposition may be associated with CTS in secondary amyloidosis. In brief, most amyloid disorders encountered are acquired.

REFERENCES

Adams, R. D., Asbury, A. K. and Michelson, J. J. (1965). Multifocal pseudohypertrophic neuropathy. *Trans. Am. Neurol. Assoc.*, **90**, 30–34

Albin, R. L., Albers, J. W., Greenberg, H. S. *et al.* (1987). Acute sensory neuropathy – neuronopathy from pyridoxine overdose. *Neurology*, **37**, 1729–1732

Asbury, A. K. (1983). New aspects of disease of the peripheral nervous system. In *Harrison's Textbook of Internal Medicine*; *Update IV*, pp. 211–229, New York: McGraw-Hill

Baba, M., Fowler, C. J., Jacobs, J. M. and Gilliatt, R. W. (1982). Changes in peripheral nerve fibres distal to a constriction. *J. Neurol. Sci.*, **54**, 197–208

Bendixen, B. H., Younger, D. S., Hair, L. S. *et al.* (1992). Cholesterol emboli neuropathy. *Neurology*, **42**, 428–430

Bilboa, J. M., Khoury, N. J. S., Hudson, A. R. and Briggs, S. J. (1984). Perineurioma (localized hypertrophic neuropathy). *Arch. Path. Lab. Med.*, **108**, 557–563

Birch, R. (1993). Peripheral nerve tumors. In *Peripheral Neuropathy*, 3rd edn (P. J. Dyck, P. K. Thomas, J. W. Griffin, P. A. Low and J. F. Poduslo, eds), pp. 1623–1640, W. B. Saunders Co., Philadelphia

Bolton, C. F., Driedger, A. A. and Lindsay, R. M. (1979). Ischaemic neuropathy in uraemic patients caused by bovine arteriovenous shunt. *J. Neurol. Neurosurg. Psychiatry*, **42**, 810–814

Brown, W. F. and Bolton, C. F. (1993). *Clinical Electromyography*, 2nd edn, Boston: Butterworth-Heinemann

Brownlee, M., Cerami, A. and Vlassara, H. (1988). Advanced glycosylation end products in tissue and the biochemical basis of diabetic complications. *N. Engl. J. Med.*, **318**, 1315–1321

Brushart, T. M. E. (1991). Central course of digital axons within the median nerve of Macaca mulatta. *J. Comp. Neurol.*, **311**, 197–207

Chalk, C. H. and Dyck, P. J. (1993). Ischemic Neuropathy. In *Peripheral Neuropathy*, 3rd edn (P. J. Dyck, P. K. Thomas, J. W. Griffin, P. A. Low and J. F. Poduslo, eds), pp. 980–989, W. B. Saunders Co., Philadelphia

Chalk, C. H., Dyck, P. J. and Conn, D. L., (1993). Vasculitic Neuropathy. In *Peripheral Neuropathy*, 3rd edn (P. J. Dyck, P. K. Thomas, J. W. Griffin, P. A. Low and J. F. Poduslo, eds), pp. 1424–1436, W. B. Saunders Co., Philadelphia

Chanard, J., Lavaud, S. and Toupance, O. (1986). Carpal tunnel syndrome and type of dialysis membrane used in patients undergoing long-term haemodialysis. *Arthritis Rheum.* **29**, 1170–1178

Cornblath, D. R., Sumner, A. J., Daube, J. *et al.* (1991). Issues and opinions: conduction block in clinical practice. *Muscle Nerve*, **14**, 869–871

Cusimano, M. D., Bilboa, J. M. and Cohen, S. M. (1988). Hypertrophic brachial plexus neuritis: a pathological study of two cases. *Ann. Neurol.*, **24**, 615–622

Dalmau, J., Graus, F., Rosenblum, M. K. and Posner, J. B., (1992). Anti-Hu-associated paraneoplastic encephalomyelitis/sensory neuronopathy. *Medicine*, **71**, 59–72

Dawson, D. M., Hallett, M. and Millender, L. H. (1990). *Entrapment Neuropathies*, 2nd edn, Little Brown and Co., Boston

Diabetes Control and Complications Research Group (1993). The effect of intensive treatment of diabetes on the development and progression of long-term complications in insulin-dependent diabetes mellitus. *N. Engl. J. Med.*, **329**, 977–986

Donaghy, M. (1993). Lumbosacral plexus lesions. In *Peripheral Neuropathy*, 3rd edn. (P. J. Dyck, P. K. Thomas, J. W. Griffin, P. A. Low and J. F. Poduslo, eds), pp. 951–961, W. B. Saunders Co., Philadelphia

Dyck, P. J., Johnson, W. J., Lambert, E. H. and O'Brien, P. C. (1971). Segmental demyelination secondary to axonal degeneration in uremic neuropathy. *Mayo Clin. Proc.*, **46**, 400–431

Dyck, P. J., Lais, A. C., Karnes, J. L. *et al.* (1981). Permanent axotomy, a model of axonal atrophy and secondary segmental demyelination and remyelination. *Ann. Neurol.*, **9**, 575–583

Dyck, P. J., Benstead, T. J., Conn, D. L. *et al.* (1987). Nonsystemic vasculitic neuropathy. *Brain*, **110**, 843–853

Dyck, P. J., Kratz, K. M., Karnes, M. S. *et al.* (1993). The prevalence by staged severity of various types of diabetic neuropathy, retinopathy, and nephropathy in a population-based cohort: The Rochester Diabetic Neuropathy Study. *Nerulogy*, **43**, 817–824

Faes, T. J., Yff, G. A., DeWeerdt, O. *et al.* (1993). Treatment of diabetic autonomic neuropathy with an aldose reductase inhibitor. *J. Neurol.*, **240**, 156–160

Fagius, J. and Wallin, B. G. (1980). Sympathetic reflex latencies and conduction velocities in patients with polyneuropathies. *J. Neurol. Sci.*, **47**, 499–507

Florkowski, C. M., Rowe, B. R., Nightingale, S. *et al.* (1991). Clinical and neurophysiological studies of aldose reductase inhibitor ponalrestat in chronic symptomatic diabetic peripheral neuropathy. *Diabetes*, **40**, 129–133

Fujimura, A., Lacroix, C. and Said, G. (1991). Vulnerability of nerve fibres to ischaemia. A quantitative light and electron microscopic study. *Brain*, **114**, 1929–1942

Giannini, C. and Dyck, P. J. (1994). Ultrastructural morphometric abnormalities of sural nerve endoneurial microvessels in diabetes mellitus. *Ann Neurol.*, **36**, 408–415

Gilliatt, R. W. and Harrison, M. J. G. (1984). In *Peripheral Nerve Disorders*, Vol. 1 (A. K. Asbury and R. W. Gilliatt, eds), pp. 243–286, Butterworths, London

Griffin, J. W., Cornblath, D. R., Alexander, E. *et al.* (1990). Ataxic sensory neuropathy and dorsal root ganglionitis associated with Sjögren's syndrome. *Ann. Neurol.*, **27**, 304–315

Hallin, S. G. (1990). Microneurography in relation to intraneural topography: somatotopic organisation of median nerve fascicles in humans. *J. Neurol. Neurosurg. Psychiatry*, **53**, 736–744

Harding, A. E. and Lefanu, J. (1977). Carpal tunnel syndrome related to antebrachial Cimino–Brescia fistula. *J. Neurol. Neurosurg. Psychiatry*, **40**, 511–513

Harding, A. E. and Thomas, P. K. (1980). The clinical features of hereditary motor and sensory neuropathies types I and II. *Brain*, **103**, 259–280

Jabaley, M. R., Wallace, W. H. and Heckler, F. R. (1980). Internal topography of major nerves of the forearm and hand. A current review. *J. Hand Surg.*, **5**, 1–8

Johnson, P. C. and Kline, D. G. (1989). Localized hypertrophic neuropathy: possible focal perineurial barrier defect. *Acta Neuropathologica*, **77**, 514–518

Kakigi, R., Shibasaki, H. and Ikeda, A. (1989). Pain-related somatosensory evoked potentials following CO_2 laser stimulation in man. *EEG Clin. Neurophysiol.*, **74**, 139–146

Kakigi, R., Shibasaki, H., Kuroda, Y. *et al.* (1991). Pain-related somatosensory evoked potentials in syringomyelia. *Brain*, **114**, 1881–1890

Katifi, H. A. and Sedgwick, E. M. (1987). Evaluation of the dermatomal evoked potential in the diagnosis of lumbo-sacral root compression. *J. Neurol. Neurosurg. Psychiatry*, **50**, 1204–1210

Keen, H., Payan, J., Allawi, J. *et al.* (1993). Treatment of diabetic neuropathy with gamma-linolenic acid. *Diabetes Care*, **16**, 8–15

Kimura, J. (1989). *Electrodiagnosis in Diseases of Nerve and Muscle. Principles and Practice*, 2nd edn, Philadelphia: F. A. Davis

Kimura, J., Machida, M., Ishida, T. *et al.*, (1986). Relation between size of compound sensory or muscle action potentials and length of nerve segment. *Neurology*, **36**, 674–681

King, R. H. M., Llewelyn, J. G., Thomas, P. K. *et al.* (1989). Diabetic neuropathy: abnormalities of Schwann cell and perineurial basal laminae. Implications for diabetic vasculopathy. *Neuropathol. Appl. Neurobiol.*, **15**, 339–355

Kissel, J. T., Slivka, A. P., Warmolts, J. R. and Mendell, J. R. (1985). The clinical spectrum of necrotizing angiopathy of the peripheral nervous system. *Ann. Neurol.*, **18**, 251–257

Kissel, J. T., Riethman, J. L., Omerza, J. *et al.* (1989). Peripheral nerve vasculitis: immune characterization of the vascular lesions. *Ann. Neurol.*, **25**, 291–297

Kocen, R. S., Lloyd, J. K., Lascelles, P. T. *et al.* (1967). Familial alpha-lipoprotein deficiency (Tangier disease) with neurological abnormalities. *Lancet*, **1**, 1341–1342

Kurer, M. H. J., Baillod, R. A. and Madgwick, O. C. A. (1991). Musculoskeletal manifestations of amyloidosis. A review of 83 patients on haemodialysis for at least 10 years. *J. Bone Joint Surg.*, **73B**, 271–276

Kyle, R. A. and Dyck, P. J. (1993). Amyloidosis and neuropathy. In *Peripheral Neuropathy*, 3rd edn (P. J. Dyck, P. K. Thomas, J. W. Griffin, P. A. Low and J. F. Poduslo, eds), pp. 1294–1308, W. B. Saunders Co., Philadelphia

Landymore, R. W. and Howell, F. (1990). Pulmonary complications following myocardial revascularization with the internal mammary artery graft. *Eur. J. Cardiothorac. Surg.*, **4**, 156–162

Levin, K. H. (1989). Ischemic monomelic neuropathy. *Muscle Nerve*, **12**, 791–795

Lisak, R. P. and Levinson, A. I. (1984). Neuropathy in connective tissue disorders: In *Peripheral Nerve Disorders: A Practical Approach* (A. K. Asbury and R. W. Gilliatt, eds) pp. 154–183, Butterworth, London

Long, R. R., Griffin, J. W., Stanley, E. F. and Price, D. L. (1980). Myelin sheath responses to alterations in axon caliber. *Neurology*, **30**, 435 (abstract)

Max, M. B., Lynch, S. A., Muir, J., Shoaf, S. E. *et al.* (1992). Effects of desipramine, amitriptyline, and fluoxetine on pain in diabetic neuropathy. *N. Engl. J. Med.*, **326**, 1250–1256

McAlister, V. C., Grant, D. R., Roy, A. *et al.* (1993). Right phrenic nerve injury in orthotopic liver transplantation. *Transplantation*, **55**, 826–830

McKhann, G. M., Cornblath, D. R., Griffin, J. W. *et al.* (1993). Acute motor axonal neuropathy: a frequent cause of acute flaccid paralysis in China. *Ann. Neurol.*, **33**, 333–342

Mitosumoto, H., Levin, K. H., Wilbourn, A. J. and Chou, S. M. (1990). Hypertrophic mononeuritis presenting with painful legs and moving toes. *Muscle Nerve*, **13**, 215–221

Moore, P. M. (1989). Immune mechanisms in the primary and secondary vasculitides. *J. Neurol. Sci.*, **93**, 129

O'Brien, J. W., Johnson, S. H. and Van Steyn, S. J. (1991). Effect of internal mammary artery dissection on phrenic nerve perfusion and function. *Ann. Thorac. Surg.*, **52**, 182–188

Ochoa, J. (1980). Nerve fiber pathology in acute and chronic compression. In *Management of Peripheral Nerve Problems* (G. E. Omer and M. Spinner, eds), pp. 487–501, W. B. Saunders Co., Philadelphia

Ochoa, J. and Neary, D. (1975). Localized hypertrophic neuropathy, intraneural tumour or chronic nerve entrapment. *Lancet*, **1**, 632–633

Panegyres, P. K., Blumbergs, P. C., Leong, A. S. Y. and Bourne, A. J. (1990). Vasculitis of peripheral nerve and skeletal muscle: clinicopathological correlation and immunopathic mechanisms. *J. Neurol. Sci.*, **100**, 193

Pirart, J. (1978). Diabetes mellitus and its degenerative complications: a prospective study of 4,400 patients observed between 1947 and 1973. *Diabetes Care*, **1**, 168–188, 252–263

Purves, A. M. (1994). The application of the CO_2 laser in analysis of small fibre function in clinical neurophysiology. M.D. Thesis, University of Cambridge

Said, G., Lacroix-Ciaudo, C., Fujimura, H. *et al.* (1988). The peripheral neuropathy of necrotizing arteritis: a clinicopathological study. *Ann. Neurol.*, **23**, 461–465

Said, G., Goulon-Goeau, C., Slama, G. and Tchobroutsky, G. (1992). Severe early-onset polyneuropathy in insulin-dependent diabetes mellitus. *N. Engl. J. Med.*, **326**, 1257–1263

Schady, W., Ochoa, J. L. and Torelbjörk, H. E. (1983). Peripheral projections of fascicles in the human median nerve. *Brain*, **106**, 745–760

Schaumburg, H., Kaplan, J., Windebank, A. *et al.* (1983). Sensory neuropathy from pyridoxine abuse: a new megavitamin syndrome. *N. Engl. J. Med.*, **309**, 445–448

Setina, M., Cerny, S., Grim, M. and Pirk, J. (1993). Anatomical interrelation between the phrenic nerve and the internal mammary artery as seen by the surgeon. *J. Cardiovasc. Surg. (Torino)*, **34**, 499–502

Shirahama, T., Skinner, M. and Cohen, A. S. (1985). Histochemical and immunohistochemical characterization of amyloid associated with chronic hemodialysis as β_2 microglobulin. *Lab. Invest.*, **53**, 705–709

Simpson, D. A. and Fowler, M. (1966). Two cases of localized hypertrophic neurofibrosis. *J. Neurol. Neurosurg. Psychiatry*, **29**, 80–87

Sladky, J. T., Tschoepe, R. L., Greenberg, J. H. and Brown, M. J. (1991). Peripheral neuropathy after chronic endoneurial ischemia. *Ann. Neurol.*, **29**, 272–278

Sorbinil Retinopathy Trial Research Group (1993). The Sorbinil Retinopathy Trial: neuropathy results. *Neurology*, **43**, 1141–1149

Stålberg, E. and Trontelj, J. V. (1979). *Single Fibre Electromyography*. Old Woking, Surrey: Miravelle Press

Sterman, A. B., Schaumburg, H. H. and Asbury, A. K. (1980). Acute sensory neuronopathy – a distinct clinical entity. *Ann. Neurol.*, **7**, 354–360

Stewart, J. D. (1993). *Focal Peripheral Neuropathies*, 2nd edn, New York: Raven Press

Sunderland, S. (1978). *Nerves and Nerve Injuries*, 2nd edn, Edinburgh: Churchill Livingstone

Thomas, P. K. and Tomlinson, D. R. (1993). Diabetic and hypoglycemic neuropathy. In *Peripheral Neuropathy*, 3rd edn (P. J. Dyck, P. K. Thomas, J. W. Griffin, P. A. Low and J. F. Poduslo, eds), pp. 1219–1250, W. B. Saunders Co., Phildelphia

Upton, A. R. M. and McComas, J. (1973). The double-crush in nerve entrapment syndrome. *Lancet*, **2**, 359–362

Wilbourn, A. J. (1993). Brachial plexus disorders. In *Peripheral Neuropathy*, 3rd edn (P. J. Dyck, P. K. Thomas, J. W. Griffin, P. A. Low and J. F. Poduslo, eds), pp. 911–950, W. B. Saunders, Co., Philadelphia

Wilbourn, A. J., Furlan, A. J., Hulley, W. and Ruschhaupt, W. (1983). Ischemic monomelic neuropathy. *Neurology*, **33**, 447–451

Wytrzes, L., Markley, H. G., Fisher, M. *et al.* (1987). Brachial neuropathy after brachial artery–antecubital vein shunts for chronic hemodialysis. *Neurology*, **37**, 1398–1402

Xu, Y., Sladky, J. T. and Brown, M. J. (1989). Dose-dependent expression of neuronopathy after experimental pyridoxine intoxication. *Neurology*, **39**, 1077–1083

Yiannikas, C., McLeod, J. G. and Walsh, J. C. (1983). Peripheral neuropathy associated with polycythemia vera. *Neurology*, **33**, 139–143

Ziegler, D., Mayer, P., Rathmann, W. and Gries, F. A. (1991). One-year treatment with the aldose reductase inhibitor, ponalrestat, in diabetic neuropathy. *Diabetes Res. Clin. Pract.*, **4**, 67–75

2
Positive motor symptoms in neuropathy: mechanisms and treatment

P. D. Thompson

POSITIVE MOTOR PHENOMENA

Most positive motor symptoms and signs that accompany peripheral nerve disease appear in the setting of an established and clinically evident neuropathy. Some motor phenomena however may be the only manifestation of a neuropathy. For example, fasciculation, fibrillation and myokymia are features of denervating motor neuropathies along with muscle wasting and weakness, while neuromyotonia and neuropathic tremor may be the presenting and predominant feature of some peripheral nerve diseases. The wide spectrum of these motor phenomena illustrates the diversity of pathophysiological mechanisms recruited by abnormal peripheral nerve function. At one end of the spectrum, fasciculations and neuromyotonia seem to be generated by peripheral nerve alone, while hemifacial spasm, neuropathic tremor and the syndrome of painful legs and moving toes are derived from a complex interaction between the abnormal peripheral nervous system and an otherwise intact central nervous system (CNS). Most of these mechanisms are poorly or incompletely understood. These issues are addressed in this chapter.

Fasciculation

Fasciculations are visible spontaneous twitches of muscle. They represent a cardinal sign of a lesion of the motor neuron at any site from the anterior horn cell to the terminal motor axon. The precise mechanism responsible for fasciculations remains unknown. The electromyographic similarity of fasciculations to voluntary muscle action potentials led Denny Brown and Pennybacker (1938) to speculate that fasciculations were due to spontaneous excitation of motor axons, resulting in activation of motor units. Fasciculations are abolished by curare but persist after nerve block and are intensified by acetyl choline or anticholinesterase drugs. Fasciculations are particularly pronounced in anterior horn cell disease, and to a lesser extent motor radiculopathies, but the above observations indicate they also arise from diseased distal axons.

Although fasciculations are recognized as a sign of motor neuron damage, they may occur during fatigue in normal subjects, as a benign familial condition, and in thyrotoxicosis. In these cases there are no other signs of a motor neuropathy suggesting mechanisms involving terminal intramuscular axons or changes in the release of acetyl choline at the neuromuscular junction.

Fibrillation

Fibrillation refers to the spontaneous discharge of a group of single muscle fibres. These are recorded electromyographically and the resulting muscle twitches are too small to be visible to the naked eye. They are thought to be due to spontaneous contraction of unstable, denervated muscle fibres. Positive sharp waves may have a similar pathophysiology. Their different morphology probably represents differences in the orientation of the electromyography needle in relation to the damaged muscle fibres.

Myokymia

Myokymia is defined clinically as a wave-like rippling of muscle. The term is used in an electromyographic sense to denote regular groups of motor **unit** discharges, especially, though not exclusively, doublets and triplets. Myokymia occurs in diseases of motor axons at any site from the ventral roots to terminal axons. It may also be seen in facial muscles in multiple sclerosis and other brain stem lesions.

Neuromyotonia

Neuromyotonia refers to the clinical syndrome of myokymia with impaired muscle relaxation. It also is used to describe trains of high frequency muscle discharges recorded by needle electromyography. These often have an abrupt crescendo–decrescendo sound, with a sudden onset and offset (lacking the waxing and waning of myotonia). Most high frequency discharges consist of stereotyped sequences of muscle **fibre** activation (Trontelj and Stålberg, 1983). Complex repetitive discharges and bizarre high frequency discharges also probably represent sequences of muscle fibre activation.

These abnormal muscle fibre discharges occur in diseases of the motor axons, but the site of origin of nerve excitation and the physiological mechanisms responsible for the distinctive patterns of muscle activity are the subject of debate. Among the theories are (1) ephaptic excitation across a peripheral nerve trunk leading to multiple orthodromic discharges in adjacent nerve fibres, (2) local circuits of re-excitation with orthodromic and antidromic passage of impulses, particularly among terminal motor axons, (3) hyperexcitability of nerve fibres and terminal motor axons which generate multiple impulses after activation and (4) prolongation of end-plate potentials at the neuromuscular junction.

ISAACS' SYNDROME – THE SYNDROME OF CONTINUOUS MUSCLE ACTIVITY

This rare but distinctive clinical syndrome comprises symptoms of muscle twitching, rippling, stiffness and cramps with electromyographic evidence of myokymia and after-discharges following nerve stimulation or voluntary contraction (Isaacs, 1961). Continuous rippling (myokymia) and fasciculations are present at rest and intensified by muscle contraction. Muscle wasting and weakness or even hypertrophy may be present (Hughes and Matthews, 1969; Valenstein *et al.*, 1978; Zisfein *et al.*, 1983). Persistence of discharge after contraction leads to delay in muscle relaxation, cramps and abnormal postures of the hands and feet resembling carpopedal spasm. Cranial and axial muscle groups are also involved and the gait may be stiff and slow. The spontaneous muscle activity persists during sleep, and after peripheral nerve, spinal nerve root or general anaesthesia but is abolished by neuromuscular block with curare and disappears locally after muscle infiltration with procaine (Isaacs, 1961). Hyperventilation and ischaemia increase the activity. Tendon reflexes are often absent and, in some cases, return after successful treatment (Isaacs and Heffron, 1974; Zisfein *et al.*, 1983; McGuire *et al.*, 1984) suggesting the areflexia was due to occlusion or inhibition of spinal monosynaptic reflexes by the continuous muscular activity.

The majority of cases reported have had no evidence or only subtle signs of an underlying peripheral neuropathy (Rowland, 1985). The disorder may be inherited (Sheaff, 1952; Ashizawa *et al.*, 1983; Auger *et al.*, 1984) or sporadic (Gardner-Medwin and Walton, 1969; van den Burgh *et al.*, 1983).

Associations of Isaacs' syndrome

Association with thymoma and intrathoracic malignancy

Neuromyotonia and continuous muscle activity have been reported in patients with intrathoracic malignancy (Wearness, 1974; Walsh, 1976) and oat cell carcinoma of the lung (Partanen *et al.*, 1980) and thymoma. The cases associated with thymoma are of considerable interest because of the known association with anti-acetyl choline receptor antibodies and impaired neuromuscular junction transmission. Among the cases associated with thymoma, elevated anti-acetyl choline receptor antibodies without myasthenia gravis (Halbach *et al.*, 1987), elevated anti-acetyl choline receptor antibodies with myasthenia gravis (Garcia-Merino *et al.*, 1991), and thymoma alone (Garcia-Merino *et al.*, 1991; Ho and Wilson, 1993) have been described. The latter three patients also had evidence of a mild neuropathy.

Association with autoimmune disease

An autoimmune cause for neuromyotonia was proposed by Newsom-Davis and Mills (1993) in a report of five patients, three of whom had oligoclonal IgG in spinal fluid. In one case IgG antibodies were demonstrated, which they suggested might enhance end-plate excitability.

Continuous muscle activity and peripheral neuropathy

Hereditary motor and sensory neuropathy (Gamstorp and Wohlfart, 1959; Lance *et al.*, 1979; Vasilescu *et al.*), chronic demyelinating neuropathy (Valenstein *et al.*, 1978), toxic neuropathies (Wallis *et al.*, 1970; Mitsumoto *et al.*, 1982), and neuropathies of unknown cause (Gamstorp and Wohlfart, 1959; Greenhouse *et al.*, 1967;

Negri *et al.*, 1977; Lubin *et al.*, 1979) have all been described in association with neuromyotonia.

Other associations

Continuous motor unit activity of peripheral nerve origin may be associated with paroxysmal ataxia with myokymia (Van Dyke *et al.*, 1975; Brunt and Van Weerden, 1990) and familial dystonic choreoathetosis (Byrne *et al.*, 1991).

Electrophysiology

The characteristic electrophysiological findings in this syndrome are continuous motor unit activity which persists during sleep, and after-discharges following voluntary contraction or peripheral nerve stimulation. The continuous activity consists of a variety of abnormal motor unit discharges including fasciculations, myokymia, long bursts of motor units of normal appearance and stereotyped high frequency discharges of muscle fibres (Figure 2.1). Continuous muscle activity may persist after peripheral nerve block, implying that the activity is driven by discharges originating in distal nerves. In some cases however, muscle activity is reduced by nerve block implying the generation of abnormal discharges at multiple, both proximal and distal, sites along the peripheral nerve (Irani *et al.*, 1977; Ashizawa *et al.*, 1983). Stimulation of peripheral motor nerves and voluntary muscle contraction are followed by after-discharges (Figure 2.2). Gentle percussion of peripheral nerves also may elicit discharges.

Pathology

Biopsy evidence of muscle denervation (Welch *et al.*, 1972; Ono *et al.*, 1989) and of segmental demyelination (Welch *et al.*, 1972) and axonal degeneration (Wallis *et al.*, 1970) have been reported in cases associated with peripheral neuropathy. A single case with a severe demyelinating neuropathy was shown to have a primary abnormality of Schwann cells (Askanas *et al.*, 1981). In some hereditary (Ashizawa *et al.*, 1983; Auger *et al.*, 1984) and sporadic (Greenhouse *et al.*, 1967; Nakanishi *et al.*, 1975) cases nerve biopsies have been normal. Abnormalities of terminal motor nerve fibre morphology (Isaacs, 1967; Lublin *et al.*, 1979) and the neuromuscular junction (Sroka *et al.*, 1975; Lütschg *et al.*, 1978; Ono, 1989) also have been demonstrated.

Possible mechanisms for continuous motor unit activity

A disorder of membrane transport was postulated by Auger *et al.* (1984) to explain familial peripheral nerve hyperexcitability (with myokymia, muscle stiffness and after-discharges) in the absence of pathological change on nerve biopsy. A reduction in the number of functional potassium channels, leading to an increase in peripheral nerve excitability (Bostock and Baker, 1988), is one physiological mechanism whereby an inherited defect or an autoimmune mechanism might result in

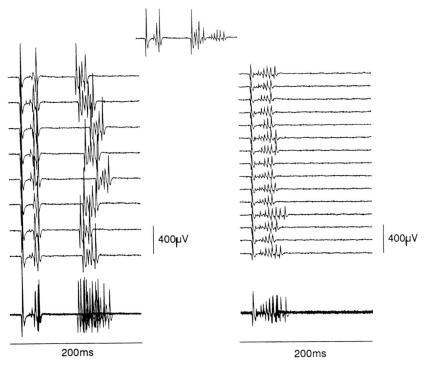

Figure 2.1 Spontaneous muscle activity recorded by needle electromyography in the tibialis anterior of a 66-year-old man with muscle cramps, stiffness and absent tendon reflexes associated with oat cell carcinoma of the lung. The uppermost trace shows a brief segment of ongoing muscle activity in which a fasciculation and a myokymic discharge are followed by a smaller high frequency discharge. These discharges were spontaneous and seemingly occurred at random in relationship to each other. Each discharge was analysed in detail in the lower traces by adjusting a trigger to collect one discharge or the other. A raster plot of eight consecutive trials is shown and these are superimposed in the bottom trace. In the lower left panel, a complex of **motor units** is shown with amplitudes up to 0.75 mV. The timing of discharge of the second group of motor units after the first shows considerable variation. In the lower right panel 15 individual trials of the smaller **muscle fibre** discharges (~0.2 mV) are shown in a raster plot and superimposed in the lowest trace. These discharges represent stereotyped sequences of muscle fibre activation. The length of the discharge varies from one trial to the next but the timing of each individual component is remarkably constant. This stereotyped nature of high frequency discharges has been interpreted as indicating ephaptic spread of activation among muscle fibres (Trontelj and Stålberg, 1983).

neuromyotonia (Newsom-Davis and Mills, 1993). This argument can be extended to those cases with an overt peripheral neuropathy. In this situation, alterations in membrane channels caused by structural damage to the axon or myelin might also lead to increased nerve excitability.

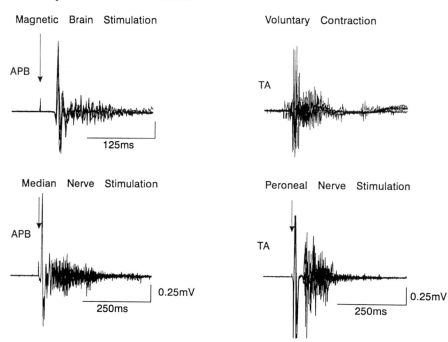

Figure 2.2 After-discharges to various forms of muscle activition from the patient illustrated in Figure 2.1. Five trials superimposed in each panel. Note that the after-discharge in this patient seems to begin immediately after the direct muscle action potential in abductor pollicis brevis (APB) following (a) brain stimulation and (b) after the burst of voluntary muscle activity in tibialis anterior (TA). However, following (c) median and (d) peroneal peripheral nerve stimulation there is a small interval between the direct muscle action potential and the F wave followed by the after-discharge. This suggests that the abnormal hyperexcitable segments of the peripheral nerves that generated the after-discharges were proximal to the stimulating electrodes (and not in the terminal motor axons or beyond).

Treatment

Carbamazepine and phenytoin are successful in abolishing symptoms in most patients with this syndrome. Muscle stiffness resolves and tendon reflexes may return to normal. Diazepam is not helpful. Plasma exchange has been reported to help two patients, one of whom had thyroid microsomal antibodies (Sinha *et al.*, 1991; Newsom-Davis and Mills, 1993), and the patient reported by Ho and Wilson (1993) improved after treatment with gamma globulin.

Prognosis

A striking feature in the majority of cases without evidence of an underlying neuropathy (or other disease) has been the benign course. Isaacs treated his original two cases with phenytoin for several years but later reported that treatment was no longer necessary some 14 years after presentation (Isaacs and Heffron, 1974).

Table 2.1 Positive motor phenomena associated with peripheral neuropathy

---

Peripheral mechanism
   Fasciculation
   Fibrillation
   Myokymia
   Neuromyotonia
   Continuous muscle activity
   Cramps
   Minipolymyoclonus

Combined peripheral – central mechanism
   Neuropathic tremor
   Sensory ataxia, pseudoathetosis
   Dyskinesias
      Painful legs and moving toes
      Painful arm and moving fingers
      Spasms of amputation stumps
   Dystonia
      Focal
      With spasms, tremor and causalgia
      Fixed dystonia with causalgia
   Myoclonus
   Hemifacial spasm
   Hemimasticatory spasm

Similar improvements over long periods of observation have been described in other cases (Hughes and Matthews, 1969; Irani *et al.*, 1977; Wilton and Gardner-Medwin, 1990).

BENIGN (PHYSIOLOGICAL) CRAMPS

Painful nocturnal muscle cramps are common in healthy people without apparent predisposing factors. Cramps may occur in association with a number of conditions such as dehydration, salt depletion and other electrolyte disturbances, pregnancy and denervation. Painful progressive muscle cramps also have been described in association with autoimmune diseases and malabsorption (Satoyoshi, 1978), and myasthenia gravis (Satoh *et al.*, 1983).

    Benign, physiological cramps occur abruptly at rest, while asleep or during exercise. They are extremely painful and may force the cessation of any activity. The muscle contraction during a cramp forces the affected limb into an abnormal posture. A distinguishing feature of benign cramps is the capacity of muscle stretch to overcome and terminate the painful cramp. Cramps are thought to originate from spontaneous activity in the terminal fibres of motor nerves. Electromyography during cramp discloses variable recruitment of normal motor units (Norris *et al.*, 1957). This finding also distinguishes cramps from other syndromes of spontaneous muscle activity of peripheral nerve origin, and from myotonia or contracture.

THE SCHWARTZ–JAMPEL SYNDROME

This rare autosomal recessive condition is characterized by muscle stiffness due to continuous motor fibre activity associated with a variety of skeletal abnormalities. These include spondylo-epiphyseal dysplasia, short stature, and dysmorphic facies with blepharophimosis, puckered mouth and dimpled chin. The latter are probably due to continuous facial muscle contraction. Percussion myotonia may be present. Electromyography reveals continuous high frequency complex repetitive muscle discharges of sudden onset and offset, often with abrupt changes in discharge frequency. After-discharges follow voluntary muscle activation or peripheral motor nerve stimulation.

Muscle activity persists after peripheral nerve block and limb ischaemia; however, the effects of curare have been variable (Taylor *et al.*, 1972; Spaans *et al.*, 1990). Persistence of activity after curare suggests a muscular origin (Spaans *et al.*, 1990), a finding supported by the demonstration of abnormal opening of sodium channels in muscle fibres (Lehmann-Horn *et al.*, 1900). Procainamide, which blocks sodium channels in nerve, abolished both the spontaneous activity and after-discharges (Lehmann-Horn *et al.*, 1990). Phenytoin and carbamazepine are less effective in this condition.

NEUROPATHIC TREMOR AND SENSORY ATAXIA

Neuropathic tremor

This has the clinical characteristics of essential tremor with a postural and kinetic tremor and a frequency of 3–6 Hz produced by alternating bursts of muscle activity in agonist and antagonist muscles. Tremors in the lower frequency have a coarse appearance similar to severe essential tremor. Neuropathic tremors typically affect the arms. Involvement of the legs is unusual, and may give the appearance of orthostatic tremor (Gabellini *et al.*, 1990). Neuropathic tremor may be the presenting symptom of an IgM paraproteinaemic neuropathy (Smith *et al.*, 1983) or chronic relapsing demyelinating neuropathies particularly when entering a relapse (Dalakas *et al.*, 1984). Peripheral sensation, in particular joint position sense is usually preserved or only mildly impaired in the tremulous limbs, and the tremor is unrelated to muscle weakness or fatigue (Dalakas *et al.*, 1984).

In IgM paraproteinaemic neuropathy a correlation has been described between tremor frequency and nerve conduction velocity (Smith *et al.*, 1984). Selective loss of large sensory fibres conveying proprioceptive input from muscle has also been implicated in a group of patients with chronic relapsing neuropathies and tremor (Adams *et al.*, 1972). These findings and the clinical observation that this type of neuropathic tremor is seen only in demyelinating neuropathies suggest peripheral nerve demyelination is in some way related to the generation of tremor. A simple delay in transmission of preserved afferent sensory information through spinal or supraspinal routes due to pure slowing of conduction seems unlikely to account for neuropathic tremor. Similarly, though there may be co-existing CNS lesions (Ormerod *et al.*, 1990, Léger *et al.*, 1992), such lesions would not explain the variation in tremor with peripheral nerve function. An interaction between degraded sensory afferent signals and potential central nervous oscillators within the motor system is another possible explanation. An example would be mismatch between kinaesthetic and proprioceptive sensory information, caused by disparate involvement of sensory fibres conveying this information to the CNS for computation of ongoing motor performance (Shahani *et al.*, 1973). This argument has been invoked to explain ataxia in peripheral nerve disease (Ropper and Shahani, 1983). Implicit in these arguments is the requirement that components of the abnormal sensory information are relayed through the cerebellum (in addition to other supraspinal centres). Evidence in support of abnormal cerebellar function, possibly related to the processing of abnormal peripheral sensory inputs and subsequent generation of oscillatory motor behaviour, comes from positron emission tomographic studies of patients with IgM associated neuropathic tremor which reveal abnormal cerebellar activation, similar to that seen in patients with essential tremor (Jenkins *et al.*, 1992).

Mention should also be made of the **Roussy–Lévy syndrome** in which a tremor resembling essential tremor occurs in the setting of type I (demyelinating) hereditary motor and sensory neuropathy. The mechanism of this tremor may be similar to that described above for other demyelinating neuropathies though genetic linkage of the two conditions also has been proposed.

These tremors are to be distinguished from the fine small amplitude and faster postural tremors similar to **exaggerated physiological tremor** that may accompany axonal peripheral neuropathies with chronic denervation and re-innervation (Said *et al.*, 1982). Tremor in these cases is attributed to enhancement of physiological tremor by weakness and fatigue leading to motor unit discharge with a greater degree of synchrony. Physiological tremor is composed of co-contracting bursts of agonist and antagonist muscle activity in contrast to the alternating tremors described above. A postural tremor may also be caused by the voluntary recruitment of enlarged motor units following denervation with re-innervation (**contraction fasciculations**, Denny-Brown and Pennybacker, 1938), or **contraction pseudotremor of chronic denervation** (Riggs *et al.*, 1983). The large motor units have the effect of amplifying normal physiological tremor, particularly during muscle fatigue. In some patients with spinal muscular atrophy, recruitment of markedly enlarged 'giant' re-innervated motor units during voluntary contraction may give rise to a jerky or myoclonic quality to the movement. This has been referred to as **minipolymyoclonus** (Spiro, 1970).

Neuropathic tremor is difficult to treat. Some benefit may be derived from propranolol, particularly in tremors resembling exaggerated physiological tremor, and primidone. In general the coarse slow tremors respond poorly to medication. The most useful strategy is treatment of the underlying neuropathy which may have a dramatic effect on tremor in chronic relapsing neuropathy.

Sensory ataxia

This differs from neuropathic tremor in that there is often pseudoathetosis of the outstretched fingers, the result of deafferentation of the affected limb, in contrast to the usual preservation of sensation on clinical testing in neuropathic tremor, and an intention tremor in addition to postural and kinetic tremors. Although a surprising degree of skill may be retained, fine tasks are performed in a clumsy fashion and the normal grading and fractionating of the control of muscle strength is lost, particularly when vision is removed.

PAINFUL LEGS AND MOVING TOES AND ITS VARIANTS

The original description of this syndrome emphasized the combination of rather slow, rhythmic sinuous abduction–adduction and flexion–extension movements of the toes with intense pain in the leg (Spillane *et al.*, 1971). The movements could be suppressed momentarily by voluntary effort, but were difficult to imitate, and modified or interrupted by voluntary movement of the affected limb (Spillane *et al.*, 1971; Dressler *et al.*, 1994). The commonest antecedents of the syndrome are spinal nerve root injury and peripheral neuropathy or peripheral limb trauma (Montagna *et al.*, 1983; Schoenen *et al.*, 1984; Léger *et al.*, 1985; Gastaut, 1986; Dressler *et al.*, 1994). Electromyographic analysis reveals long bursts of normal motor units with normal recruitment patterns. These findings suggest the movements are generated within the CNS, rather than in the periphery. A number of clinical features such as the spread of movements and pain from one segment to another, support this concept.

Theories about the origin of the moving toes have focused on the role of subtle alterations in the transmission of sensory afferent information and sympathetic input to the CNS as the result of the peripheral nerve or soft tissue injury (Nathan, 1978; Schott, 1981). This is analogous to the role of aberrant peripheral afferent sensory information in the development of causalgia via central nervous mechanisms (Schott, 1986). The excitability of segmental motor networks including interneurons within the spinal cord may be influenced by subtle changes in the character of afferent discharge (Nathan, 1978). Such reorganization of sensorimotor interaction may extend beyond segmental levels to higher centres within the nervous system. Similarly, the interaction of descending motor signals with segmental interneurons and motor neurons could also be influenced by subtle changes in sensory feedback. The end result of these complex, and speculative, interactions is the release of involuntary movements in response to corruption of normal peripheral sensory feedback.

Analogous to this syndrome is the **painful arm and moving fingers syndrome**, reported following radiation injury to the brachial plexus (Verhagen *et al.*, 1985) and the involuntary **spasms of amputation stumps** (Marion *et al.*, 1989, Kulisevsky *et al.*, 1992).

DYSTONIA

There appear to be at least three clinically identifiable groups of dystonic syndromes that develop in the wake of peripheral nerve and soft tissue injury or trauma. In the first, typical focal dystonia develops at the site of trauma (Sheehy and Marsden, 1980; Schott, 1986). In the second group, causalgia, tremor, spasms and dystonic posturing, accompanied by Sudeck's atrophy and elements of reflex sympathetic dystrophy develop after trauma to the affected body part (Marsden *et al.*, 1984; ter Bruggen and Tijssen 1988; Jankovic and Van der Linden, 1988). A third group develop fixed dystonic posturing associated with causalgia following often minor trauma (Schwartzman and Kerrigan, 1990; Bhatia *et al.*, 1993). The mechanisms underlying these phenomena are not known, though arguments similar to those described above have been invoked. In some patients, peripheral trauma is thought to precipitate dystonia in those at genetic risk for dystonia (Fletcher *et al.*, 1991). The causalgia–dystonia syndromes of the third group exhibit several differences from idiopathic dystonia (Bhatia *et al.*, 1993). Fixed dystonic postures with contractures, severe pain and a preponderance of women distinguish this syndrome from idiopathic dystonia (Bhatia *et al.*, 1993). These differences, unusual patterns of spread and the absence of any overt pathological change on extensive investigation have raised the question of whether some of these patients are suffering from conversion hysteria.

MYOCLONUS

Segmental myoclonus consists of rhythmic or semi-rhythmic brisk contractions of muscles innervated by adjacent spinal segments. Typically this persists throughout sleep and is not modified by external stimuli. Segmental myoclonus is usually considered to be spinal in origin (spinal segmental myoclonus) but a small number of cases have been described in association with lesions of the peripheral nervous system. These have included rhythmic myoclonus of the quadriceps associated with sarcomatous infiltration of the femoral nerve (Said and Bathien, 1977), rhythmic myoclonus of muscles innervated by the axillary and radial nerves due to a lesion of the posterior cord of the brachial plexus (Banks *et al.*, 1985), mid-thoracic paraspinal myoclonus due to a thoracic radicular tumour (Sotaniemi, 1985) and myoclonus of the legs and buttocks in association with lumbosacral radiculopathy (Jankovic and Pardo, 1986).

EKBOM'S SYNDROME, NOCTURNAL MYOCLONUS AND PERIODIC MOVEMENTS OF SLEEP

The sensory symptoms of the restless legs syndrome have been described in a variety of graphic ways (Ekbom, 1945). Ekbom used the terms 'creeping' and 'crawling' to describe the unpleasant, deep sensations felt bilaterally between the knees and the feet and accompanied by an intense and irresistible desire to move the feet. These overwhelming sensations appeared a short time after going to bed and would interfere with sleep. Patients would find it quite impossible to keep their legs still. They would pace the floor at night, or immerse their feet in hot and cold water in an effort to relieve these symptoms. Such symptoms have been described in association with pregnancy and iron-deficient anaemia. Subsequently it has emerged that many patients with restless legs have an extended syndrome associated with periodic movements of sleep and nocturnal myoclonus (Coleman *et al.*, 1980). In some this is dominantly inherited and responds to treatment with opiates (Walters *et al.*, 1986).

Ekbom was careful to point out that the symptoms reported in this syndrome were different from paraesthesiae, dysaesthesia, hyperpathia and cutaneous sensory disturbances such as formication that occur in sensory neuropathies. Restless legs can occasionally be a feature of peripheral neuropathies and has been described as a presenting complaint of familial amyloid neuropathy (Salvi *et al.*, 1990).

Treatment with clonazepam may afford relief from both the subjective discomfort and the nocturnal myoclonus or periodic movements of sleep.

CRANIAL NERVE LESIONS AND MOVEMENT DISORDERS

Hemifacial spasm is perhaps the most common movement disorder of peripheral origin. The brief repetitive unilateral facial movements beginning in orbicularis oculi, and later spreading to orbicularis oris, frontalis, nasalis and platysma produce a distinctive clinical picture. Though in most cases the disorder is idiopathic and no cause is found, occasionally ectatic arteries or tumours are found compressing the facial nerve in the posterior fossa. A small number of cases follow Bell's palsy. Facial muscle activity consists of high frequency discharges spreading throughout to adjacent muscle groups at short intervals (synkinesis). This activity is thought to be derived from ectopic excitation of the facial nerve near the root entry zone (where the nerve is most excitable) with ephaptic cross-activation of adjacent facial nerve fibres (Nielsen, 1984; Sanders, 1989). Synkinetic activation of facial muscles in hemifacial spasm can be demonstrated after electrical stimulation of the facial nerve. Electrophysiological recordings of synkinesis following stimulation of the intracranial portion of the facial nerve (Møller and Jannetta, 1984) and enhanced excitability of the blink reflex (Valls-Sole and Tolosa, 1989) suggest involvement of the facial nucleus in the generation of hemifacial spasm. Whether the peripheral ectopic facial nerve discharge alters facial nuclear excitability by ectopic sensory activation or antidromic discharge of motor fibres is not known.

Reinforcing this importance of ectopic generators in the pathophysiology of hemifacial spasm is the success of microvascular decompression in alleviating symptoms in a high percentage of cases. Similar relief can be obtained by injection of facial muscles with small quantities of botulinum toxin, thereby avoiding the need for posterior fossa craniotomy.

Hemimasticatory spasm may occur in isolation (Thompson and Carroll, 1983) or in association with facial hemiatrophy, a localised form of scleroderma (Kaufman, 1980; Cruccu *et al.*, 1994). Unilateral peripheral, paroxysmal activation of the motor fibres of the trigeminal nerve produce repetitive brief spasms of the muscles of mastication, predominantly masseter and temporalis. Prolonged spasms also occur with high frequency discharges of motor units. There is usually evidence of a peripheral trigeminal nerve lesion with unilateral absence of the jaw jerk and masseter silent period, slowing of conduction in the affected trigeminal nerve and after discharges in masseter following direct stimulation of the motor root of the trigeminal nerve (Cruccu *et al.*, 1994). Injection of botulinum toxin into masseter may help relieve spasms in some cases (Cruccu *et al.*, 1994).

REFERENCES

Adams, R. D., Shahani, B. T. and Young, R. R. (1972). Tremor in association with polyneuropathy. *Trans. Am. Neurol. Assoc.*, **97**, 44–48

Ashizawa, T., Butler, I. J., Harati, Y. and Roongta, S. M. (1983). A dominantly inherited syndrome with continuous motor neurone discharges. *Ann. Neurol.*, **13**, 285–290

Askanas, V., Engel, W. K., Berginer, V. M. *et al.* (1981). Lysosomal abnormalities in cultured Schwann cells from a patient with peripheral neuropathy and continuous muscle fibre activity. *Ann. Neurol.*, **10**, 238–242

Auger, R. G., Daube, J. R., Gomez, M. R. and Lambert, E. H. (1984). Hereditary form of sustained muscle activity of peripheral nerve origin causing generalized myokymia and muscle stiffness. *Ann. of Neurol.*, **15**, 13–21

Banks, G., Nielsen, V. K. Short, M. P. and Kowal, C. D. (1985). Brachial plexus myoclonus. *J. Neurol. Neurosurg. Psychiatry*, **48**, 582–584

Bhatia, K. P., Bhat, M. H. and Marsden, C. D. (1993). The causalgia–dystonia syndrome. *Brain*, **116**, 843–51

Bostock, H. and Baker, M. (1988). Evidence for two types of potassium channel in human motor axons in vivo. *Brain Res.*, **462**, 354–358

Brunt, E. R. P. and van Weerden, T. W. (1990). Familial paroxysmal kinesigenic ataxia and continuous myokymia. *Brain*, **113**, 1361–1382

Byrne, E., White, O. and Cook, M. (1991). Familial dystonic choreoathetosis with myokymia: a sleep responsive disorder. *J. Neurol. Neurosurg. Psychiatry*, **54**, 1090–1092

Coleman, R. M., Pollak, C. P. and Weitzmann, E. D. (1980). Periodic movements in sleep (nocturnal myoclonus): relation to sleep disorders. *Ann. Neurol.*, **8**, 416–421

Cruccu, G., Inghilleri, M., Berardelli, A. *et al.* (1994). Pathophysiology of hemimasticatory spasm. *J. Neurol. Neurosurg. Psychiatry*, **57**, 43–50

Dalakas, M. C., Teravainen, H. and Engel, W. K. (1984). Tremor as a feature of chronic relapsing dysgammaglobulinemic polyneuropathies. *Arch. Neurol.*, **41**, 711–714

Denny Brown, D. and Pennybacker, J. B. (1938). Fibrillation and fasciculation in voluntary muscle. *Brain*, **61**, 311–332

Dressler, D., Thompson, P. D., Gledhill, R. F. and Marsden, C. D. (1994). The syndrome of painful legs and moving toes. *Movement Disorders*, **9**, 13–21

Ekbom, K. (1945). Restless legs: a clinical study. *Acta Med. Scand.*, **158**, 1–123

Fletcher, N. A., Harding, A. E. and Marsden, C. D. (1991). The relationship between trauma and dystonia. *J. Neurol. Neurosurg. Psychiatry*, **54**, 713–717

Gabellini, A. S., Martinelli, P., Gulli, M. R. *et al.* (1990). Orthostatic tremor: essential and symptomatic cases. *Acta Neurol. Scand.*, **81**, 113–117

Gamstorp, I. and Wohlfart, G. (1959). A syndrome characterised by myokymia, myotonia, muscular wasting and increased perspiration. *Acta Psychiatr. Scand.*, **34**, 181–194

Garcia-Merino, A., Cabello, A., Mora, J. S. and Liano, H. (1991). Continuous muscle fibre activity, peripheral neuropathy and thymoma. *Ann. Neurol.*, **29**, 215–218

Gardner-Medwin, D. and Walton, J. (1969). Myokymia with impaired muscle relaxation. *Lancet*, **i**, 127–130

Gastaut, J. L. (1986). Jambes douloureuses et orteils instables. *Rev. Neurol. (Paris)*, **142**, 641–642

Greenhouse, A. H., Bicknell, J. M., Pesch, R. N. and Seelinger, D. F. (1967). Myotonia, myokymia, hyperhidrosis and wasting of muscle. *Arch. Neurol.*, **17**, 263–268

Halbach, M., Homberg, V. and Freund, H.-J. (1987). Neuromuscular, autonomic and central cholinergic hyperactivity associated with thymoma and acetylcholine receptor-binding antibody. *J. Neurol.*, **234**, 433–436

Ho, W. K. W. and Wilson, J. F. (1993). Hypothermia, hyperhidrosis, myokymia and increased urinary excretion of catecholamines associated with a thymoma. *Med. J. Aust.*, **158**, 787–788

Hughes, R. C. and Matthews, W. B. (1969) Pseudomyotonia and myokymia. *J. Neurol. Neurosurg. Psychiatry*, **32**, 11–14

Irani, P. F., Purohit, A. V. and Wadia, N. H. (1977). The syndrome of continuous muscle fibre activity. *Acta Neurol. Scand.*, **55**, 273–288

Isaacs, H. (1961). A syndrome of continuous muscle-fibre activity. *J. Neurol. Neurosurg. Psychiatry*, **24**, 319–325

Isaacs, H. (1967). Continuous muscle fibre activity in an Indian male with additional evidence of terminal motor fibre abnormality. *J. Neurol. Neurosurg. Psychiatry*, **30**, 126–133

Isaacs, H. and Heffron, J. J. A. (1974). The syndrome of "continuous muscle fibre activity" cured: further studies: *J. Neurol. Neurosurg. Psychiatry*, **37**, 1231–1235

Jankovic, J. and Pardo, R. (1986). Segmental myoclonus. *Arch. Neurol.*, **43**, 1025–1031

Jankovic, J. and Van der Linden, C. (1988). Dystonia and tremor induced by peripheral trauma: predisposing factors. *J. Neurol. Neurosurg. Psychiatry*, **51**, 1512–1519

Jenkins, I. H., Bain, P., Colebatch, J. G. *et al.* (1992). Neuropathic and essential tremor are both associated with abnormally increased activity in cerebellar pathways. *J. Neurol. Neurosurg. Psychiatry*, **55**, 1216

Kaufman, M. D. (1980). Masticatory spasm in facial hemiatrophy. *Ann. Neurol.*, **7**, 585–587

Kulisevsky, J., Marti-Fabregas, J. and Grau, J. M. (1992). Spasms of amputation stumps. *J. Neurol. Neurosurg. Psychiatry*, **55**, 626–627

Lance, J. W., Burke, D. and Pollard, J. (1979). Hyperexcitability of motor and sensory neurones in neuromyotonia. *Ann. Neurol.*, **5**, 523–532

Léger, J. M., Lubetzki, C., Bouche, P. *et al.* (1985). Jambes douloureuses et orteils instables, *Rev. Neurol. (Paris)*, **141**, 296–304

Léger, J. M., Younes-Chennoufi, A. B., Zuber, M. *et al.* (1992). Frequency of central lesions in polyneuropathy associated with IgM monoclonal gammopathy: an MRI, neurophysiological and immunochemical study. *J. Neurol. Neurosurg. Psychiatry*, **55**, 112–115

Lehmann-Horn, F., Iaizzo, P. A., Franke, C. *et al.* (1990). Schwartz–Jampel syndrome 2. Na^+ channel defect causes myotonia. *Muscle Nerve*, **13**, 528–535

Lublin, F. D., Tsiaris, P., Streletz, L. J. *et al.* (1979). Myokymia and impaired muscular relaxation with continuous motor unit activity. *J. Neurol. Neurosurg. Psychiatry*, **42**, 557–562

Lütschg, J., Jerusalem, F., Ludin, H. P. *et al.* (1978). The syndrome of continuous muscle fibre activity. *Arch. Neurol.*, **35**, 198–205

Marion, M. H., Gledhill, R. F. and Thompson, P. D. (1989). Spasms of amputation stumps: a report of 2 cases. *Movement Disorders*, **4**, 354–358

Marsden, C. D., Obeso, J. A., Traub, M. M. *et al.* (1984). Muscle spasms associated with Sudeck's atrophy after injury. *Br. Med. J.*, **288**, 173–176

McGuire, S. A., Tomasvovic, J. J. and Ackerman, N. J. R. (1984). Hereditary continuous muscle fibre activity. *Arch. Neurol.*, **41**, 395–396

Mitsumoto, H., Wilbourn, A. J. and Subramony, S. H. (1982). Generalised myokymia and gold therapy. *Arch. Neurol.*, **39**, 449–450

Møller, A. R. and Jannetta, P. J. (1984). On the origin of synkinesis in hemifacial spasm: results of intracranial recording. *J. Neurosurg.*, **61**, 569–576

Montagna, P., Cirignotta, F., Sacquegna, T. *et al.* (1983). Painful legs and moving toes associated with polyneuropathy. *J. Neurol. Neurosurg. Psychiatry*, **46**, 399–403

Nakanishi, T., Sugita, H., Shimada, Y. and Toyokura, Y. (1975). Neuromyotonia. A mild case. *J. Neurol. Sci.*, **26**, 599–604

Nathan, P. W. (1978). Painful legs and moving toes: evidence on the site of the lesion. *J. Neurol. Neurosurg. Psychiatry*, **41**, 934–939

Negri, S., Caraceni, T. and Boardi, A. (1977). Neuromyotonia. *Eur. Neurol.*, **16**, 35–41

Newsom-Davis, J. and Mills, K. R. (1993). Immunological associations of acquired neuromyotonia (Isaac's syndrome). *Brain*, **116**, 453–469

Nielsen, V. K. (1984). Pathophysiology of hemifacial spasm. I. Ephaptic transmission and ectopic excitation. *Neurology*, **34**, 418–426

Norris, F. H., Gasteiger, E. L. and Chatfield, P. O. (1957). An electromyographic study of induced and spontaneous muscle cramps. *Electroencephalogr. Clin. Neurophysiol.*, **9**, 139–147

Ono, S., Munakata, S., Kagao, K. and Shimizu, N. (1989). The syndrome of continuous muscle fibre activity: light and electron microscopic studies in muscle and nerve biopsies. *J. Neurol.*, **236**, 377–381

Ormerod, I. E. C., Waddy, H. M., Kermode, A. G. *et al.* (1990). Involvement of the central nervous system in chronic inflammatory demyelinating neuropathy: a clinical, electrophysiological and magnetic resonance imaging study. *J. Neurol. Neurosurg. Psychiatry*, **53**, 789–793

Partanen, V. S. J., Soininen, H., Saska, M. and Riekkinen, P. (1980). Electromyographic and nerve conduction findings in a patient with neuromyotonia, normocalcaemic tetany and small-cell lung cancer. *Acta Neurol. Scand.*, **61**, 216–226

Riggs, J. E., Gutmann, L. and Schochet, S. S. (1983). Contraction pseudotremor of chronic denervation. *Arch. Neurol.*, **40**, 518–519

Ropper, A. H. and Shahani, B. (1983). Proposed mechanism of ataxia in Fisher's syndrome. *Arch. Neurol.*, **40**, 537–538

Rowland, L. P. (1985). Cramps and stiffness. *Rev. Neurol. (Paris)*, **141**, 261–273

Said, G. and Bathien, N. (1977). Myoclonies rhythmées du quadriceps en relation avec un envalessment sarcomateux du nerf crural. *Rev. Neurol. (Paris)*, **133**, 191–198

Said, G., Bathien, N. and Cesaro, P.(1982). Peripheral neuropathies and tremor. *Neurology*, **8**, 480–485

Salvi, F., Montagna, P., Plasmati, R. *et al.* (1990). Restless legs syndrome and nocturnal myoclonus: initial clinical manifestation of familial amyloid neuropathy. *J. Neurol. Neurosurg. Psychiatry*, **53**, 522–525

Sanders, D. B. (1989). Ephaptic transmission in hemifacial spasm: a single fiber EMG study. *Muscle Nerve*, **12**, 690–694

Satoh, A., Tsujihat, M., Yoshimura, T. *et al.* (1983). Myasthenia gravis associated with Satoyoshi syndrome: muscle cramps, alopecia and diarrhea. *Neurology*, **33**, 1209–1211

Satoyoshi, E. (1978). A syndrome of progressive muscle spasm, alopecia and diarrhoea. *Neurology*, **28**, 458–471

Schoenen, J., Gonce, M. and Delwaide, P. J. (1984). Painful legs and moving toes: a syndrome with different pathophysiologic mechanisms. *Neurology*, **34**, 1108–1112

Schott, G. D. (1981). Painful legs and moving toes: the role of trauma. *J. Neurol. Neurosurg. Psychiatry*, **44**, 344–346

Schott, G. D. (1986). Induction of involuntary movements by peripheral trauma: an analogy with causalgia. *Lancet*, **ii**, 712–716

Schwartzman, R. J. and Kerrigan, J. (1990). The movement disorder of reflex sympathetic dystrophy. *Neurology*, **40**, 57–61

Shahani, B., Young, R. R. and Adams, R. D. (1973). The tremor in Roussy–Levy syndrome. *Neurology*, **23**, 425–426

Sheaff, H. M. (1952). Hereditary myokymia. *Arch. Neurol. Psychiatry*, **68**, 236–247

Sheehy, M. P. and Marsden, C. D. (1980). Trauma and pain in spasmodic torticollis. *Lancet*, **i**, 777–778

Sinha, S., Newsom-Davis, J., Mills, K. *et al.* (1991). Autoimmune aetiology for acquired neuromyotonia. *Lancet*, **338**, 75–77

Smith, I. S., Kahn, S. N., Lacey, B. W. *et al.* (1983). Chronic demyelinating neuropathy associated with benign IgM paraproteinaemia. *Brain*, **106**, 169–195

Smith, I. S., Furness, P. and Thomas, P. K. (1984). Tremor in peripheral neuropathy. In *Movement Disorders: Tremor* (L. J. Findley and R. Capildeo, eds) pp. 399–406, London: MacMillan Press

Sotaneimi, K. (1985). Paraspinal myoclonus due to a spinal root lesion. *J. Neurol. Neurosurg. Psychiatry*, **48**, 722–723

Spaans, F., Theunissen, P., Reekers, A. D. *et al.* (1990). Schwartz–Jampel syndrome: 1 Clinical, electromyographic and histologic studies. *Muscle Nerve*, **13**, 516–527

Spillane, J. D., Nathan, P. W., Kelly, R. E. and Marsden, C. D. (1971). Painful legs and moving toes. *Brain*, **94**, 541–556

Spiro, A. J. (1970). Minipolymyoclonus: a neglected sign of childhood spinal muscular atrophy. *Neurology*, **20**, 1124–1126

Sroka, H., Bornstein, M. and Sandbank, U. (1975). Ultrastructure of the syndrome of continuous muscle fibre activity. *Acta Neuropathol.*, **31**, 85–90

Taylor, R. G., Layzer, R. B., Davis, H. S. and Fowler, W. M. (1972). Continuous muscle fibre activity in the Schwartz–Jampel syndrome. *Electroencephalogr. Clin. Neurophysiol.*, **33**, 497–509

ter Bruggen, J. P. and Tijssen, C. C. (1988). Crural and axial myclonic dystonia following meralgia paraesthetica. *Movement Disorders*, **3**, 176–178

Thompson, P. D. and Carroll, W. M. (1983). Hemimasticatory spasm: a peripheral paroxysmal cranial neuropathy? *J. Neurol. Neurosurg. Psychiatry*, **46**, 274–276

Trontelj, J. and Stålberg, E. (1983). Bizarre repetitive discharges recorded with single fibre EMG. *J. Neurol. Neurosurg. Psychiatry*, **46**, 310–316

Valenstein, E., Watson, R. T. and Parker, J. L. (1978). Myokymia, muscle hypertrophy and percussion "myotonia" in chronic recurrent polyneuropathy. *Neurology*, **28**, 1130–1134

Valls-Sole, J. and Tolosa, E. S. (1989). Blink reflex excitability cycle in hemifacial spasm. *Neurology*, **39**, 1061–1066

van den Burgh, P., De Meirsman, J., Dom, R. and Bulcke, J. (1983). Motor neurone ridigity. *J. Neurol.*, **230**, 183–192

Van Dyke, D. H., Griggs, R. C., Murphy, J. M. and Goldstein, M. N. (1975). Hereditary myokymia and periodic ataxia. *J. Neurol. Sci.*, **25**, 109–118

Vasilescu, C., Alexianu, M. and Dan, A. (1984). Neuronal type of Charcot–Marie–Tooth disease with a syndrome of continuous motor unit activity. *J. Neurol. Sci.*, **63**, 11–25

Verhagen, W. I. M., Horstink, M. W. I. M. and Notermans, S. L. H. (1985). Painful arm and moving fingers. *J. Neurol. Neurosurg. Psychiatry*, **48**, 384–385

Wallis, W. E., van Poznack, A. and Plum, F. (1970) Generalised muscular stiffness, fasciculations and myokymia of peripheral nerve origin. *Arch. Neurol.*, **22**, 430–439

Walsh, J. C. (1976) Neuromyotonia: an unusual presentation of intrathoracic malignancy. *J. Neurol. Neurosurg. Psychiatry*, **39**, 1086–1091

Walters, A., Hening, W., Cote, L. and Fahn, S. (1986) Dominantly inherited restless legs with myoclonus and periodic movements of sleep: a syndrome related to enogenous opiates? *Adv. Neurol.*, **43**, 309–319

Wearness, E. (1974). Neuromyotonia and bronchial carcinoma. *Electromyogr. Clin. Neurophysiol.*, **14**, 527–535

Welch, L. K., Appenzeller, O. and Bicknell, J. M. (1972). Peripheral neuropathy with myokymia, sustained muscular contraction and continuous motor unit activity. *Neurology*, **22**, 161–169

Wilton, A. and Gardner-Medwin, D. (1990). 21-year follow-up of myokymia with impaired muscle relaxation. *Lancet*, **ii**, 1138–1139

Zisfein, J., Sivak, M., Aron, A. and Bender, A. N. (1983). Isaacs' syndrome with muscle hypertrophy reversed by phenytoin therapy. *Arch. Neurol.*, **40**, 241–242

3
Positive sensory symptoms in neuropathy: mechanisms and aspects of treatment

J. L. Ochoa

INTRODUCTION

In human neuropathy, the occurrence of positive somatosensory complaints reasonably indicates dysfunction of the nerve fibres of diseased primary sensory units. It is conceivable, however, that secondary pathophysiological events of clinical significance might develop in central sensory pathways as a consequence of primary nerve dysfunction. This alternative – abundantly examined in experimental animals – has been enthusiastically but uncritically extrapolated to explain atypical and perpetuating positive sensory symptoms that may emerge and grow after focal tissue injury, even when careful investigation reveals absence of 'organic' peripheral or central nervous system (CNS) dysfunction. It is safe to keep in mind that, even in the presence of documented organic nerve disease, it may be impossible to ascertain whether positive sensory symptoms are genuinely derived from abnormal nerve physiology. This doubt, which seldom arises for cases of polyneuropathy, is justified for chronic positive sensory complaints following actual or presumed focal nerve trauma. The doubt is an imperative for cases of chronic regional painful 'neuropathic' symptoms, in the absence of nerve injury, fulfilling current criteria laid for reflex sympathetic dystrophy (RSD) by the International Association for the Study of Pain, IASP (1986) and others (Jänig et al., 1991).

Positive sensory symptoms may arise from disorders affecting somatosensory function anywhere between sensory receptors and the brain–mind (cognition). Determination of the precise origin of these symptoms may acquire challenging proportions. The commonest positive somatosensory symptoms experienced by patients with organic or psychogenic 'nerve' disease, be it focal or generalized, are **paraesthesias** and **pains**. These abnormal sensations may occur spontaneously or may arise in response to the application of gentle mechanical or thermal stimuli which normally just evoke natural sensations of touch, pressure, warmth or cold.

CEREBRAL DECODING OF SUBJECTIVE ATTRIBUTES OF SOMATIC SENSATION

Much of our current knowledge about finer aspects of normal and abnormal physiology of the human sensory unit has been contributed through application of **microneurography** (Vallbo and Hagbarth, 1968; Hagbarth, 1979; Vallbo et al.,

1979). **Intraneural microstimulation,** a method of more recent advent (Torebjörk and Ochoa, 1980), has allowed researchers to interrogate the human brain as to how it decodes messages conveyed by identified primary sensory units, in terms of magnitude, subjective quality and localization of the projected sensation. Subjective somatosensory **quality** is specific for particular kinds of afferent channels and magnitude of somatic sensation can be resolved from the contents of afferent messages conveyed, even by single sensory units, in the absence of spatial summation. Finally, **locognosis,** the cortical function of localization of stimuli, can match precisely, at the millimetre level, a cutaneous locus of stimulation and the locus where the sensation is projected on the psychophysical body map. This function may also be resolved in the absence of spatial summation. Metaphorically, it has been stated 'the brain knows the address of cutaneous mechanoreceptors, at least in the fingers' (Ochoa and Torebjörk, 1983). It has been demonstrated directly that excitation of primary cutaneous nociceptors elicits either a dull burning pain (C nociceptors), or a sharp pricking pain (A delta myelinated nociceptors) (Torebjörk and Ochoa, 1980; Ochoa and Torebjörk, 1989). By contrast, excitation of nociceptors from muscle evokes a distinct cramp-like pain projected to the muscle belly and, not uncommonly, pains projected to remote body parts which may mislead the clinician (Torebjörk and Ochoa, 1980; Torebjörk *et al.*, 1984b; Marchettini *et al.*, 1990; Simone *et al.*, 1994). Human studies correlating subjective quality of somatic sensations against identified kinds of primary afferent channels which are selectively activated, have yielded a handful of practical clinical rules. For example, paraesthetic sensations consisting of tingling or 'pins and needles' relate to activity in somatosensory channels supplying the skin; burning pain and itch are also affairs of cutaneous sensation and relate to activity in C nociceptor channels; pains of a cramping quality, but without tingling or itch, emanate from muscle afferents.

DEFINITIONS

Whereas pains are commonplace experiences that do not require, and actually defy, definition, paraesthesias are defined in various ways. In his manual of *Diseases of the Nervous System*, Gowers (1886, page 8) proposed a number of definitions pertinent to the present subject:

'A painful sensation is often felt more acutely than normal; this is called "hyperaesthesia", or, more correctly "hyperalgesia". Occasionally a touch on the skin gives rise to pain, but it is probable that this is due to the stimulation of the over-sensitive nerves of common sensibility, and is not an intensification of a tactile sensation. Both tactile and painful impressions may produce sensations that are abnormal in character, described as "thrilling", "tingling", etc. This perverted sensation has been termed "paraesthesiae", or "dysaesthesia", words that have also been applied to purely subjective sensations'.

An inventory of somatosensory symptoms, as well as the indulgence that characterizes our choice of terms to define subjective neuropathic sensations, is exemplified by the descriptions and dicta of Dejerine (1901, p. 900):

'Under the name "Paresthésies" are defined in France all modifications of objective perception other than "anesthésie" and "hyperesthésie". In Germany, the word "Paresthesien" defines non-painful subjective sensations, such as "engourdissements, fourmillements", etc., which I will describe under the title of abnormal sensations or "dysesthésies"'.

Dejerine (1901, p. 897) defined **hyperalgesia** with rare insight:

'"Hyperesthésie" rarely relates to any of the specialized qualities of tactile sensibility [touch, pressure, localization]. Increased refinement of touch ["hyperpilaphésie"] results from particular dispositions or exercise [as in the blind], but is not a pathological phenomenon. Therefore, hyperesthesia does not result from augmentation of tactile faculties, but from a tendency towards rapid transformation of tactile sensations into painful sensations and towards an exaggeration of painful sensibility: it is synonymous of "hyperalgésie"'.

Although a symptom that fulfills Dejerine's definition of hyperalgesia is described classically in the thalamic syndrome caused by organic disease of the brain (Dejerine–Roussy syndrome) and therefore logically biases the mind toward central explanations for hyperalgesia in disease of the nervous system, there should be no doubt that primary peripheral nerve dysfunction can readily cause hyperalgesia (Koltzenburg *et al.*, 1993; Ochoa and Yarnitsky, 1993).

PARAESTHESIAS

Paraesthesias as symptoms of dysfunction of peripheral nerve fibres have been shown indirectly and directly to be due to ectopic nerve impulses generated in dysfunctional nerve fibres (Merrington and Nathan, 1949; Ochoa and Torebjörk, 1980; Burke, 1993). The unnatural subjective character of neuropathic paraesthesias, relative to sensations evoked by natural stimulation of receptors of primary sensory units, should not detract from acceptance of their primary peripheral origin. Neuropathic paraesthesias simply reflect unphysiological evocation of elementary physiological sensations (Ochoa and Torebjörk, 1980, 1983), as discerned through experimental selective intraneural stimulation of discrete types of primary afferents. Experimental studies (Ochoa *et al.*, 1984) have provided insights for understanding the abnormal subjective character of neuropathic paraesthesias, as follows: firstly, the abnormal quality of buzzing, tingling, prickling, etc., is due to the fact that sensations evoked by random chaotic activation of primary sensory units evoke pure elementary sensations which are foreign to us. Normally we feel blends of sensations due to co-activation of units of different types, whenever a suprathreshold stimulus is applied naturally to receptors. The localization of paraesthesias is also chaotic because the various units discharging are not being recruited more or less contiguously by a natural stimulus but are recruited randomly within the nerve trunk from where they project randomly to the cortical map. Therefore, during paraesthesias an erratic succession of various qualities of sensations projected to various points of the skin is felt. Finally, the magnitude of the multifocal succession of elementary sensations which constitute the paraesthesias is often disproportionate as a result of very high frequency discharge. A useful conceptual point is that the abnormal subjective characteristics of paraesthesias are not determined by an anomaly introduced into an operant **pattern theory**; they simply reflect an unnatural recruitment of **specific sensations**. It would also be unjustified to invoke **secondary centralization** to explain neuropathic paraesthesias, a concept which has strongly pervaded the interpretation of the mechanisms of neuropathic pains. Equally, there would be no reason to invoke sympathetic dependence of neuropathic paraesthesias, a concept which has also pervaded theory on neuropathic pains. And yet it is likely that in a subpopulation of individuals complaining of 'neuropathic' paraesthesias, sympathetic blocks uncontrolled for placebo might abolish the symptom through placebo effect.

Neuropathic paraesthesias may become exaggerated, or revived, by interjection of natural stimuli. This is clearly due to multiplication, somewhere along the hyperexcitable sensory fibres, of receptor-generated afferent impulses. This 'peripheral windup' was shown directly by microneurography in experimentally induced postischaemic paraesthesias in volunteers. Hyperventilation may cause a similar effect (Ochoa and Torebjörk, 1980).

NEUROPATHIC PAINS

For neuropathic pains, the hypothetical pathogenic mechanisms appear to be more complex than for paraesthesias and theory has become progressively convoluted over the last decade (Ochoa, 1993a). The separate denomination of paraesthesias and pains tacitly implies an essential difference. However, there is nothing magical about neuropathic pains as compared with neuropathic paraesthesias. It is most likely that, in the context of neuropathy, the mechanisms of causation of spontaneous pains, tingling, pins and needles, itching, etc., are broadly similar. The qualitative differences are predictably determined by the specific type of primary afferent channel that generates the input evoking those abnormal sensations (Ochoa *et al.*, 1990; Ochoa, 1992b; Thomas and Ochoa, 1993; Ochoa, 1995).

While more than one mechanism might explain the symptom **spontaneous pain** in neuropathy, until proven otherwise, spontaneous ectopic discharge in nociceptor fibres must be a key factor. Researchers should not be disconcerted by the frequent burning quality of neuropathic pains; again, it need not reflect the operation of the pattern theory, secondary centralization or sympathetic mediation. Burning is an intrinsic subjective characteristic of elementary, pure C nociceptor pain. Its expression tends to be buried through modulatory influences exerted by simultaneous afferent input from other types of afferent units which are unavoidably co-activated by natural stimulation. The answer to 'what happened to the burning component' of C pain is addressed elsewhere (see Discussion in Ochoa and Yarnitsky, 1994).

As for tactile paraesthesias, neuropathic pains may become exaggerated or revived by natural stimulation of symptomatic parts. This **allodynia** or **hyperalgesia** (for definitions, see Ochoa, 1992a) may be explained either by sensitization of primary nociceptors or by multiplication of impulses along nociceptor axons, both phenomena having been clearly documented in symptomatic patients (Cline and Ochoa, 1986; Cline *et al.*, 1989; J. L. Ochoa, J. Serra and M. Campero, unpublished results).

Basic hypothetical mechanisms of pain in neuropathy

Sensitization of receptor endings of nociceptor units

This may abnormally lower the threshold for pain in response to natural stimulation. This biophysical anomaly was originally described following experimental animal injury (Bessou and Perl, 1969; Perl *et al.*, 1976) and also after physical or chemical injury to human nociceptors (Torebjörk and Hallin, 1977; Torebjörk *et al.*, 1984a).

Nociceptor sensitization was also described as the basis for chronic hyperalgesia in clinical neuropathy (Cline *et al.*, 1989). It probably underlies erythralgia or the 'ABC syndrome' (Lewis, 1936; Ochoa, 1986).

Spontaneous ectopic impulse generation

This, in sensory nerve fibres, is a proven abnormal mechanism behind spontaneous neuropathic paraesthesias, also likely to operate as a mechanism of spontaneous pain. Loci of hyperexcitability within nerve fibres are prone to discharge with low threshold to mechanical energy applied to them. This is the basis for tactile paraesthesias (and probably pains) provoked by passive stretch or compression of focal pathological sources during elicitation of standard clinical manoeuvres (Tinel, Lasègue, Lhermitte). In an outstandingly investigated series of patients experiencing such signs, due to injury of somatosensory pathways, electrical nerve impulses generated ectopically from proximal sources were recorded antidromically in skin nerve fascicles of distal nerves. The abnormal activity was time-locked to the manoeuvre-evoked positive sensory symptoms. The primary disorders were peripheral nerve injuries, plexus entrapment, radiculopathy, and even demyelinating disease of the posterior columns of the spinal cord. An excellent correlation was established between the amount and time course of abnormal neural activity and the positive sensory symptoms (Nordin *et al.*, 1984). Similar observations have been recorded at the single unit level for the sign of Spurling (Ochoa *et al.*, 1987).

Ephapses

Abnormal electrical cross-excitation between axons may develop as a consequence of acute focal trauma to nerves (Katz and Schmitt, 1942). Rasminsky (1982) documented comparable phenomena through refined single-fibre electrophysiological techniques in an animal model of natural nerve pathology. Ephapses were a vintage explanation for causalgia (Granit *et al.*, 1944). Although theory on causalgia has proliferated imaginatively, it remains very likely that ephapses contribute not only to motor (Nielsen, 1984; Sanders, 1989) but also to sensory symptomatology in neuromuscular disease. Direct demonstration of ephapses in human sensory nerves remains an unsurmounted technical challenge.

Multiplication of primary afferent impulses in nociceptor channels

Exaggeration of pain magnitude is the predictable psychophysical consequence of abnormal multiplication of nociceptor input. This phenomenon has been documented in single C nociceptors in painful diabetic neuropathy (J. L. Ochoa, J. Serra and M. Campero, unpublished results).

Release of primary nociceptor input due to defective co-activation of modulatory non-nociceptor input

'Removal of epicritic sensibility exposes the activity of the protopathic system in its full nakedness' (Head, 1921). This concept has been popularized by Melzack and

Wall (1965) in the gate control theory. It is likely that these abnormal mechanisms may explain some forms of stimulus-induced hyperalgesia, for example the exaggeration of mechanically induced pain or of low temperature-induced pain during selective block of myelinated fibre input (Wahrén *et al.*, 1989; Yarnitsky and Ochoa, 1990) (See also the triple cold syndrome in Ochoa and Yarnitsky, 1994.)

Possible histopathological correlates for positive sensory nerve fibre phenomena

Fine molecular and ionic mechanisms may break down in the excitable apparatus of nerve fibres causing nerve impulse dysfunction without recognizable ultramicroscopic change. Certain recognized structural anomalies of nerve fibres may evidently make axons liable to ectopic generation of impulses. Immature axon sprouts in experimental animals have achieved a reputation as mechanosensitive and chemosensitive structures potentially capable of spontaneous nerve impulse generation (Wall and Gutnick, 1974; Brown *et al.*, 1976; Ochoa and Noordenbos, 1979). Probable examples of this are given by Sivak *et al.* (1993, pp. 140–142) in the context of traumatic neuromas associated with spontaneous pain, Tinel's sign and hyperalgesia. In those neuroma patients both electrophysiological and pathological findings supported the likely assumption that immature nerve sprouts might serve as ectopic sources of propagated nerve impulses.

Demyelinated nerve fibres have also been singled out as probable sources of ectopic impulse generation. Evidence for this was provided by Rasminsky (1982) on the basis of his animal model of dysmyelination and ectopic nerve impulse generation. Calvin (1982) made a strong theoretical proposal for nodes of demyelinated or thinly remyelinated intercalated nerve segments being capable of such behaviour. Morphophysiological evidence raised in experimental animals by Smith and McDonald (1980, 1982) directly proves that locally demyelinated fibres in the posterior columns may behave as spontaneous and mechanosensitive generators of ectopic impulses. The combined clinical and electrophysiological evidence generated by Nordin *et al.* (1984) proves indirectly that in their patients the substrate for abnormal sensory nerve impulses correlating with paraesthesias must be myelinated nerve fibres with local lesions in continuity, since those impulses were recorded antidromically, distal to the site of injury.

A case has been made (Ochoa, 1981) for the '**myelin balloon**' as potentially capable of ectopic impulse generation. This is a non-specific anomaly of nerve fibres, sometimes seen in paranodal regions. These focal varicosities (illustrated in Figures 1 and 2 of Ochoa, 1981), involve accumulation of amorphous fluid between myelin lamellae or between the axon and the myelin sheath. Bubbles of this kind have been described ultrastructurally in a variety of other conditions.

THE HYPOTHETICAL ISSUE OF 'CENTRALIZATION' OF NEUROPATHIC PAIN MECHANISMS

Fascination with secondary central mechanisms to explain much of the chronic sensory symptoms and even some of the motor phenomena in chronic neuropathic pain patients is currently in vogue. Fashion is sustained by evidence raised in experimental animals for cytological and physiological anomalies in central sensory neurons following acute trauma to peripheral nerves. Many clinicians are persuaded by clinical opinions issued by basic scientists who have conducted these fashionable experiments. Experimental interest in hypothetical secondary central changes was originally motivated by relatively concrete clinical observations following presumed nerve trauma, such as the territorial expansion of sensory, motor and autonomic symptoms, particularly the hyperalgesia. Livingston (1947) imagined that 'the internuncial pool' would develop an abnormal 'irritable state' in the spinal cord following nociceptive input which would explain the non-anatomical distribution of symptoms in 'causalgia' patients. In turn, Evans (1946) imagined that 'a prolonged bombardment of pain impulses sets up a vicious circle of reflexes spreading through a pool of many neuronal connections upward, downward, and even across the spinal cord, and perhaps reaching as high as the thalamus itself . . . . Depending on the wide spread of the pool we detect the phenomenon of pain and sympathetic disturbances observed a long distance from the injured area in the limb and occasionally even spread to a contralateral limb'. In turn, Loh and Nathan (1978) imagined that 'the abnormal state (of the CNS) is kept going by mechanoreceptors and large afferent fibres . . . which causes a state of disinhibition or facilitation spreading from the original site of input'. The observation that transcutaneous electrical nerve stimulation (TENS) might relieve pain in 'causalgia' (Wall and Sweet, 1967), supported apparently the concept of secondary 'centralization'. However, the TENS unit is a powerful placebo agent and its development and routine use were never placebo controlled (Deyo *et al.*, 1990; Shealy *et al.*, 1993; Verdugo and Ochoa 1994b). The concept of centralization was also supported apparently by the disappointing outcome of ablative neurectomy as a therapy addressed to patients with chronic 'neuropathic' pains following local truama. 'It is therefore not unreasonable to suggest these patients had transferred the source of their processing of nerve impulses from the periphery to the center' (Noordenbos and Wall, 1981). The idea appeared to be further strengthened because in many such patients the type of primary nerve fibres that carry the impulses which are eventually decoded centrally as a painful response are **tactile** myelinated fibres (Lindblom and Verrillo, 1979; Campbell *et al.*, 1988).

The grounds for scepticism about the relevance of secondary central changes in the genesis of chronic neuropathic symptoms are solid and include the following:

(1) Thorough neurological and refined laboratory investigation of patients who express expansive chronic 'neuropathic' symptoms that cannot be explained through primary nerve damage, and which are theoretically explicable through secondary sensitization and expansion of receptive fields of central neurons, reveal not only evidence of absence of nerve dysfunction, but that the positive and negative sensory and motor phenomena are best explained through a hysterical conversion–somatization process (Charcot, 1889; Adler *et al.*, 1959; Weintraub, 1988; Voiss, 1993; Ochoa, 1993a; Ochoa *et al.*, 1994). These patient's painful syndrome may be curable by psychotherapy (J. L. Ochoa *et al.*, unpublished results).

Dans l'hystérie il existe souvent des zones d'hyperesthésie superficielle ou profonde qui atteignent, soit les téguments sous forme de plaques plus ou moins étendues ou de points limités comme le vertex, soit des régions anatomiques comme les regions mammaire, cardiaque, rachidienne, soit des organes, l'ovaire, le testicule. Ces points d'hyperesthésie apparaissent spontanément, mais, très souvent aussi, ils sont le résultat d'une suggestion inconsciente de l'observateur qui les recherche.

Des sensations ordinairement indifferéntes, comme celles qui résultent du contact de corps neutres, produisent chez ces sujets des impressions douloureuses très pénibles; mais ici on est en présence de faits suggérés inconsciemment et, pour ma part, il ne m'a pas encore été donné de les observer. Du reste, les troubles de la sensibilité des hystériques défient toute description complète et précise: ils peuvent varier à l'infini sous l'influence de la suggestion et on ne s'est pas toujours assez méfié de l'influence de cette dernière, dans l'étude des troubles de la sensibilité chez ces malades.

Généralement l'hyperesthésie est totale, c'est-à-dire qu'elle atteint tous les modes de la sensibilité; elle peut cependant être inégale chez un même malade pour des excitations de même nature mais d'intensités différentes (Dejerine, 1901, pp. 899–900).

(2) In patients with unquestionable evidence of focal nerve injury of the kind that has inspired animal experimental models of painful neuropathy, the chronic symptomatology is usually explicable through bona fide primary nerve fibre mechanisms. In them, expansion of the areas of hyperalgesia, a typical 'centralized' phenomenon, is very rare (M. Campero and J. L. Ochoa, unpublished results).

(3) The apparent support lent to centralization theory by the fact that many chronic neuropathic pain patients can be subclassified into the category of **sympathetically maintained pain (SMP)** is fallacious. The concept of SMP includes the premise that primary input triggered by sympathetic events is processed centrally by secondarily sensitized neurons. The concept is negated by overwhelming evidence that SMP is a mirage. Indeed, throughout its history, the whole concept of SMP has relied critically on subjective relief of pain in 'reflex sympathetic dystrophy' by a medical intervention intended to block the sympathetic system, but without proper placebo control. Adequate placebo control of these patients proves that such response is entirely explicable through an inert or active placebo effect (Verdugo and Ochoa, 1994a,b; Verdugo *et al.*, 1994).

(4) An exposé of historical and intellectual reasons that explain candid misunderstanding (or denial) of evidence that disproves current concepts relating the sympathetic system and chronic neuropathic pain, is given elsewhere (Ochoa, 1991a,b; 1992a,b,c; 1993a,b; Ochoa and Verdugo 1993a,b; Ochoa *et al.*, 1994).

TESTS

Certain new tests that prove useful in the evaluation of 'neuropathic' pain syndromes are (1) the quantitative sensory thermotest (QST); (2) thermography; (3) local anaesthetic nerve blocks combined with thermography; and (4) microneurography.

Quantitative sensory thermotest (QST)

The QST (Fruhstorfer *et al.*, 1976; Verdugo and Ochoa, 1992) assesses the function of afferent channels concerned with sensory submodalities served by small-calibre fibres. Measured ramps of ascending or descending temperature are applied to the skin through a Peltier contact thermode, and detection thresholds are recorded as the subject signals the onset of a particular sensation. Thermal specific hypoaesthesias and thermal hyperalgesias may be detected separately or in combination. These anomalies may occur in the absence of hypoaesthesia for tactile submodalities served by large-calibre afferents. Thus a negative routine sensory examination and unimpaired sensory nerve action potentials do not exclude possible somatosensory dysfunction. This psychophysical test does not specify the level within the afferent channels, between skin and brain-mind (cognition), where the primary abnormality resides. Purely psychogenic disorders often account for abnormal patterns which may closely resemble patterns caused by peripheral nerve dysfunction. Certain atypical features of an abnormal pattern may be suggestive of psychogenic disorder (Verdugo and Ochoa, 1992). This test is essential for understanding the basis of painful neuropathic syndromes (Ochoa 1992a,b).

Thermography

Thermography sensitively detects, and precisely delineates, areas of deviation of cutaneous temperature caused by neurosecretory derangement, either affecting sympathetic efferent vasoconstrictor units, or somatic afferent nociceptor units capable of eliciting antidromic vasodilatation. In the evaluation of patients with small-calibre nerve fibre disorders, thermography is an essential tool in that it helps in understanding the pathophysiological basis of neuropathic syndromes and in classifying clinical conditions (Cline *et al.*, 1989; Culp *et al.*, 1989, Lindblom and Ochoa 1992; Ochoa 1992a,b). (See also colour plate I in Dyck *et al.*, 1993.)

Local anaesthetic nerve blocks combined with thermography

Local anaesthetics block somatic and sympathetic vasoconstrictor fibres, which explains vasodilatation in the cutaneous distribution of the sympathetic fibres. Such distribution matches the area of hypoaesthesia because vasomotor fibres cover the same area of skin as cutaneous nerve fibres. Thus determination of the area of sympathetic supply reflects the area of sensory distribution. This technique is more objective than other methods of delineating sensory patterns, such as mapping paraesthesias following percutaneous electrical stimulation, or mapping sensory deficit following nerve block, both of which rely on the patient's subjective sensory witnessing (Campero *et al.*, 1993; see Chapter 10, Rosenbaum and Ochoa, 1993). This combined method helps assess the pathophysiology of cold painful limbs and also helps to differentiate organic versus psychogenic sensory profiles. (See colour plates 16-2 and 16-4 in Rosenbaum and Ochoa, 1993.)

Microneurography in 'neuropathic pain patients'

Microneurography may help to clarify the pathophysiological basis for pains in patients with polyneuropathy or mononeuropathy, and also in those without demonstrable organic disease, typically labelled 'reflex sympathetic dystrophy'. Like spontaneous paraesthesias of peripheral nerve origin, shown to be due to recordable ectopic impulse generation in myelinated tactile mechanoreceptors (Ochoa and Torebjörk, 1980; Burke, 1993), pains in natural or experimental disease of the peripheral nervous system may be due to anomalous discharge in primary sensory units. This is the case for sensitized nociceptors: their threshold is abnormally reduced and they may respond with repetitive discharge to receptor stimulation. Microneurography has not enlightened mechanisms of pains that reflect 'release' of stimulus-induced multimodality input due to impaired central gating, as for example the triple cold syndrome (Ochoa and Yarnitsky, 1994). However, microneurography has shown normal absence of ongoing discharge in nociceptors; therefore spontaneous neuropathic pain is unlikely to reflect gate release due to defective non-nociceptor input. In pseudoneuropathic 'reflex sympathetic dystrophy' patients, generally believed to have sympathetically mediated pains, microneurography has provided evidence against that concept (Dotson, 1993; M. Campero and J. L. Ochoa, unpublished results).

A strategy to assess possible pathophysiological mechanisms of neuropathic pains based on microneurography and intraneural microstimulation has been proposed (Ochoa, 1985).

NEUROPATHIC PAINFUL SYNDROMES OF RENEWED INTEREST

The ABC syndrome

'There is a redness of the skin associated with tenderness . . . the gentlest manipulation elicits pain . . . pain is also provoked by warming . . . cooling abolishes the pain . . . the pain burns . . .' (Lewis, 1936). This syndrome, which Lewis termed 'erythralgia', is experimentally replicated in a dose-dependent way by acute application of capsaicin to skin (Culp *et al.*, 1989). It was termed the ABC syndrome (Angry Backfiring C Nociceptor syndrome) after demonstrating the presence of sensitized C nociceptors as its pathophysiologic basis (Ochoa, 1986; Cline and Ochoa, 1986; Cline *et al.*, 1989). Although by definition this syndrome fits descriptive features of 'reflex sympathetic dystrophy' (IASP, 1986), the sympathetic system is neither responsible for the abnormal temperature of the symptomatic skin in these patients, nor for the pain. If anything, engagement of sympathetic vasoconstrictor tone relieves pain and heat hyperalgesia in these patients through **cross-modality receptor threshold modulation** (Ochoa, 1986; Culp *et al.*, 1989).

The triple cold syndrome

In the triple cold syndrome (Ochoa and Yarnitsky, 1994) there is also burning pain and some mechanical hyperalgesia. However, the skin is cold and pale, and pain is provoked by cooling while warming may abolish the pain. Strikingly, triple cold syndrome patients have loss of cold sensation. This defect is likely to be pathophysiologically significant because selective blockade of cold-specific afferent input disinhibits pain induced by low temperature and the subjective quality of pain thus evoked is converted from cold pain into burning pain (Wahrén *et al.*, 1989; Yarnitsky and Ochoa, 1990). The small-calibre fibre neuropathy affecting these patients may cause enough sympathetic denervation to make the skin vasoconstricted due to denervation supersensitivity of the smooth muscle of arterioles. Again, the pain in these patients is not due to exaggerated sympathetic activity.

Psychogenic pseudoneuropathy

Unfortunate patients with primary psychological dysfunction may express a clinical picture that combines positive and negative sensory, motor and vasomotor manifestations. Very commonly these patients are misconstrued as having peripheral nerve disease. When a nerve lesion is excluded, these patients are typically relegated to the descriptive diagnostic category of 'reflex sympathetic dystrophy.' The possibility that they may have a respectable health disorder with a psychogenic basis is usually dismissed on cultural or pseudoscientific grounds. It is regularly possible to demonstrate, through properly placebo-controlled sympathetic block, that the clinical picture is not dependent on the sympathetic system. Actually, the concept of sympathetically maintained pain disappears when these placebo responder patients undergo sympathetic blocks which are properly controlled for placebo (Verdugo and Ochoa, 1994a; Verdugo et al., 1994). When rigorously assessed, it becomes possible to demonstrate, explicitly rather than by default, that the clinical symptomatology in these pseudoneuropathy patients derives from dysfunction at a psychological level rather than from disease of the peripheral nervous system (see Ochoa 1991a,b; 1992b,c; 1993a).

NOTES ON THERAPY

Therapy for neuropathic paraesthesias is seldom a consideration since the symptom tends not to be annoying. On the other hand, therapy for neuropathic pain is a very sought-after commodity and its results are disappointing more often than not. There are two main reasons for our failure to relieve patients effectively with neuropathic pain. First is the reality that the fine abnormal mechanisms which alter membrane excitability in primary nociceptors currently escape effective therapeutic manipulation. The second reason is that an important proportion of the overall population of 'neuropathic pain patients' in reality do not have organic neuropathic damage but a primary psychogenic somatoform **pseudoneuropathy syndrome** (Ochoa, 1993a,b). In a vast and representative population of chronic neuropathic pain patients evaluated rigorously in an academic neurological centre in the USA, the subpopulation of psychogenic pseudoneuropathy patients amounted to a majority (Ochoa et al., 1994).

Sadly, the drug industry's interest in pain relief has been side-tracked by seductive theories prioritizing the development of agents that might control secondary central hyperexcitability of unproven relevance (Woolf and Thompson, 1991; Kristensen et al., 1992) or development of new approaches to block an unjustly blamed sympathetic system (Ochoa, 1993a; Ochoa and Verdugo, 1993a). There is a huge market of patients suffering the consequences of nociceptor membrane hyperexcitability who await development of new and better membrane stabilizers. There is also a market of patients with neuropathy causing pain and neurotrophic dysfunction through inappropriately triggered neurogenic inflammation (Ochoa, 1986, 1992a). Elements of pathophysiological identity between this particular neuropathic painful syndrome and migraine have been reported in the past (Cline et al., 1989). It is encouraging that the drug industry has recently developed an agent which effectively controls nociceptor-induced pain and inflammation in migraine. An appropriate analogue for the extracranial nociceptor target is keenly awaited.

The **placebo issue** is paramount in the context of management of neuropathic pains. Past and current neglect of the placebo phenomenon practically nullifies every test or therapy ritual, as well as every theory, based upon subjective response to the administration of such rituals, when not controlled for inert placebo effect through administration of a control substance (Verdugo and Ochoa, 1994b). Neglect of both inert and active placebo effect and lack of appreciation of the importance of the length of time required for establishment of the placebo effect, has led to the uncritical elaboration of the concept of sympathetically maintained pain (Verdugo and Ochoa, 1994a,b; Verdugo *et al.*, 1994). When the practitioner misconstrues an inert or an active placebo response as though it were a specific response to a test or a therapy, the patient is hurt on two scores: the correct therapy is postponed, and an inappropriate therapy (or even an invasive procedure such as sympathectomy) will erroneously be implemented.

REFERENCES

Adler, E., Weiss, A. A. and Zohari, D. A. (1959). Psychosomatic approach to sympathetic reflex dystrophy. *Psychiat. Neurol.*, **138**, 256–271

Bessou, P. and Perl, E. R. (1969). Response of cutaneous sensory units with unmyelinated fibers to noxious stimuli. *J. Neurophysiol.*, **32**, 1025–1043

Brown, M. J., Martin, J. R. and Asbury, A. K. (1976). Painful diabetic neuropathy. *Arch. Neurol.*, **33**, 164–171

Burke, D. (1993). Microneurography, impulse conduction and paresthesias. *Muscle Nerve*, **16**, 1025–1032

Calvin, W. H. (1982). To spike or not to spike? Controlling the neuron's rhythm, preventing the ectopic beat. In *Abnormal Nerves and Muscles as Impulse Generators* (W. J. Culp and J. L. Ochoa, eds), pp. 295–321. New York: Oxford University Press

Campbell, J. N., Raja, S. N., Meyer, R. A. and Mackinnon, S. E. (1988). Myelinated afferents signal the hyperalgesia associated with nerve injury. *Pain*, **32**, 89–94

Campero, M., Verdugo, R. J. and Ochoa, J. L. (1993). Vasomotor innervation of the skin of the hand. A contribution to the study of human anatomy. *J. Anat.*, **182**, 361–368

Charcot, J. M. (1889). *Clinical Lectures on the Diseases of the Nervous System*, Vol. 3, The New Sydenham Society

Cline, M. and Ochoa, J. (1986). Chronically sensitized C nociceptors in skin: patient with hyperalgesia, hyperpathia and spontaneous pain. *Soc. Neurosci Abstracts*, **12**, 331

Cline, M. A., Ochoa, J. L. and Torebjörk, E. (1989). Chronic hyperalgesia and skin warming caused by sensitized C nociceptors. *Brain*, **112**, 621–647

Culp, W. J., Ochoa, J. L., Cline, M. A. and Dotson, R. (1989). Heat and mechanical hyperalgesia induced by capsaicin: cross modality threshold modulation in human C nociceptors. *Brain*, **112**, 1317–1331

Deyo, R. A., Walsh, N. E., Martin, D. C. *et al.* (1990). A controlled trial of transcutaneous electrical nerve stimulation (TENS) and exercise for chronic low back pain. *N. Engl. J. Med.*, **16**, 1049–1055

Dejerine, J. (1901). Sémiologie du système nerveux. In *Traité de Pathologie Générale* (Ch. Bouchard, ed.), Vol. 5, pp. 559–1168, Paris: Masson

Dotson, R. M. (1993). Causalgia–reflex sympathetic dystrophy – sympathetically maintained pain: myth and reality. *Muscle Nerve*, **16**, 1049–1055

Dyck, P. J., Thomas, P. K., Griffin, J. W. *et al.* (1993). *Peripheral Neuropathy*, 3rd edn. Philadelphia: W. B. Saunders

Evans, J. A. (1946). Reflex sympathetic dystrophy. *Surg. Gynecol. Obstet.*, **82**, 36–43

Fruhstorfer, H., Lindblom, U. and Schmidt, W. G. (1976). Method for quantitative estimation of thermal thresholds in patients. *J. Neurol. Neurosurg. Psychiatry*, **39**, 1071–1075

Gowers, W. R. (1886). *A Manual of Diseases of the Nervous System*, Vol. I. London: J. and A. Churchill

Granit, R., Leksell, L. and Skoglund, C. R. (1944). Fibre interaction in injured or compressed region of nerve. *Brain*, **67**, 125–140

Hagbarth, H. E. (1979). Exteroceptive, proprioceptive and sympathetic activity recorded with microelectrodes from human peripheral nerves. *Mayo Clin. Proc.*, **54**, 353–365

Head, H. (1921). Release of function in the nervous system. *Proc. R. Soc. Lond.*, [B], **92**, 184–209

International Association for the Study of Pain, IASP (1986). Classification of chronic pain. Description of chronic pain syndromes and definition of pain terms. Prepared by the subcommittee on taxonomy. *Pain, 3* (suppl.), 529–530

Jänig, W., Blumberg, H., Boas, R. A. and Campbell, J. N. (1991). The reflex sympathetic dystrophy syndrome: consensus statement and general recommendations for diagnosis and clinical research. In *Proceedings of the VIth World Congress on Pain* (M. R. Bond, J. E. Charlton and C. J. Woolf, eds), pp. 373–376, Amsterdam: Elsevier Science Publishers

Katz, B. and Schmitt, O. H. (1942). A note on interaction between nerve fibres. *J. Physiol.*, **100**, 369–371

Kristensen, J. D., Svensson, B. and Gordh, T. J. (1992). The NMDA-receptor antagonist Cpp abolishes neurogenic 'wind-up pain', after intrathecal administration in humans. *Pain*, **51**, 249–253

Koltzenburg, M., Lundberg, L. E. R. and Torebjörk, H. E. (1993). Significant addendum, dynamic and static components of mechanical hyperalgesia in human hairy skin. *Pain*, **53**, 363

Lewis, T. (1936). *Vascular Disorders of the Limbs, Described for Practitioners and Students.* London & New York: MacMillan

Lindblom, U. and Verrillo, R. T. (1979). Sensory functions in chronic neuralgia. *J. Neurol. Neurosurg. Psychiatry*, **42**, 422–435

Lindblom, U. and Ochoa, J. L. (1992). Somatosensory function and dysfunction. In *Diseases of the Nervous System. Clinical Neurobiology*, Vol. 1 (A. K. Asbury, G. M. McKhann and I. W. McDonald, eds), pp. 213–228, Philadelphia: W. B. Saunders Co

Livingston, W. K. (1947). *Pain Mechanisms*, pp. 209–223, New York: MacMillan Company

Loh, L. and Nathan, P. W. (1978). Painful peripheral states and sympathetic blocks. *J. Neurol. Neurosurg. Psychiatry*, **41**, 664–671

Marchettini, P., Cline, M. and Ochoa, J. L. (1990). Innervation territories for touch and pain afferents of single fascicles of the human ulnar nerve. *Brain*, **113**, 1491–1500

Melzack, R. and Wall, P. D. (1965). Pain mechanisms: a new theory. *Science*, **150**, 971–979

Merrington, W. R. and Nathan, P. W. (1949). A study of post-ischaemic paraesthesiae. *J. Neurol. Neurosurg. Psychiatry*, **12**, 1-18

Nielsen, V. K. (1984). Pathophysiology of hemifacial spasm. I. Ephaptic transmission and ectopic excitation. *Neurology*, **34**, 418–426

Noordenbos, W. and Wall, P. D. (1981). Implications of the failure of nerve resection and graft to cure chronic pain produced by nerve lesions. *J. Neurol. Neurosurg. Psychiatry*, **44**, 1068–1073

Nordin, M., Nyström, B., Wallin, V. and Hagbarth, K.-E. (1984). Ectopic sensory discharges and paresthesiae in patients with disorders of peripheral nerves, dorsal roots and dorsal columns. *Pain*, **20**, 231–245

Ochoa, J. L. (1981). Some aberrations of nerve repair. In *Posttraumatic peripheral nerve regeneration; experimental basis and clinical implications* (A. Gorio, H. Millesi and S. Mingrino, eds), pp. 147–155, New York: Raven Press

Ochoa, J. L. (1985). Pain and paresthesiae from neuropathy: intraneural microrecording and microstimulation studies and proposed strategy for pathophysiological assessment. In *Clinical Neurophysiology in Peripheral Neuropathies* (P. J. Delwaide and A. Gorio, eds), pp. 57–65, Elsevier Science Publications

Ochoa, J. L. (1986). The newly recognized painful ABC syndrome: thermographic aspects. *Thermology*, **2**, 65–107

Ochoa, J. L. (1991a). A dangerous diagnosis to be given. *Eur. J. Pain*, **12**, 3–63 (editorial)

Ochoa, J. L. (1991b). Afferent and sympathetic roles in chronic 'neuropathic' pains: confessions on misconceptions. In *Lesions of Primary Afferent Fibers as Tool for Study of Clinical Pain* (J. M. Besson and G. Guilbaud, eds), pp. 25–44, Amsterdam: Elsevier Science Publishers

Ochoa, J. L. (1992a). Thermal hyperalgesia as a clinical symptom. In *Hyperalgesia and Allodynia* (W. Willis, ed.), pp. 151–165, New York: Raven Press

Ochoa, J. L. (1992b). Peripheral Pain. The Cleveland Clinic Foundation, International Symposium on Pain Management. Official video recording. New Jersey: CME Conference Video Inc

Ochoa, J. L. (1992c). Reflex sympathetic dystrophy: a disease of medical understanding. *Clin. J. Pain*, **8**, 363–366

Ochoa, J. L. (1993a). Essence, investigation and management of "neuropathic" pains. Hopes from acknowledgement of chaos. *Muscle Nerve*, **16**, 997–1008

Ochoa, J. L. (1993b). The human sensory unit and pain. New concepts, syndromes and tests. *Muscle Nerve*, **16**, 1056–1062.

Ochoa, J. L. (1995). Human nociceptors in health and disease. In *Neurobiology and Disease: Contributions from Neuroscience to Clinical Neurology* (H. Bostock, P. A. Kirkwood and A. H. Pullen, eds), Cambridge University Press (in press)

Ochoa, J. L. and Noordenbos, W. (1979). Pathology and disordered sensation in local nerve lesions: an attempt at correlation. In *Advances in Pain Research and Therapy*, Vol. 3, (J. J. Bonica, J. C. Liebeskind and D. G. Albe-Fessard, eds), pp. 67–90, New York: Raven Press

Ochoa, J. and Torebjörk, E. (1980). Paresthesiae from ectopic impulse generation in human sensory nerves. *Brain*, 103, 835–853

Ochoa, J. L. and Torebjörk, H. E. (1983). Sensations evoked by intraneural microstimulation of single mechanoreceptor units innervating the human hand. *J. Physiol.*, 342, 633–654

Ochoa, J. L. and Torebjörk, H. E. (1989). Sensations evoked by intraneural microstimulation of C nociceptor fibres in human skin nerves. *J. Physiol.*, 415, 583–599

Ochoa, J. L. and Verdugo, R. J. (1993a). Reflex sympathetic dystrophy. Definitions and history of the ideas. A critical review of human studies. In *The Evaluation and Management of Clinical Autonomic Disorders* (P. A. Low, ed.), pp. 473–492, Boston: Little, Brown and Co

Ochoa, J. L. and Verdugo, R. J. (1993b). The mythology of reflex sympathetic dystrophy and sympathetically maintained pains. *Physical Medicine and Rehabilitation Clinics of North America*, 4, 151–163

Ochoa, J. L. and Yarnitsky, D. (1993). Mechanical hyperalgesias in neuropathic pain patients: dynamic and static subtypes. *Ann. Neurol.*, 33, 465–472

Ochoa, J. L. and Yarnitsky, D. (1994). The triple cold syndrome: cold hyperalgesia, cold hypoaesthesia and cold skin in peripheral nerve disease. *Brain*, 117, 185–197

Ochoa, J., Torebjörk, E. and Culp, W. (1984). Determinants of subjective attributes of normal cutaneous sensation and of paresthesiae from ectopic nerve impulse generation. In *Somatosensory Mechanisms* (C. Von Euler, O. Franzén, U. Lindblom and D. Ottoson, eds), pp. 379–389, Wenner-Gren Center International Symposium 41

Ochoa, J. L., Cline, M. A., Dotson, R. and Marchettini, P. (1987). Pain and paresthesias provoked mechanically in human cervical root entrapment (sign of Spurling). Single sensory unit antidromic recording of ectopic, bursting, propagated nerve impulse activity. In *Effects of Injury on Trigeminal Somatosensory Systems* (L. M. Pubols and B. J. Sessle, eds), pp. 389–397, Alan R. Liss Publishers, Inc

Ochoa, J. L., Marchettini, P. and Cline, M. (1990). Lessons from human research on the pathophysiology of neuropathic pains. In *Management of Pain in the Hand and Wrist* (C. B. Wynn-Parry, ed.), pp. 28–33, London: Churchill Livingstone

Ochoa, J. L., Verdugo, R. J. and Campero, M. (1994). Pathophysiological spectrum of organic and psychogenic disorders in 270 "neuropathic" pain patients fitting the description of "Causalgia" and or "RSD". In *Proceedings of the 7th World Congress on Pain* (G. F. Gebhart, D. L. Hammond and T. S. Jensen, eds), Amsterdam: Elsevier Science Publishers

Perl, E. R., Kumazawa, T., Lynn, B. and Kenins, P. (1976). Sensitization of high threshold receptors with unmyelinated (C) afferent fibers. In *Progress in Brain Research*. Somatosensory and Visceral Receptor Mechanisms (A. Iggo and O. B. Iyinsky, eds), 43, 263–277

Rasminsky, M. (1982). Ectopic excitation, ephaptic excitation and autoexcitation in peripheral nerve fibers of mutant mice. In *Abnormal Nerves and Muscles as Impulse Generators* (W. J. Culp and J. L. Ochoa, eds.), pp. 344–362, New York: Oxford University Press

Rosenbaum, R. and Ochoa, J. L. (1993). *The Carpal Tunnel Syndrome and other Disorders of the Median Nerve*. Boston: Butterworth-Heinemann

Sanders, D. B. (1989). Ephaptic transmission in hemifacial spasm: a single-fiber EMG study. *Muscle Nerve*, 12, 690–694

Shealy, C. N. and Maulsden, C. C. (1993). Modern medical electricity in the management of pain. In *Physical Medicine and Rehabilitation Clinics of North America* (G. H. Kraft, M. T. Andary and M. A. Tomski, eds), pp. 175–186, Philadelphia: W. B. Saunders Co

Simone, D. A., Marchettini, P., Caputi, G. and Ochoa, J. L. (1994). Identification of muscle afferents subserving sensation of deep pain in humans. *J. Neurophysiol.*, 72, 888–889

Sivak, M., Ochoa, J. and Fernández, J. M. (1993). Positive manifestations of nerve fiber dysfunction: clinical, electrophysiologic and pathologic correlates. In *Clinical Electromyography*, 2nd edn (W. F. Brown, C. F. Bolton, eds), pp. 117–147, Boston: Butterworth-Heinemann

Smith, K. J. and McDonald, W. I. (1980). Spontaneous and mechanically evoked activity due to central demyelinating lesion. *Nature*, 286, 154–155

Smith, K. J. and McDonald, W. I. (1982). Spontaneous and evoked electrical discharges from central demyelinating lesion. *J. Neurol. Sci.*, 55; 39

Thomas, P. K. and Ochoa, J. L. (1993). Clinical features and differential diagnosis. In *Peripheral Neuropathy*, 3rd edn (P. Dyck, P. K. Thomas, J. W. Griffin, P. A. Low and J. F. Poduslo, eds), pp. 749–774, New York: W. B. Saunders

Torebjörk, H. E. and Hallin, R. G. (1977). Sensitization of polymodal nociceptors with C fibres in man. *Proc. Int. Un. Physiol. Sci.*, **13**, 758 (abstract)

Torebjörk, H. E. and Ochoa, J. L. (1980). Specific sensations evoked by activity in single identified sensory units in man. *Acta Physiol. Scand.*, **110**, 445–447

Torebjörk, H. E., LaMotte, R. H. and Robinson, C. J. (1984a). Peripheral neural correlates of magnitude of cutaneous pain and hyperalgesia: simultaneous recordings in human sensory judgements of pain and evoked responses in nociceptors with C-fibers. *J. Neurophysiol.*, **51**, 325–339

Torebjörk, H. E., Ochoa, J. L. and Schady, W. (1984b). Referred pain from intraneural stimulation of muscle fascicles in the median nerve. *Pain*, **18**, 145–156

Vallbo, A. B. and Hagbarth, K. E. (1968). Activity from skin mechanoreceptors recorded percutaneously in awake human subjects. *Exp. Neurol.*, **21**, 270–289.

Vallbo, A. B., Hagbarth, K. E., Torebjörk, H. E. *et al.* (1979). Somatosensory proprioceptive and sympathetic activity in human peripheral nerve. *Physiol. Rev.*, **59**, 919–957

Verdugo, R. J. and Ochoa, J. L. (1992). Quantitative somatosensory thermotest. A key method for functional evaluation of small caliber afferent channels. *Brain*, **115**, 893–913

Verdugo, R. J. and Ochoa, J. L. (1994a). Sympathetically maintained pain. I. Phentolamine block questions the concept. *Neurology*, **44**, 1003–1010

Verdugo, R. J. and Ochoa, J. L. (1994b). Placebo response in chronic, causalgiform, "neuropathic" pain patients. Study and Review. *Pain Rev.*, **1**, 33–46

Verdugo, R. J., Campero, M. and Ochoa, J. L. (1994). Phentolamine sympathetic block in painful polyneuropathies. Further questioning of the concept of "sympathetically maintained pain". *Neurology*, **44**, 1010–1014

Voiss, D. V. (1993). The problem patient with pain: from myth to mayhem. *Phys. Med. Rehabil. Clin. N. Am.*, **4**, 27–40

Wahrén, L. K., Torebjörk, H. E. and Jörum, E. (1989). Central suppression of cold-induced C fibre pain by myelinated fibre input. *Pain*, **38**, 313–319

Wall, P. D. and Gutnick, M. (1974). Ongoing activity in peripheral nerves: the physiology and pharmacology of impulses originating from neuroma. *Exp. Neurol.*, **43**, 580

Wall, P. D. and Sweet, W. H. (1967). Temporary abolition of pain in man. *Science*, **155**, 108–109

Weintraub, M. I. (1988). Regional pain is usually hysterical. *Arch. Neurol.*, **45**, 914–918

Woolf, C. J. and Thompson, W. N. (1991). The induction and maintenance of central sensitization is dependent on N-methyl-D-aspartic acid receptor activation; implications for the treatment of post-injury pain hypersensitivity states. *Pain*, **44**, 293–299

Yarnitsky, D. and Ochoa, J. L. (1990). Release of cold-induced burning pain by block of cold-specific afferent input. *Brain*, **113**, 893–902

4
Neuropathies predominantly affecting sensory or motor function
P. K. Thomas and J. W. Griffin

INTRODUCTION

Most neuropathies simultaneously affect motor, sensory and sometimes also autonomic function. Others have a relatively selective effect on these different modalities. This chapter will consider those neuropathies that predominantly implicate motor and sensory function separately. Disorders that are considered primarily to affect anterior horn cells (motor neuronopathies or 'spinal muscular atrophies') will not be considered. Pure sensory neuropathies sometimes represent sensory ganglionopathies whereas in others, the peripheral sensory fibres are selectively involved. This distinction is not absolute. Thus in the sensory neuropathy produced by pyridoxine, experimental studies have shown that whether an axonopathy or a ganglionopathy occurs depends upon dosage (Xu *et al.*, 1989; see also Chapter 1). The differing environments of anterior horn and dorsal root ganglion neurons could well underlie some selective motor neuronopathies and sensory ganglionopathies but the reasons for differential involvement of motor and sensory axons are more difficult to envisage. The recent demonstration that sensory axons survive longer than motor axons following axotomy in the C57BL/Ola mouse (Glass *et al.*, 1994) indicates that these two types of nerve fibre can show differential responses to injury. In acute experimental studies in the rat it has been found that dorsal spinal roots show evidence of damage from hyperglycaemic hypoxia as indicated by a lack of posthypoxic recovery whereas this is not exhibited by ventral roots (Schneider *et al.*, 1993a).

Motor involvement in the Guillain–Barré syndrome and in chronic inflammatory demyelinating polyneuropathy is considered in Chapter 9. Sensory neuropathies related to HIV infection are considered in Chapter 11 and those related to toxic agents in Chapter 12. Leprosy is covered in Chapter 10.

SENSORY NEUROPATHIES

An early and evocative recognition of selective disease of sensory nerves was provided by Thomas Willis, the great Oxford physician and anatomist of the late seventeenth century, who included the following in a description *Of the Palsy*:

In a certain species of the palsy the sensitive faculty is hurt by itself, motion being still entire . . . the touch perishes, the locomotive power being without hurt . . . (the) members deprived of sense do not wither as those of motion, but continue full and fleshy.

(Willis, 1685)

Willis specified leprosy as an example of a selective disorder of the 'sensible fibres'. Today, there is a long list of disorders (Table 4.1) that potentially might be included under the designation 'pure sensory neuropathies', although the 'purity' of most of these disorders should be thought of as 'reagent grade' rather than 'analytical grade'.

Table 4.1 Predominantly sensory neuropathies

Infectious disorders
  Sensory neuropathy of AIDS (see Chapter 11)
  Some cases of Lyme disease
  Some cases of diphtheritic neuropathy
  Tabes dorsalis

Immune-mediated neuropathies
  Some dysproteinaemic neuropathies (e.g. IgM monoclonal gammopathies with anti-myelin-associated glycoprotein reactivity)
  Amyloidosis associated with paraproteinaemia
  Sensory ganglionitides
    idiopathic sensory neuronopathy
    carcinomatous sensory neuronopathy
    sensory ganglionitis associated with features of Sjögren syndrome

Hereditary disorders
  Hereditary sensory neuropathies
  Hereditary amyloidoses

Metabolic disorders
  Diabetes mellitus
  Some cases of uraemia
  Some cases of hypothyroidism

Neurotoxic disorders
  Cisplatin
  Metronidazole and misonidazole
  Pyridoxine
  N-3-pyridylethyl N'-p-nitrophenyl urea (Vacor)
  Taxol

DIABETIC SENSORY NEUROPATHIES

A variety of different syndromes may affect the peripheral nerves in patients with diabetes mellitus. Some give rise to pure or predominantly sensory manifestations.

'Hyperglycaemic neuropathy'

Patients with poorly controlled diabetes may complain of distal paraesthesias and sometimes pain distally in the lower extremities, unassociated with demonstrable sensory loss. These symptoms rapidly resolve with correction of the hyperglycaemia. In such patients nerve conduction velocity is usually reduced (Gregerson, 1967; Ward *et al.*, 1971) and there is increased tolerance to ischaemic conduction failure (Seneviratne and Peiris, 1968; Christensen and Ørskov, 1969). These phenomena are again rapidly corrected by the establishment of euglycaemia and the reduced nerve conduction velocity by aldose reductase inhibitors (Judzewitsch *et al.*, 1983). They may be equivalent to the early changes observed in experimental diabetic neuropathy in rodents. Such animals also show reduced nerve conduction velocity and increased tolerance to ischaemic conduction failure that is corrected by treatment with insulin, aldose reductase inhibitors and other manoeuvres (see Thomas and Tomlinson, 1993). Changes in K^+ conductance in rat spinal sensory root nerve fibres secondary to experimental hyperglycaemic but not normoglycaemic hypoxia have been demonstrated (Schneider *et al.*, 1993b). These could contribute to the occurrence of positive sensory symptoms. It has also been shown that under conditions of hyperglycaemic hypoxia, anaerobic glycolysis is enhanced in rat spinal roots. This could provide an explanation for the observed resistance to ischaemic conduction failure shown by diabetic nerve (Schneider *et al.*, 1993a). Peripheral nerve is known to be hypoxic in rats with streptozotocin-induced diabetes (Tuck *et al.*, 1984). It is possible that hypoxia could account for these various phenomena that are reversed by correction of hyperglycaemia in humans. Increased plasma viscosity, reduced red cell deformability and reduced O_2 dissociation from red cells could provide an explanation for reversible nerve hypoxia. Whether these acute changes bear any causal relationship to the more persistent diabetic polyneuropathy associated with structural changes is still uncertain.

Diabetic sensory and autonomic polyneuropathy

The commonest type of diabetic neuropathy is a symmetric distal sensory neuropathy that predominantly affects the lower limbs. As with other length-related neuropathies, with increasing severity the sensory loss advances up the limbs and later may involve the anterior aspect of the trunk and the vertex of the head. It is usually of insidious onset. There may be mild distal motor involvement. Autonomic dysfunction frequently co-exists. The neuropathy affects all sensory modalities, but there is some evidence from quantitative sensory testing that small-fibre modalities are affected selectively, possibly in the initial stages, giving rise to predominant pain and temperature sensory loss. Guy *et al.* (1985) examined thermal sensation as a measure of small-fibre involvement and vibration sense as indicative of large-fibre damage. From quantitative testing they found that temperature sensation could be affected in isolation or in combination with impaired vibration sense. Selective loss of vibration sense was not encountered. Longitudinal studies on individual patients have not been reported but would be of considerable interest. A pseudosyringomyelic picture may be encountered (Said *et al.*, 1983) and in such cases of 'small-fibre neuropathy' spontaneous pain can be a feature (Brown *et al.*, 1976). It is difficult to establish the pattern of sensory loss from morphometric studies on nerve biopsies because of the prominent regenerative activity which results in the presence of large numbers of small fibres (Llewelyn *et al.*, 1991).

Foot ulceration

The most troublesome consequence of diabetic polyneuropathy is chronic foot ulceration. This is rarely encountered as a consequence of ischaemia alone and is usually seen either as a result of sensory/autonomic neuropathy or neuropathy with ischaemia. Two syndromes are thus identifiable (Edmonds and Foster, 1994). In cases with neuropathy alone, the foot is usually warm, dry and painless and the pulses are present. The neuropathic ulcers may be associated with Charcot joints, neuropathic oedema and digital necrosis. In the neuroischaemic foot the pulses are absent and rest pain may occur. Ulceration occurs as a result of localized pressure necrosis and gangrene may supervene.

Neuropathic ulcers, although commonly believed to be most frequent under the heads of the metatarsal bones, are most often encountered on the toes, particularly on the plantar aspect of the hallux or on the tips of the other toes. Heel ulceration is not infrequent (Edmonds *et al.*, 1986). Ulcers are often associated with callus and are usually painless. Infected ulcers on the toes can lead to thrombotic occlusion of the digital arteries and digital necrosis (Edmonds and Foster, 1994).

The most important factor leading to neuropathic ulceration is sensory loss, resulting in unrecognized injury that can be mechanical, thermal or chemical. Studies from the UK and the USA, both from cross-sectional data (Edmonds, 1987; Thompson *et al.*, 1991) and prospective studies (Boulton *et al.*, 1986; Sosenko *et al.*, 1990; Rith-Najarian *et al.*, 1992; Young *et al.*, 1992), have established a strong association between sensory loss in the feet and foot ulceration. Abnormal areas of high pressure on the plantar aspect of the foot related to foot deformity or other factors are highly important (Boulton *et al.*, 1983; Veves *et al.*, 1992). Pressure from tight-fitting shoes may lead to ulceration, particularly in the presence of neuropathic oedema, a manifestation of autonomic neuropathy (Edmonds *et al.*, 1983). A further consequence of autonomic neuropathy is anhidrosis which can produce dry, fissured skin that predisposes to ulceration: there is a strong correlation between anhidrosis and the occurrence of foot ulceration (Boulton *et al.*, 1983).

Diabetic neuroarthropathy (Charcot joints)

These have similar radiological features to those of tabes dorsalis but tend to affect more distal joints, consistent with the peripheral accentuation of the sensory loss (Bailey and Root, 1947). The prevalence of diabetic neuroarthropathy is uncertain. In a recent study by Cavanagh *et al.* (1994), the prevalence in a series of neuropathic patients was 9.6%. All had a history of foot ulceration. As is true for neuropathic ulcers, the most important measure in treatment is the prevention of further mechanical trauma, although there are promising early results with the use of intravenous biphosphonates (Selby *et al.*, 1994).

Unrecognized fractures, usually of the shafts of the metatarsal bones, also occur in patients with diabetic sensory neuropathy (Cundy *et al.*, 1985). Cavanagh *et al.* (1994) compared patients with diabetic neuropathy with and without a previous history of foot ulceration with non-neuropathic diabetic and non-neuropathic subjects. When assessed radiologically, evidence of foot fractures, usually of the metatarsal shafts, was found in 22.2% of the neuropathic patients with a history of foot ulceration, but this was rare in the other three groups. The precise pathogenesis of neuroarthropathy is still not established. Loss of pain sensation is clearly fundamental, but other factors such as autonomic neuropathy leading to hyperaemia, osteolysis and ligamentous laxity may be important.

Sensory ataxia

Lower-limb incoordination leading to unsteadiness of gait, particularly in the dark, can be a feature in patients with severe diabetic neuropathy affecting proprioceptive afferents. Falls can result in fractures and contribute to the development of Charcot arthropathy. In milder cases, measurements of body sway show increased instability of posture, the severity of the abnormality being correlated with the degree of neuropathy (Ojala *et al.*, 1985).

Acute painful diabetic neuropathy

Although spontaneous pain may be a feature of the insidiously developing diabetic sensory polyneuropathy, acute painful diabetic neuropathy constitutes a distinct and uncommon syndrome, probably originally recognized by Ellenberg (1974) and termed 'diabetic neuropathic cachexia'. Archer *et al.* (1983) described a series of nine cases who were all male, although the condition is not restricted to males. In all there was an initial, precipitous and profound weight loss followed by severe, unremitting burning pain distally in the lower limbs which was most troublesome at night. Cutaneous hyperaesthesia was a prominent feature so that contact with clothing and the bedclothes at night was highly unpleasant. Motor function was preserved as were the tendon reflexes and sensory loss was only slight. There were minor autonomic features. Nerve biopsies showed acute axonal degeneration affecting fibres of all sizes. Slow recovery occurred over the course of some months with institution of strict diabetic control.

Precipitation of acute painful diabetic neuropathy in females with anorexia nervosa has been described (Steele *et al.*, 1987). It can also occur with establishment of strict diabetic control in patients with poorly controlled diabetes (Llewelyn *et al.*, 1986).

The nature of diabetic neuropathy

The selective involvement of sensory and autonomic function in diabetic neuropathy with the relative preservation of motor function is suggestive of a neuronal system degeneration in which particular sets of neurons are affected because of differential metabolic vulnerability. The teased fibre studies undertaken by Said *et al.* (1983, 1992) have indicated that the underlying pathological process is a distal axonal degeneration of dying-back pattern, accompanied by secondary demyelination central to the site of axonal degeneration. Loss of dorsal root ganglion cells is relatively modest (Dolman, 1963). Many distal axonopathies are of the central–peripheral type (Spencer and Schaumburg, 1976). As they affect the primary sensory neurons, they involve a distal degeneration of the peripherally directed axons and a rostrally accentuated degeneration of the centrally directed axons entering the spinal cord. Previous studies have demonstrated loss of axons in the dorsal columns (Dolman, 1963; Greenbaum *et al.*, 1964), but whether this shows a rostral accentuation has not yet been established. Multifocal fibre loss related to ischaemia could summate to produce a distally accentuated neuropathy (Sugimura and Dyck, 1982), but it is difficult to explain a predominantly sensory/autonomic neuropathy on this basis. In general, ischaemic neuropathies affect motor fibres to a greater extent than sensory or autonomic function (Fujimura *et al.*, 1991).

The nature of the pathological changes outlined above focuses attention on the dorsal root ganglion cells, where the synthetic mechanisms on which axonal integrity depends are sited, or on a disturbance of axonal transport. Non-enzymatic glycation of cytoskeletal proteins leading to the formation of advanced glycosylation–end products has been shown to occur (Ryle and Donaghy, 1995) and could interfere with axonal transport, although correlations with neuropathy have not been shown. The possibility of an interference with neurotrophic factors is also being explored (Thomas, 1994).

A major metabolic abnormality in diabetic nerve is increased flux in the polyol pathway leading to the accumulation of sorbitol and fructose (Gabbay, 1973). A pointer towards sorbitol accumulation being relevant to the causation of diabetic neuropathy is that, in sural nerve biopsies, sorbitol concentrations have been found to be negatively correlated with myelinated fibre density (Dyck *et al.*, 1988), although this could merely reflect a correlation with hyperglycaemia. On the other hand, increased regenerative sprouting has been reported in serial sural nerve biopsies in patients treated with the aldose reductase inhibitor sorbinil, which prevents the accumulation of sorbitol, in comparison with placebo (Sima *et al.*, 1988).

Once diabetic sensory polyneuropathy is established, significant recovery usually does not occur (Watkins, 1990) even with good glycaemic control. Nerve biopsies show that initially regenerative activity is profuse but that it later fails (Llewelyn *et al.*, 1991). The reason for this is uncertain. As indicated above, it is not because of loss of dorsal root ganglion cells. It will be important to establish whether the failure is because of a disturbance affecting the capacity of the axons to regenerate or whether the intraneural environment becomes unfavourable in some way for the support of nerve fibre elongation secondary to the diabetic state. In addition, if diabetic sensory polyneuropathy is a central–peripheral distal axonopathy, the lack of regenerative capacity in the central nervous system (CNS) would preclude recovery.

NUTRITIONAL DEFICIENCY AND SENSORY NEUROPATHIES

Predominantly sensory neuropathies in association with changes in the CNS occur as a result of a deficiency of vitamins B_{12} and E and are also seen in Strachan's syndrome. Recent advances in knowledge concerning these disorders will now be reviewed.

Cobalamin (vitamin B_{12}) deficiency

A symmetric distal sensory neuropathy may develop as a consequence of vitamin B_{12} deficiency, accompanied or preceded by a myelopathy (subacute combined degeneration) and sometimes optic atrophy and cognitive changes. In contradistinction to most neuropathies the symptoms may begin in the upper limbs which can be misleading diagnostically. Lhermitte's symptom can be encountered. The neuropathy predominantly affects large fibre modalities and nerve conduction and nerve biopsy studies indicate that it is predominantly an axonopathy (Kosik *et al.*, 1980;

McCombe and McLeod, 1984). Recordings of spinal somatosensory evoked responses suggest that the earliest changes are in the posterior columns, i.e. affecting the centrally directed axons of the primary sensory neurons (Fine and Hallett, 1980).

The metabolic explanation for the neurological dysfunction in cobalamin deficiency remains uncertain. One metabolic role of cobalamin is in the conversion of methylmalonyl CoA to succinyl CoA by methylmalonyl CoA mutase. This requires the participation of deoxyadenosylcobalamin (ado-B_{12}) (Figure 4.1). Patients with vitamin B_{12} deficiency excrete increased quantities of methylmalonic acid (MMA) in the urine because of the block in this conversion (Flavin *et al.*, 1955). It was reported that patients with neurological involvement excrete greater quantities of MMA than those with haematological involvement alone (Vivaqua *et al.*, 1966). On the other hand they tend to have a more severe deficiency of vitamin B_{12}. Nevertheless, this observation led to the proposal that this is the relevant pathway for the development of neurological complications. This now seems unlikely as in hereditary transcobalamin II deficiency, urinary MMA excretion may not be elevated even in the presence of severe neurological disorder (Burman *et al.*, 1979; Thomas *et al.*, 1982). Transcobalamin II is the most important of the three B_{12}-binding proteins in the serum. Children with transcobalamin II deficiency develop a neurological disorder dominated by ataxia and seizures. This conclusion was also reached by Carmel *et al.* (1988) from studies on a patient with subacute combined degeneration with a hereditary defect of cobalamin metabolism associated with defective methionine synthetase activity. This enzyme converts homocysteine to methionine with the participation of methyl-B_{12}.

Methyl-B_{12} was implicated in the causation of subacute combined degeneration by the observation that both a megaloblastic anaemia and this neurological syndrome can be produced by nitrous oxide inhalation (Layzer, 1978). Nitrous oxide is known to inactivate methyl-B_{12} but not ado-B_{12}. A very similar neurological disorder can be produced experimentally in monkeys by exposure to an atmosphere containing nitrous oxide (Dinn *et al.*, 1978). The observation that this can be prevented by the administration of methionine (Scott *et al.*, 1981) led to the formulation of the '**methyl group deficiency' hypothesis**. Methionine is converted to S-adenosyl

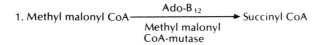

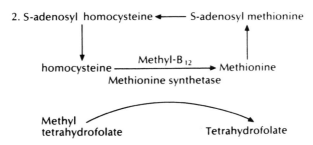

Figure 4.1 Metabolic reactions subserved by vitamin B_{12} in humans.

methionine which is the main methyl group donor in transmethylation reactions. This occurs when it is converted to S-adenosyl homocysteine. The S-adenosyl homocysteine is then converted to homocysteine which, in nervous tissue, is recycled back to methionine by receiving a methyl group from methyl tetrahydrofolate (CH_3H_4 folate) (Figure 4.1). This raised the possibility that deficiency of S-adenosyl methionine and impaired methylation underlie the neurological disorder of vitamin B_{12} deficiency (Scott *et al.*, 1981). Support for this came from the observation of Weir *et al.* (1988) that S-adenosyl homocysteine concentrations in cobalamin-deficient pig brain were increased. However, this observation was not confirmed by Viera-Makings *et al.* (1990) in cobalamin-deficient fruit bats. Moreover, incorporation of labelled methyl groups into brain components in deficient animals has been found to be normal (Deacon *et al.*, 1986; McLoughlin and Cantrill, 1986). It therefore seems improbable that impaired transmethylation is the cause of the neurological disorder related to vitamin B_{12} deficiency.

Cobalamin and folate metabolism are intimately linked. Folates are necessary for the transfer of single carbon (1-C) units in the provision of bases for DNA synthesis and in the synthesis of methionine. These single carbon units are formate, methylene and methyl groups used in purine, thymidine and methionine synthesis, respectively. Cobalamin, with folate, is needed for methionine synthesis, but cobalamin is not required for the production of the bases necessary for the manufacture of DNA. Despite this, synthesis of these bases is markedly impaired in vitamin B_{12} deficiency. This is the result of the part cobalamin plays in the supply of 1-C units.

Methyl folate is produced by the reduction of the methylene group of CH_2H_4 to CH_3H_4 folate by methylene H_4 reductase. The reaction does not occur in the opposite direction to any important extent. This led to the development of the '**methyl folate trap' hypothesis**. In this, the methyl group of CH_3H_4 folate cannot be donated to homocysteine to produce methionine and, in addition, the methyl group cannot be oxidized back to methylene to form CH_2H_4 folate. The H_4 folate is therefore 'trapped', interfering with 1-C unit transfer and depressing thymidine and purine synthesis. However, injected CH_3 folate has been found to be removed from plasma more rapidly in patients with cobalamin deficiency (Chanarin and Perry, 1968). In addition, Deacon *et al.* (1990a), in incubated bone marrow cells from cobalamin-deficient rats, followed the incorporation of a 1-C unit delivered as [^{14}C]formate into methionine, purines and thymine and detected no accumulation of [^{14}C]methyl folate. The methyl folate trap hypothesis can thus be discounted.

A further suggestion is the '**formate starvation' hypothesis** to account for the consequences of vitamin B_{12} deficiency (see Chanarin *et al.*, 1992). This hypothesis proposes that cobalamin is involved in the supply of formyl H_4 folate and has largely been derived from studies on cobalamin-deficient rats exposed to nitrous oxide. Formate is linked to H_4 folate by formyl H_4 folate synthetase. This enzyme is induced by cobalamin deficiency (Deacon *et al.*, 1990b).

The active folate coenzyme is H_4 folate polyglutamate. Cobalamin-deficient rats are unable to use H_4 folate to synthesize folate polyglutamate but can use formyl H_4 folate (Perry *et al.*, 1983). This is also true for the synthesis of thymidine (Deacon *et al.*, 1981). Methionine is able to reverse the impairment of polyglutamate synthesis in rats exposed to nitrous oxide (Perry *et al.*, 1983) and it is likely that this is by the provision of formate (see Chanarin *et al.*, 1992). It was therefore suggested that the role of cobalamin is either in the supply or the use of formate by the folate coenzyme and that cobalamin deficiency leads to 'formate starvation'. This proposal requires further support.

Strachan's syndrome

The combination of amblyopia, painful neuropathy and orogenital dermatitis was first reported from Jamaica towards the end of the last century by Strachan (1888, 1897) and attributed to malaria. Similar cases were documented, again from Jamaica, by Scott (1918), from prisons in Singapore and Johore by Landor and Pallister (1935), from Madrid during the Spanish Civil War by Peraita (1946) and in prisoners of war in the middle and far east during World War II by Denny-Brown (1947), Spillane (1947), Miller Fisher (1966) and others. They were identified as a distinct type of nutritional deficiency by Miller Fisher (1955) and Victor (1974) and termed Strachan's syndrome. Victor considered that the essential features of the condition were optic neuropathy with bilateral central or caecocentral scotomata and a painful sensory neuropathy which could also present in the absence of the mucocutaneous manifestations (Spillane and Scott, 1945; Clarke and Sneddon, 1946). The cases of tropical nutritional amblyopia reported from Trinidad by Métivier (1941) were believed to be a partial manifestation of the syndrome. It is highly likely that Strachan's syndrome is due to nutritional deficiency but the precise micronutrients involved have not been identified.

Cuban neuropathy

During the latter part of 1991 cases of bilateral optic neuropathy began to appear in unusual numbers in the Western part of Cuba characterized by visual failure with bilateral central or caecocentral scotomata. Later cases were associated with a painful sensory neuropathy with manifestations predominantly distally in the legs (Lincoff *et al.*, 1993). Nerve conduction studies and nerve biopsy findings indicated an axonopathy. Some patients had accompanying deafness, ataxia and mild long tract signs. These symptoms developed on a background of weight loss and were sometimes associated with angular stomatitis. The number of cases reached epidemic proportions but the outbreak subsided in 1993 when B vitamins were administered to the whole population of Cuba. The features resembled those of Strachan's syndrome (Thomas *et al.*, 1994). The Cuban patients were identical to others that are currently being investigated in coastal Tanzania (G. Plant, personal communication).

Vitamin E deficiency

A neurological syndrome related to severe and prolonged vitamin E deficiency has been recognized over the past few years. The clinical features, which were reviewed by Harding (1987), are remarkably stereotyped and combine a spinocerebellar syndrome with a predominantly sensory neuropathy. A pigmentary retinopathy may occur. Limb and gait ataxia is prominent and dysarthria may be present. The tendon reflexes are depressed or absent. The plantar responses are usually extensor. Proprioceptive and vibration sensory loss are prominent but loss of pain and temperature sensibility is less often encountered. Generalized muscle weakness is sometimes evident and skeletal deformity may be present in cases with onset in childhood. The syndrome has been described most often in children with congenital biliary atresia and cystic fibrosis, but it has also been reported in adults with extensive intestinal resection. It is also now clear that vitamin E deficiency is the explanation for the neurological syndrome of abetalipoproteinaemia (see later).

Nerve conduction studies demonstrate normal motor conduction velocity but depressed or absent sensory action potentials (Harding *et al.*, 1982; Alvarez *et al.*, 1983; Sokol *et al.*, 1985). There may be electromyographic evidence of denervation, mainly in distal muscles, but minor myopathic changes may be evident, seen also in muscle biopsies (Neville *et al.*, 1983). Experimental vitamin E deficiency in monkeys (Nelson *et al.*, 1981) and rats (Towfighi, 1981; Southam *et al.*, 1991), shows a distal axonopathy in sensory nerve fibres that particularly affects the centrally directed axons of the primary sensory neurons. This appears to be due to free radical damage because of the lack of antioxidant effect of vitamin E, possibly affecting mitochondrial function (Thomas *et al.*, 1993).

Clinical improvement may follow vitamin E supplementation (Harding *et al.*, 1982; Guggenheim *et al.*, 1993; Landrieu *et al.*, 1985; Sokol *et al.*, 1985).

HEREDITARY SENSORY NEUROPATHIES

The hereditary sensory neuropathies (HSN) have not shared in the conspicuous recent advances in the molecular genetics of the hereditary demyelinating motor and sensory neuropathies (see Chapter 6). Current classifications therefore necessarily have to be based on patterns of inheritance and clinical and pathological features. Nevertheless, the delineation of definite genetic entities is vital for clinical management and an important preliminary to the elucidation of the underlying gene defects. A classification devised on these principles is given in Table 4.2.

Table 4.2 Genetic classification of the hereditary sensory neuropathies (HSN)

Autosomal dominant inheritance
  Dominantly inherited sensory neuropathy
  HSN with spastic paraplegia
  Sensory neuropathy with deafness and dementia

Autosomal recessive inheritance
  Autosomal recessive sensory neuropathy
    Congenital non-progressive
    Progressive
  Congenital sensory neuropathy with anhidrosis
  Familial dysautonomia (Riley–Day syndrome)
  HSN with spastic paraplegia
  HSN with predominant loss of small myelinated fibres
  Others

X-linked recessive inheritance
  X-linked recessive sensory neuropathy

Autosomal dominant hereditary sensory neuropathy

Early descriptions of this disorder are probably recognizable as familial ulceromutilating acropathy (Thévenard, 1942) or similar designations and sometimes referred to as familial lumbosacral syringomyelia because of the greater involvement of pain and temperature sensation. Its recognition as a sensory neuropathy dates from the studies by Jughenn *et al.* (1949) and Denny-Brown (1951). It corresponds to type I hereditary sensory and autonomic neuropathy (HSAN I) in the classification proposed by Dyck *et al.* (1983). The onset is most commonly during the second or third decades and is often with chronic foot ulceration because of undetected loss of pain and temperature sensation in the feet. Neuropathic joint degeneration may occur. Spontaneous pain either of an aching nature or as lanciating stabs felt mainly in the feet and lower legs frequently occurs and 'burning feet' has been described as a presenting symptom (Dyck and Bastron, 1983). Other sensory modalities, and the upper limbs, are affected later. There may be minor distal motor manifestations. Autonomic involvement is lacking or only slight. Deafness occurs in some families (Hicks, 1922; Denny-Brown, 1951) related to end-organ failure.

The autopsy study by Denny-Brown (1951) revealed loss of dorsal root ganglion cells. The later nerve biopsy investigation by Lambert and Dyck (1975) demonstrated by *in vitro* electrophysiological recordings and morphometric analysis that in the earlier stages there is a predominant depletion of unmyelinated and small myelinated axons. The condition probably also involves a distal axonopathy as fibre loss was found to be greater at ankle than calf level in the sural nerve. This presumably precedes the loss of dorsal root ganglion cells.

The condition is slowly progressive. With respect to management the main consideration is to educate the patients to protect their anaesthetic feet from injury.

Autosomal dominant hereditary sensory neuropathy with spastic paraplegia

Four families with an autosomal dominant disorder originally reported as familial lumbosacral syringomyelia (Van Epps and Kerr, 1940) combined a childhood onset of spastic paraplegia with lower-limb sensory loss predominantly affecting pain and temperature sensibility. This led to a mutilating acropathy. One of the families was later investigated by Khalifeh and Zellweger (1963). A further family with autosomal dominant spastic paraplegia and sensory neuropathy was reported by Koenig and Spiro (1970). No descriptions of this condition have appeared in recent years and results for nerve conduction studies or nerve biopsies are not available. In an additional family documented by Van Epps and Kerr the inheritance was possibly autosomal recessive.

Hereditary sensory neuropathy with sensorineural hearing loss and early onset dementia

A kindred spanning six generations with a disorder of probable autosomal dominant inheritance has recently been described (Wright and Dyck, 1995). This combined a sensory neuropathy affecting all modalities and progressive sensorineural hearing loss and dementia beginning at the age of 30–40 years. Neuropathic ulcers and arthropathy developed in the feet. Sensory nerve action potentials were lost and sural nerve biopsy showed an almost total loss of myelinated axons and some loss of unmyelinated axons.

Autosomal recessive sensory neuropathy

Although it is likely that some of the early reports described such cases, the existence of autosomal recessive sensory neuropathy was first established by Ogryzlo (1946) in four members of a sibship of 12 from Newfoundland who had normal parents. This was shown by nerve biopsy. Other families with sensory neuropathy from Canada were recorded by Heller and Robb (1955) and Ohta *et al.* (1973). The latter authors designated the disorder as type II hereditary sensory neuropathy (HSN). The segregation analysis of reported cases of HSN in which the disorder was confined to a single sibship that was undertaken by Kondo and Horikawa (1974) was consistent with autosomal recessive inheritance, giving a segregation ratio of 0.26. Parental consanguinity was common. These authors concluded that the condition was genetically heterogeneous.

The disorder described by Ohta *et al.* (1973) is congenital or has a presentation in infancy or early childhood. All forms of sensation are affected, the sensory loss being maximal distally in the limbs. The tendon reflexes are depressed or absent. Autonomic manifestations are slight but distal anhidrosis may be evident in the limbs (Ohta *et al.*, 1973) and tonic pupils may occur (Miller *et al.*, 1976). Distal acrodystrophic changes with chronic ulceration, tissue loss, neuropathic joint degeneration and osteomyelitis are frequently severe.

The question as to whether the disorder is progressive or whether it represents a static congenital sensory deficit on which progressive acrodystrophic changes are superimposed had given rise to discussion (Murray, 1973). The finding of fibrillation potentials in the small foot muscles during adolescence (Ohta *et al.*, 1973) suggests progression which was also concluded from nerve biopsy studies (Nukada *et al.*, 1982). It seems likely that a congenital and substantially non-progressive form and a progressive form which may be of later onset (Jedrzejowska and Milczarek, 1976) both exist.

The over-riding consideration in management, as for dominantly inherited sensory neuropathy, is to prevent accumulated damage to the feet and hands. This poses particular problems in this form because of the early onset of the disease.

Hereditary anhidrotic sensory neuropathy

This disorder was first recognized by Swanson (1963) and Swanson *et al.* (1965). Similar kinships were reported by Pinsky and Di George (1966) and Brown and Podosin (1966). It is probably of autosomal recessive inheritance and distinguishable on clinical and pathological grounds from autosomal recessive sensory neuropathy and familial dysautonomia, although confirmation of this is required by gene mapping. It has been designated by HSAN IV in the classification of Dyck *et al.* (1983).

The disease presents in early infancy by the occurrence of recurrent pyrexia related to diffuse anhidrosis and elevated ambient temperature. There is also widespread loss of pain sensibility and mental retardation. The sensory loss leads to the occurrence of repeated soft tissue damage, joint injuries and painless fractures.

Pathological studies have shown a lack of smaller dorsal root ganglion cells, a depletion of small-calibre fibres in dorsal roots, an absence of Lissauer's tracts and reduced size of the spinal tract of the trigeminal nerve (Swanson *et al.*, 1965). Preservation of myelinated nerve fibres and a total absence of unmyelinated axons has been found in nerve biopsies (Pinsky and Di George, 1966; Goebel *et al.*, 1980).

Familial dysautonomia (Riley–Day syndrome)

This disorder, which is of autosomal recessive inheritance, has recently been mapped to chromosome 9q31-33 (Blumenfeld *et al.*, 1993). It has been designated as HSAN III in the classification of Dyck *et al.* (1983). The salient manifestations are those of autonomic dysfunction, but there is an accompanying sensory neuropathy. Most patients display loss of pain and temperature sensation and some also have impaired joint position and vibration sense (Pearson *et al.*, 1971). The ankle jerks are depressed or absent. Fungiform papillae are absent from the tongue. The sensory deficit probably increases with age. The patients are often of short stature and kyphoscoliosis may be present. Acrodystrophic changes are not prominent but neuropathic joint degeneration may develop. The wide range of autonomic symptoms that occurs has recently been reviewed (Dyck, 1993).

Pathological studies have shown a loss of neurons from dorsal root and trigeminal ganglia (Pearson *et al.*, 1978) and a greater loss from sural nerve biopsy in a single case showed a severe reduction in the population of unmyelinated axons. Myelinated fibre density was within normal limits, but it was considered that there was a relative reduction in those of larger and smaller diameter (Aguayo *et al.*, 1971) which might equate with the observed pattern of sensory loss.

There have been isolated reports of conditions of probable autosomal recessive inheritance that combined a congenital sensory neuropathy and autonomic dysfunction but in which the features were not typical of the Riley–Day syndrome. Thus Nordborg *et al.* (1981) reported three isolated cases of a congenital non-progressive sensory and autonomic neuropathy. The findings on nerve biopsy differed from those of the Riley–Day syndrome in that there was an almost total loss of unmyelinated fibres and a variable loss of unmyelinated axons. Axelrod *et al.* (1981) reported a case clinically similar to the Riley–Day syndrome but with an associated skeletal dysplasia. The status of such cases will remain uncertain until it is known whether they also map to the same locus on chromosome 9q.

Hereditary sensory neuropathy with predominant loss of small myelinated nerve fibres

A sensory neuropathy present in three members of two generations related to double consanguinity was described in a Kashmiri family by Donaghy *et al.* (1987). The inheritance was likely to have been autosomal recessive. The neuropathy was probably present from birth. There was widespread loss of pain sensation and the index case showed evidence of old injuries to his lips and tongue. Keratitis was a prominent feature in the family. Vibration and joint position sense were preserved as were the tendon reflexes and there was no motor involvement. Apart from widespread anhidrosis shown by the index case, autonomic function was preserved. Sural nerve biopsy showed a severe relative reduction in the numbers of small myelinated axons. The density of unmyelinated axons was increased.

Three isolated cases of what may be the same disorder have also been reported (Low *et al.*, 1978; Dyck *et al.*, 1983). All had selective loss of pain sensation dating back to infancy and one of the two cases reported by Dyck *et al.* may have had accompanying mental retardation. They were categorized as HSAN V. Nerve biopsies again showed a selective reduction in the numbers of small myelinated axons and, in the two cases reported by Dyck *et al.*, there may have been some loss of unmyelinated axons.

The question arises as to the explanation for the profound loss of pain sensibility in the face of large numbers of unmyelinated axons in the peripheral nerves. There possibly could be a selective depletion in a subpopulation of nociceptor afferents or a neurotransmitter defect, or perhaps an accompanying abnormality of central processing. The same question arises in the cases of dominantly inherited 'congenital indifference to pain' reported by Landrieu *et al.* (1990) in which the peripheral nerves were found to be morphologically normal.

Autosomal recessive sensory neuropathy with spastic paraplegia

Two pairs of siblings born to consanguineous parents, together with an isolated case with similar features, have recently been reported (Thomas *et al.*, 1994). It is likely that two of the cases reported by Cavanagh *et al.* (1979) were also of autosomal recessive inheritance with the same or a similar condition. These patients all developed symptoms in childhood and showed a combination of bilateral pyramidal signs in the legs together with a distal sensory neuropathy, maximal in the lower limbs. This affected all modalities. The condition was slowly progressive and led to the development of acrodystrophic changes. Autonomic dysfunction was not a feature.

Nerve biopsies in the cases reported by Thomas *et al.* showed a loss both of myelinated nerve fibres, particularly those of larger size, and of unmyelinated axons.

X-linked sensory neuropathy

A single family has been described with possible X-linked HSN (Jestico *et al.*, 1985). Onset was in the first or second decades. Sensory loss was restricted to the distal lower limbs and mainly affected pain and temperature sensibility. This was accompanied by foot ulceration and neuropathic joint degeneration. Apart from depression or loss of the ankle jerks, the tendon reflexes were preserved, as was autonomic function. Nerve biopsies showed a predominant loss of small myelinated fibres and a normal unmyelinated axon density.

Inherited multifocal sensory neuropathy

In most inherited sensory neuropathies the sensory loss is symmetric, as is true for the majority of inherited neuropathies. The manifestations in familial neuralgic amyotrophy, a dominantly inherited disorder, are normally predominantly motor but presentation with a multifocal painful sensory neuropathy has been described (Thomas and Ormerod, 1993).

SENSORY NEUROPATHY IN HEREDITARY ATAXIAS

The hereditary ataxias comprise a diverse group of conditions in which the salient neurological manifestation is incoordination of voluntary movement (Harding, 1984). The incoordination may be the result of a disturbance affecting the cerebellum or its pathways or reflect a sensory ataxia related to loss of the larger afferent fibres in the peripheral nerves that subserve proprioception.

Friedreich's ataxia

This disorder is of autosomal recessive inheritance, the responsible gene having been mapped to chromosome 9q (Chamberlain *et al.*, 1988). The onset of symptoms is most commonly at around the age of 11–12 years with gait difficulty and later upper-limb ataxia. The findings at an early stage are often predominantly those of a sensory neuropathy (Ouvrier *et al.*, 1982) with tendon areflexia and sensory impairment of large fibre type, i.e. for joint position, vibration and discriminative tactile sensation. Sensory nerve action potentials are depressed or absent. The other manifestations of the disorder, including pyramidal weakness in the limbs, dysarthria, cardiomyopathy and skeletal deformity become superimposed later, but a sensory neuropathy remains a prominent aspect of the clinical picture.

A salient pathological feature is loss of large dorsal root ganglion cells (Inoue *et al.*, 1979) accompanied by depletion of larger myelinated fibres in the peripheral nerves (Dyck *et al.*, 1971; McLeod, 1971; Rizzutto *et al.*, 1981). There has been discussion as to the nature of the pathological changes. Early studies indicated that the characteristic abnormality is a distal axonopathy of dying-back type, the degeneration extending centripetally towards the parent cell bodies (Mott, 1907). From studies on peripheral nerve, Dyck and Lais (1973) considered that axonal atrophy and secondary demyelination preceded axonal degeneration. The myelin sheaths were found to be abnormally thick for axon diameter. Said *et al.* (1986), on the other hand, found that myelinated fibre diameter is reduced at an early stage and that myelin sheath thickness is relatively reduced. They concluded that there is a maturational defect in specific neurons which remain hypotrophic and subsequently die back at a slow rate. More recent studies by Jitpimolmard *et al.* (1993) confirmed the presence of a distal axonopathy with no evidence that this was preceded by axonal atrophy. As had been found by Said *et al.* peripheral nerve fibres were relatively hypomyelinated. Selective loss of a 40-kDa protein from the dorsal root ganglia of patients with Friedrech's ataxia has recently been reported (Small *et al.*, 1993). The nature of the protein and the significance of this finding is still uncertain.

Autosomal dominant cerebellar ataxia

The autosomal dominant cerebellar ataxias have an onset in mid or later life. Limb ataxia and dysarthria are combined with a variety of other features including dementia, optic atrophy, disorders of ocular movement, pyramidal signs and tendon areflexia. The group is genetically complex, four gene loci having so far been detected in which involvement of the primary sensory neurons occurs. Spinocerebellar ataxia 1 (SCA 1) has been mapped to chromosome 6, SCA 2 to chromosome 12, SCA 3 to chromosome 14 and SCA 4 to chromosome 16 (see Zoghbi *et al.*, 1993). Other clinically similar disorders do not map to any of these four loci. Sensory nerve action potentials may be reduced or lost in the dominantly inherited cerebellar ataxias. Nerve biopsies have shown a predominant loss of larger myelinated nerve fibres (Wadia *et al.*, 1978; McLeod and Evans, 1981).

Benign hereditary cerebellar ataxia with extensive thermoanalgesia

A single family has been described with probable autosomal dominant inheritance of a slowly advancing late-onset cerebellar ataxia accompanied by widespread near global loss of pain and temperature sensibility (Pollock and Kies, 1990). Nerve biopsy showed severe loss of myelinated nerve fibres, particularly those of smaller size, and a less severe depletion of unmyelinated axons.

INHERITED SENSORY DISORDERS WITH VITAMIN E DEFICIENCY

Abetalipoproteinaemia and hypobetalipoproteinaemia

Abetalipoproteinaemia (Bassen–Kornzweig disease) is of autosomal recessive inheritance. The disease begins in childhood and is characterized by a progressive spinocerebellar degeneration and a predominantly sensory neuropathy, associated with a pigmentary retinopathy, fat intolerance and diarrhoea. Acanthocytes are present in the peripheral blood, The tendon reflexes tend to be depressed before the onset of ataxia and there is distal sensory loss for large fibre sensory modalities, often with foot deformity and scoliosis. External ophthalmoplegia and generalized muscle weakness occur later. Sensory nerve action potentials are depressed or absent but motor nerve conduction velocity is normal or only mildly reduced. Nerve biopsy shows a predominant loss of large myelinated nerve fibres.

The disorder is caused by an inability to synthesize apoprotein B (apo B), required for the production of chylomicrons, and low density and very low density lipoproteins which are all lacking from plasma. This lack leads to a failure to transport vitamin E across the intestinal mucosa and to impaired vitamin E transport in plasma. There is now compelling evidence that the neurological syndrome is secondary to vitamin E deficiency (Harding, 1987), although deficiency of vitamin A may also contribute to the pigmentary retinopathy. The disorder can be prevented if vitamin E is administered sufficiently early or progression can be halted or function improved in established cases (Muller *et al.*, 1970; Azizi *et al.*, 1978).

Familial hypobetalipoproteinaemia is caused by mutations in the gene for apolipoprotein B that often give rise to truncated apo B in the plasma, accompanied by reduced levels of low density lipoprotein cholesterol. Heterozygotes are asymptomatic. Homozygotes for these mutations are extremely rare. Such individuals may also be symptomatic or show a neurological disorder related to vitamin E deficiency (Hardman *et al.*, 1991; Gabelli, 1992). Whether they develop the neurological syndrome does not appear to depend simply upon the degree of truncation of the apo B molecule (Young *et al.*, 1994).

Isolated vitamin E deficiency

In recent years reports have appeared of a spinocerebellar syndrome related to vitamin E deficiency in the absence of generalized fat malabsorption (Krendel *et al.*, 1977; Burck *et al.*, 1981; Harding *et al.*, 1985; Stumpf *et al.*, 1987; Yokota *et al.*, 1987; Laplante *et al.*, 1988; Sokol *et al.*, 1988). The precise mechanism of the vitamin E deficiency has not yet been established. The age of onset has been variable, ranging from early childhood to early adult life. The condition has been described as displaying the phenotype of Friedreich's disease (Stumpf *et al.*, 1987; Ben Hamida *et al.*, 1993) but there are important differences. Head tremor is often prominent. Loss of tendon reflexes has been a feature in most cases, accompanied by distal loss of joint position and vibration sense, although preservation of the tendon reflexes was noted in the family reported by Sokol *et al.* (1988). Sensory nerve action potentials were found to be normal in the patients reported by Harding *et al.* (1985), as was motor nerve conduction velocity. Somatosensory evoked potentials, however, were markedly prolonged. This suggests that the underlying pathological process differs materially from that of Freidreich's ataxia in which it consists of a central–peripheral distal axonopathy. As already mentioned, in experimental vitamin E deficiency the initial changes are those of a central distal axonopathy in which the degenerative changes mainly affect the centrally directed axons or the primary sensory neurons (Nelson *et al.*, 1981; Southam *et al.*, 1991). The same appears to be true for inherited isolated vitamin E deficiency.

Using homozygosity mapping, inherited isolated vitamin E deficiency has recently been mapped to chromosome 8q in three Tunisian and two other families (Ben Hamida *et al.*, 1993). It is not yet certain whether the responsible genes in the reported families with slightly different phenotypes (Burck *et al.*, 1983; Sokol *et al.*, 1988) also have the same localization.

IMMUNE-MEDIATED SENSORY DISORDERS

Sensory ganglionitides

The sensory ganglionitides are acquired disorders characterized by lymphocytic inflammation of sensory ganglia and destruction of sensory neurons. The sensory ganglionitides include **idiopathic sensory neuronopathy**, **carcinomatous sensory neuronopathy**, and **sensory ganglionitis associated with features of Sjögren syndrome**. Common clinical features shared by all three include loss of kinaesthesia and joint-position sensibility, with consequent gait ataxia and loss of motor control in the arms. In all three disorders, the initial complaints are often of incoordination, unsteadiness in walking, or even 'dizziness'. There may also be paraesthesias or occasionally neuropathic pain.

On examination, the abnormalities usually include one or more of the following: defects in the localization of one or more of the limbs in space, sensory gait ataxia, Rombergism, and pseudoathetosis of the outstretched hands. In the arms, the loss of kinaesthesia is reflected in the inability to touch the thumbnail of one hand with the index finger of the other when the eyes are closed (Rothwell *et al.*, 1982; Sanes *et al.*, 1985; Griffin *et al.*, 1990). On sensory examination, there is the expected elevation of vibratory threshold and loss of joint-position sensibility in the toes, fingers, or both. More distinctive and more pertinent to the functional deficits is the frequent finding of loss of ability to identify where the static limb is in space, or to appreciate movements at the ankle, knee, or hip in the leg, or in the more proximal joints of the arm (Griffin *et al.*, 1990; Windebank *et al.*, 1990). In affected limbs, tendon reflexes are invariably absent, and often globally absent, even in limbs with relatively preserved sensory function on examination. The presence of tendon reflexes in a limb with severe loss of kinaesthesia is not compatible with a neuropathic aetiology alone, and suggests instead the possibility of myelopathy with dorsal column involvement.

In addition to the feet and hands, paraesthesias frequently involve the proximal face, the trunk, and the proximal regions of the limbs, often in a patchy and asymmetric fashion. The rates of onset and progression vary. In all of these disorders there can be an abrupt onset (Sterman *et al.*, 1980; Trapp *et al.*, 1989; Windebank *et al.*, 1990), producing a picture termed the acute sensory neuronopathy syndrome (Sterman *et al.*, 1980). The resulting inability to walk is often misinterpreted by the patient and by examiners as weakness, leading to the potential misdiagnosis of Guillain–Barré syndrome. By asking the patient to sustain a muscle contraction under visual guidance, the strength can be shown to be nearly normal. More frequently the course is either subacute (Griffin *et al.*, 1990; Windebank *et al.*, 1990), with worsening and spread from week to week, or slowly progressive (Griffin *et al.*, 1990; Windebank *et al.*, 1990). The disorder may begin focally, leading to the suspicion of either a spinal root disease or a mononeuropathy.

Pathology: in all these disorders autopsy studies or dorsal root ganglion biopsies have identified intense lymphocytic infiltration as the underlying pathology (Denny-Brown, 1948; Griffin *et al.*, 1990; Panegyres *et al.*, 1993; Smith *et al.*, 1993) (Figure 4.2). Ganglion cells are destroyed, with both lymphocytic and macrophage invasion of neurons. In some cases the fibre loss can be global, but in all three disorders the large sensory neurons and their fibres are predominantly affected. As a result there is degeneration of the large sensory fibres in the peripheral nerves (Denny-Brown, 1948; Griffin *et al.*, 1990) (Figure 4.3) and of their central processes in the dorsal columns, but the innervation of the skin by C fibres can be strikingly spared (Figure 4.4).

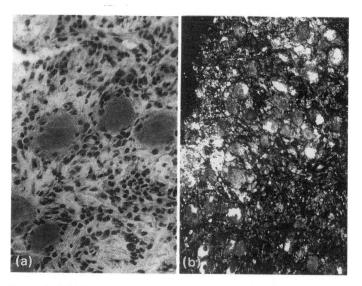

Figure 4.2 Dorsal root ganglion from a patient with sensory ganglionitis associated with features of Sjögren syndrome. The areas of lymphocytic infiltration are apparent in the haematoxylin and eosin-stained section (a) and in the section immunostained for T cells and photographed in dark-field, so that the lymphoctyes appear white (b). Note lymphocytes are present within some degenerating sensory neurons.

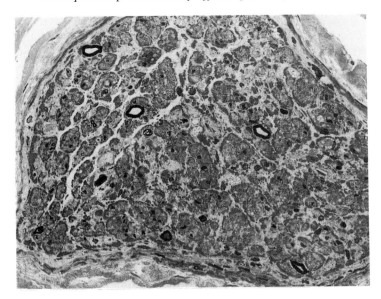

Figure 4.3 Transverse section of peripheral nerve from a patient with sensory ganglionitis associated with features of Sjögren syndrome. This biopsy was taken 6 weeks after acute onset of ataxic neuropathy. Note the ongoing Wallerian-like degeneration of large myelinated fibres.

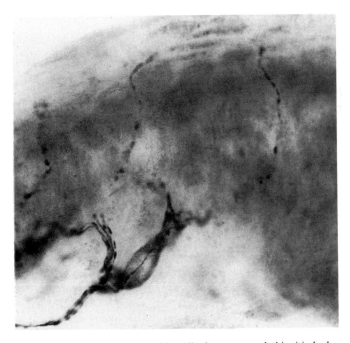

Figure 4.4 Skin biopsy stained with antibody to neuronal ubiquitin hydrolase, demonstrating the relative preservation of unmyelinated C-fibre terminals in the epidermis in skin from a patient with ataxic neuropathy associated with Sjögren syndrome. This patient had severe loss of large myelinated fibres. (Courtesy of Dr Justin C. McArthur).

Idiopathic sensory ganglionitis

Sterman and colleagues (Sterman *et al.*, 1980) initially identified the acute ataxic sensory neuronopathy syndrome. They raised the possibility that the disorder might involve antibiotic toxicity, because their first case had been receiving penicillin shortly before onset of the neuropathy. Since that time most cases have occurred without antecedent antibiotic use (Windebank *et al.*, 1990), and the presence of inflammation in the dorsal root ganglia of the rare autopsied cases suggests that this is an autoimmune disorder (Smith *et al.*, 1993). Acute sensory neuropathy most often occurs without association with other disorders or antecedent events, and is therefore termed **idiopathic**. A much smaller proportion of the acute sensory neuronopathy cases occur in the setting of underlying carcinoma or in association with features of Sjögren syndrome. Conversely, a higher proportion of patients with a subacute or chronically evolving sensory ganglionitis have underlying carcinoma or Sjögren syndrome, but a significant proportion remain idiopathic.

Electrodiagnostic studies in the first 7–10 days may be normal (Griffin *et al.*, 1990). Such normal studies can be seen at the stage when sensory neurons have degenerated, but before Wallerian-like degeneration has resulted in loss of sensory nerve fibres (Griffin *et al.*, 1990). Follow-up studies a week later are usually sufficient to demonstrate extensive loss of sensory nerve action potentials. In one patient with loss of sensation over the face the short latency (R1) somatosensory evoked potentials were lost while the long latency (R2) potentials remained, suggesting selective loss of large-diameter sensory neurons (Knazan *et al.*, 1990). During the initial stages, the spinal fluid protein may be elevated, but routine haematological and serological studies for evidence of collagen–vascular or inflammatory disease are normal. Varying degrees of autonomic dysfunction may be noted. Although some residual disability remains (Windebank *et al.*, 1990), most individuals return to a high level of function with time. A short course of high-dose corticosteroids is widely prescribed (Windebank *et al.*, 1990), but its value is undetermined.

Carcinomatous sensory neuropathy

Sensory ganglionitis with degeneration of primary sensory neurons in the dorsal root ganglion was recognized by Denny-Brown (1948). Subsequent series have confirmed the association of sensory neuropathy with oat cell carcinoma of the lung and, less frequently, carcinomas of the breast, ovary, oesophagus, kidney and liver. Evaluation for carcinomatous sensory neuropathy is an important aspect of differential diagnosis in any patient with ataxic nerve disease.

Clinical features: this disorder presents in a subacute fashion, often beginning with apparently abrupt onset of paraesthesias in one site (Horwich *et al.*, 1977; McLeod, 1993). The initial sites involved may affect the legs, arms, or even the face. There may be an element of neuropathic discomfort at the beginning, and the paraesthesias develop a painful character in a high proportion of individuals. Complaints of difficulty with 'coordination' and with use of the limbs usually supervene. These complaints reflect the loss of proprioception and kinaesthetic sensibility that characterizes the disorder. Usually within a matter of weeks other regions become involved, and in most individuals the neuropathy comes to affect both arms and both legs within a few months. Gait ataxia is often the most severe functional alteration.

On examination, there is little muscle wasting. Vibratory and joint-position sensibility are severely impaired and sensory ataxia with Rombergism is frequent. In the arms pseudoathetosis of the outstretched hands and inability to localize the limb in space with the eyes closed are characteristic. Adie's pupils and autonomic dysfunction may be present (Nemoto *et al.*, 1992; Liang *et al.*, 1994). In addition, there are frequently signs of CNS involvement, particularly cerebellar disease, with nystagmus, occasionally brainstem findings, and, in a proportion of individuals, manifestations of cognitive or personality change. Tendon reflexes are universally absent.

Laboratory features: electrodiagnostic testing is characterized by the absence of sensory nerve action potentials and by motor nerve conduction studies that are normal or only minimally abnormal. Electromyography typically shows only occasional scattered denervation. The cerebrospinal fluid is often abnormal, with either lymphocytic pleocytosis, elevated spinal fluid protein, or both. The finding of a distinctive antibody against a 37-kDa neuronal nuclear protein, the 'anti-Hu' antibody (Graus *et al.*, 1986) is the most specific laboratory finding. The specificity of this test is good; no positive studies were found in patients with idiopathic sensory neuronopathy, whereas 91% of 67 seropositive patients had small-cell lung carcinoma (Chalk *et al.*, 1993). The antibody is directed against a neuronal nuclear antigen, but also binds to tumour cells.

Pathology: the primary lesion is degeneration of dorsal root ganglion cells with consequent degeneration of both the central and peripheral processes of the primary sensory neuron (Sterman *et al.*, 1980; Yoshioka *et al.*, 1992; Panegyres *et al.*, 1993). Consequent to this, the dorsal roots and the dorsal columns show ongoing Wallerian-like degeneration and fibre loss. Our experience has been that the loss of small neurons is greater in this disorder than in the other types of sensory ganglionitis, so that in the peripheral nerves the fibre loss involves large fibres, but with small-fibre populations lost to a lesser extent. At the level of the dorsal root ganglia, there is infiltration with lymphocytes (Sterman *et al.*, 1980; Yoshioka *et al.*, 1992; Nishiyama *et al.*, 1993; Panegyres *et al.*, 1993). The degenerating sensory neurons are surrounded by proliferated satellite Schwann cells, forming nodules of Nageotte, and there is macrophage activation in the same regions (Panegyres *et al.*, 1993). The infiltrating lymphocytes include both CD4 and CD8-positive cells, but B cells are absent.

Treatment and prognosis: in most individuals, the neuropathy occurs before the carcinoma has become clinically manifest. Some reports suggest that removal or chemotherapy of the tumour can slow the progress of the neurological disease (Valldeoriola *et al.*, 1992) and occasional patients improve. However, even with resection of the underlying neoplasm the neuropathic disease persists and often progresses. Although it is presumably immunopathogenically mediated, even vigorous immunotherapy does not improve the disorder (Valldeoriola *et al.*, 1992) and in most instances it appears to progress even in the face of cytotoxic agents, plasmapheresis, administration of gamma globulin and administration of intravenous immunoglobulin. The presence of anti-Hu antibodies has been associated with spontaneous tumour regression (Zaheer *et al.*, 1993) and in some cases with prolonged survival (Darnell and DeAngelis, 1993; Zaheer *et al.*, 1993) for patients with small-cell carcinoma. It is possible that the antibodies contribute to suppression of the neoplastic disease.

The neuropathic pain can be distressing. While it may respond to high doses of tricyclic drugs, it often requires use of opiates.

Sensory ganglionitis associated with features of Sjögren syndrome

Sjögren syndrome is associated with several types of neuropathy. The pattern most frequently encountered is a distally predominant sensorimotor neuropathy (Mellgren *et al.*, 1989). This may begin in a somewhat patchy fashion but typically cumulates to produce a symmetric distally predominant disorder. Multiple mononeuropathy also occurs (Mellgren *et al.*, 1989). Both patterns of neuropathy tend to occur in individuals with well-established and previously diagnosed Sjögren syndrome. In contrast, patients with ataxic neuropathies associated with features of Sjögren syndrome (Hull *et al.*, 1984; Kennett and Harding, 1986; Malinow *et al.*, 1986; Bakchine *et al.*, 1987; Hankey and Gubbay, 1987; Graus *et al.*, 1988; Laloux *et al.*, 1988; Griffin *et al.*, 1990) often consult neurologists before the diagnosis of rheumatological disease is made, and their symptoms of xerophthalmia and xerostomia are brought out only by specific questioning. The ataxic neuropathy is substantially less common than the sensorimotor neuropathy in patients with Sjögren syndrome, but because ataxic neuropathies in general are rare disorders, this disorder is among the most frequent causes of ataxic neuropathy.

Clinical manifestations: the neurological examination is dominated by sensory ataxia and loss of kinaesthesia. Romberg's sign is frequently present. The characteristic clinical features are loss of kinaesthesia and joint-position sensibility, invariably associated with loss of vibratory sensibility (Griffin *et al.*, 1990). Small-fibre modalities, including pain and thermal sensibility, are relatively unaffected. Tendon reflexes are lost in affected limbs and are often lost globally. Patients present complaining of paraesthesias and often of unsteadiness of gait, reflecting their sensory ataxia. Usually they do not associate dry eyes and dry mouth with neuropathic symptoms, so that specific inquiry is required. Autonomic dysfunction is present in most (Font *et al.*, 1990; Griffin *et al.*, 1990; Kaplan *et al.*, 1990; Kumazawa *et al.*, 1993). The most characteristic autonomic feature on examination is Adie's pupils (Kennett and Harding, 1986; Laloux *et al.*, 1988; Font *et al.*, 1990; Griffin *et al.*, 1990; Kaplan *et al.*, 1990; Kumazawa *et al.*, 1993), often bilateral. The Adie's pupils can long antecede the development of other manifestations of ganglionitis (Griffin *et al.*, 1990).

As with idiopathic sensory ganglionitis, the course is variable, with some patients having acute onset and rapid progression. More often there is a prolonged phase of gradual progression. During the progressive phase, gait ataxia and incoordination of the hands can produce severe functional disability and consequent psychological distress. The disorder ultimately stabilizes, but often after years of progression.

Laboratory features: the spinal fluid is normal in most patients. The outstanding laboratory abnormality is the presence of high anti-nuclear antibody titres. About half the patients have elevated Ro antibody titres, and one-third have polyclonal hypergammaglobulinaemia. Schirmer and Rose-Bengal tests demonstrate xerophthalmia. Lip biopsy typically demonstrates inflammation of minor salivary glands. Taken together, these laboratory features are sufficient to satisfy rheumatological criteria for Sjögren syndrome (Fox *et al.*, 1986). However, these patients represent a distinctive subset of patients. Beyond their unusual neurological manifestations, they have very few other extraglandular manifestations of Sjögren syndrome. Thus, surveys of rheumatological clinics for patients with ataxic neuropathy produce few cases (Mellgren *et al.*, 1989), and most patients with sensory ganglionitis present to neurologists before being seen by rheumatologists.

Treatment: in patients with slowly progressing disease, the sensory nerve action potentials are frequently absent at the time the diagnosis is established. The Johns Hopkins group has evaluated over 30 patients with sensory ganglionitis associated with features of Sjögren syndrome, and most have had treatment attempts with immunosuppressive regimens. There have been no convincing responses in any individuals with severe involvement and absent sensory nerve action potentials. Two patients had clear benefit: one received intravenous methylprednisolone and one cyclosporin (the latter patient had previously received no benefit from corticosteroids, plasmapheresis, intravenous gammaglobulin or cytotoxic agents).

In spite of the ineffectiveness of immunosuppression in most patients, the long-term prognosis for substantial recovery of function is good. This functional improvement is the consequence of learned compensation for the lack of proprioception and kinaesthesia. Individuals learn to use visual and other cues to replace the lost afferent input. Patients are frequently unable to walk during the progressive phase, but recover surprisingly good gait function with time. Realistic discussions of this prognosis can relieve some of the distress these syndromes produce.

SENSORY NEUROPATHIES RELATED TO INFECTIONS

Sensory neuropathy of AIDS

The predominantly sensory neuropathy associated with AIDS is reviewed in detail in Chapter 11. From the standpoint of differential diagnosis, most individuals with AIDS-associated sensory neuropathy have severe immunosuppression (CD4 lymphocytes $< 200 \mu l$) and previous AIDS-defining illnesses; only rarely has HIV infection escaped detection by the time individuals present with sensory neuropathy. Conversely, in late stages of AIDS, sensory neuropathy is frequent, affecting at least 30% of individuals with AIDS (Cornblath and McArthur, 1988; So *et al.*, 1988; Leger, 1992), and some degree of sensory fibre degeneration is virtually universal by the time of death from AIDS. In approximately 10% of individuals with AIDS, the symptoms of the sensory neuropathy include neuropathic pain, typically on the soles of the feet (Cornblath and McArthur, 1988; So *et al.*, 1988; Fuller *et al.*, 1989, 1993). There is an element of mechanical allodynia, so that touch or walking can be painful. The painful symptoms can begin abruptly or insidiously. They occasionally spontaneously improve after several weeks or months. As association of painful sensory symptoms with systemic cytomegalovirus (CMV) infection has been suspected, based on the presence of ocular or other systemic CMV infection with painful neuropathy in many patients (Fuller *et al.*, 1989). However, typical cases occur in the absence of detectable systemic CMV infection. Similarly, an association with weight loss and presumed malnutrition has been suggested, but some cases of sensory neuropathy develop before any opportunistic infections, in patients with no weight loss or other symptoms of malnutrition.

Autopsy studies have demonstrated that some degree of sensory fibre degeneration and loss is virtually universal by the time of death from AIDS, but the severity varies widely. The predominant feature of the pathology is distal axonal degeneration in the long sensory nerves, reflected in loss of fibres in distal regions of cutaneous nerves such as the sural, as well as a variable degree of degeneration in the rostral gracile tracts of the dorsal columns (Rance *et al.*, 1988; Scaravilli *et al.*, 1992). There is also some loss of dorsal root ganglia neurons, with consequent nodules of

Nageotte, proliferated satellite cells marking degeneration of sensory neurons. The neuronal loss is always less severe than the extent of distal cutaneous fibre loss. In these regards, the sensory neuropathy of AIDS conforms to the pattern of a 'dying back' disorder or a central–peripheral distal axonopathy. In addition to fibre loss, axonal atrophy has been documented in sural nerve biopsies of individuals with painful neuropathy. Cornford and colleagues have demonstrated a variable, but usually modest, degree of inflammatory response, particularly in the epineurium (Robert *et al.*, 1989; Cornford *et al.*, 1992). There is an often prominent macrophage response in distal cutaneous nerves, and those macrophages produce a number of markers of activation, including major histocompatibility complex (MHC) class II and tumour necrosis factor-α (TNF-α). Cornford and colleagues have pointed out the frequency with which endothelial cell infection with CMV is detected, and documented a relationship between the severity of CMV infection and the degree of neuropathy (Cornford *et al.*, 1992). Only occasionally is CMV found in dorsal root ganglia.

An increasing problem is the interaction between sensory neuropathy of AIDS and toxicity of the anti-retroviral agents dideoxycytidine (ddC) and dideoxyinosine (ddI) (see Chapter 12). These agents produce a very similar painful sensory neuropathy.

PURE MOTOR NEUROPATHIES

Many neuropathies, including typical Guillain–Barré syndrome and Charcot–Marie–Tooth disease, can have a motor predominance, but have electrophysiological evidence of considerable sensory nerve involvement. Two neuropathies, multifocal motor neuropathy and the acute motor axonal neuropathy form of the Guillain–Barré syndrome, are considered here because of their very marked dissociation between severe motor and minimal sensory involvement, together with motor neuropathy in diabetes.

Multifocal motor neuropathy

Multifocal motor neuropathy (MMN), a relatively recently described disorder, has been the source of controversy with regard to its perceived relationship to amyotrophic lateral sclerosis on the one hand and to chronic inflammatory demyelinating neuropathy on the other. At the present time, because of its distinctive features and unusual pattern of response to therapy, it is appropriate to view MMN as a distinct disorder, albeit closely related to chronic inflammatory demyelinating polyneuropathy.

The short history of MMN began with a clinical description 8 years ago (Lewis *et al.*, 1982). Pestronk and colleagues (Pestronk *et al.*, 1988) subsequently found IgM anti-GM$_1$ antibodies in two patients who had almost exclusive involvement of motor nerves and evidence of multifocal conduction block. The basic features, extended in several recent series (Krarup *et al.*, 1990; Feldman *et al.*, 1991; Lange *et al.*, 1990, 1992; Pestronk *et al.*, 1990; Sadiq *et al.*, 1990; Santoro *et al.*, 1990; Chaudhry *et al.*, 1993a). The clinical features usually include asymmetric weakness, a very slow progression, and frequently loss of tendon reflexes in limbs with relatively strong muscles. The IgM anti-GM$_1$ antibodies are not essential features for the diagnosis but are present in about 70% of cases. The pathogenetic role of the anti-GM$_1$ antibodies remains to be established, but it is noteworthy that the epitope is located in nodes of Ranvier (Thomas *et al.*, 1989, 1990; Santoro *et al.*, 1990; Goldstein *et al.*, 1993), providing a potential mechanism for interference with conduction by antibody.

MMN appears, by clinical and electrophysiological criteria, to be a 'pure' motor disorder, but sural nerve biopsies in a series of 12 patients have shown definite but very mild evidence of demyelination and occasional ongoing Wallerian-like degeneration (M. A. Corse, unpublished observation). Only one case had a myelinated fibre density less than normal. Data on the pathology of the lesions in motor nerves remain fragmentary at this time. In the best-studied case there was focal demyelination with endoneurial oedema and a variable degree of lymphocytic infiltration (Kaji *et al.*, 1993).

Treatment: Multifocal motor neuropathy was initially found to improve following immunosuppression by cyclophosphamide (Pestronk *et al.*, 1988, 1990; Feldman *et al.*, 1991). Patients usually do not respond to corticosteroids or plasmapheresis (Pestronk *et al.*, 1988; Feldman *et al.*, 1991). Several groups have now observed improvement with intravenous immunoglobulin infusion (Nobile-Orazio *et al.*, 1988, 1993; Azulay *et al.*, 1992; Kaji *et al.*, 1992; Chaudhry *et al.*, 1993a,b). Multifocal motor neuropathy stands out as a disorder that is distinctive both in its clinical manifestations and its pattern of response to various immunomodulatory modalities. The relationship of the anti-GM$_1$ antibody to pathogenesis remains a matter of speculation.

Acute motor axonal neuropathy syndrome (AMAN)

From among the group of patients diagnosed clinically to have Guillain–Barré syndrome (GBS), subgroups with 'pure' motor involvement have been identified. Some such patients appear to have typical demyelinating neuropathy by electrophysiology. Others have a predominantly axonal form. Such cases have been termed 'acute motor axonal neuropathy' (AMAN) (McKhann *et al.*, 1993). These cases have been studied in a collaborative research programme involving the Second Teaching Hospital of Hebei Medical College, China; the University of Pennsylvania; and the Johns Hopkins University, working in Shijiazhuang, China. In Hebi Province, as elsewhere in northern China (Zhao *et al.*, 1981) and Korea (Coe, 1989), there are annual seasonal epidemics of a disorder diagnosed clinically as Guillain–Barré syndrome that occur in the summers. The numbers of patients involved are quite large; clinical series from just two hospitals in northern China have included over 1500 patients seen over a 15-year period (McKhann *et al.*, 1993). Many of these patients are found clinically to have normal sensation and to have electrodiagnostic patterns consistent with selective degeneration of motor axons (McKhann *et al.*, 1993). A serological survey showed that 76% of individuals with the AMAN pattern had evidence of antecedent *Campylobacter jejuni* infection (Ho *et al.*, 1994). In the AMAN pattern cases there has been an association with the presence of IgG anti-GM$_1$ antibodies (Yuki *et al.*, 1990, 1992), although this relationship remains controversial (Thomas, 1992; Enders *et al.*, 1993; Griffin and Ho, 1993; Vriesendorp *et al.*, 1993).

The pathology of the most severe AMAN cases has been studied in autopsies from Shijiazhuang (McKhann *et al.*, 1993; Griffin *et al.*, 1994a,b). The outstanding change is extensive Wallerian-like degeneration exclusively involving motor fibres

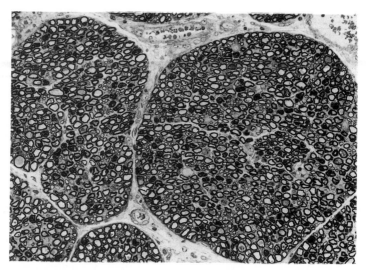

Figure 4.5 Transverse section through the ventral root of a patient with the AMAN pattern of Guillain–Barré syndrome. Note the large number of fibres undergoing Wallerian-like degeneration. (Courtesy of Dr Chun Yan Li.)

(Figure 4.5), with sparing of dorsal root and sensory nerve fibres in the periphery. The degeneration begins within a few hundred micrometres of the ventral root exit zone, but the motor neurons and intraparenchymal motor axons remain normal, except for evidence of axon reaction (McKhann *et al.*, 1993). The disorder is not purely 'axonal'; there is evidence of paranodal demyelination in many fibres and occasional examples of internodal demyelination have been identified in all cases studied (Griffin *et al.*, 1994b). Most cases have no evidence of inflammation by standard histological techniques, but both immunocytochemistry (Griffin *et al.*, 1994b) and reverse transcriptase polymerase chain reaction (PCR) probing for lymphocyte-derived cytokines, have shown a low degree of lymphocytic response. Three cases with a clinical picture consistent with AMAN, but with very mild degrees of pathology, have been studied in detail (Griffin *et al.*, 1994b). The changes identified include a small number of fibres degenerating within the spinal roots and peripheral nerves, and widespread paranodal myelin changes. These cases had very little evidence of inflammation and only rare examples of internodal demyelination. Such cases demonstrate that paralysis in the Guillain–Barré syndrome, as clinically defined, can occur with surprisingly little structural pathology. The lesion responsible for the paralysis could be motor nerve terminal degeneration (nerve terminals have not been systematically examined in any such cases), or paranodal demyelination changes, or a physiological block of the distal motor nerves by antibody. In any event, the issue is important because these cases have a time to recovery that is comparable with that of typical acute inflammatory demyelinating polyneuropathy (AIDP) cases in the same population (Ho *et al.*, 1994).

Motor syndromes in diabetic neuropathy

The most characteristic motor syndrome related to diabetes is the usually asymmetric proximal lower-limb motor neuropathy, generally of relatively acute or subacute onset and often accompanied by pain, particularly at night. This syndrome, originally recognized by Bruns (1890), was termed diabetic amyotrophy by Garland (1955). Associated sensory changes are usually slight. The prognosis for recovery is good (Watkins, 1990). The study by Raff *et al.* (1968) suggested an ischaemic basis but some of the 'infarcts' observed by these authors were later recognized to be Renaut bodies, a normal structural component of peripheral nerve (Asbury, 1973). It is of considerable interest that a recent report by Said *et al.* (1994) has documented inflammatory changes, including evidence of vasculitis, in biopsies of the intermediate cutaneous nerve of the thigh in cases of diabetic amyotrophy. In the patient reported by Raff *et al.* (1968) an epineurial inflammatory infiltrate was illustrated. How common this finding will prove to be has yet to be established.

Some patients with diabetic amyotrophy may exhibit more widespread lower-limb motor involvement, particularly of the anterolateral lower leg muscles. The simultaneous involvement of these muscles and the anterior thigh muscles led to the use of the term 'anterior compartment syndrome' by Greenfield *et al.* (1957). The patients recorded by Timperley *et al.* (1985) displayed some similarities. Proximal upper-limb involvement (Locke *et al.*, 1963) is rare and contemporary descriptions are not available.

The pattern of muscle involvement indicates that the site of the pathology in diabetic amyotrophy includes the lumbosacral plexus and probably also spinal nerves in addition to lower-limb peripheral nerves. The intercostal (or thoracic spinal nerves) may be implicated (Sun and Streib, 1981), either independently or in conjunction with a proximal lower-limb motor neuropathy, resulting in girdle pain and sometimes focal weakness of the anterior abdominal wall (Boulton *et al.*, 1984; Parry and Floberg, 1989).

A slowly progressive symmetric lower-limb motor neuropathy has been described (Asbury, 1977; Subramony and Wilbourn, 1982) which has been considered to represent a separate syndrome, perhaps with a metabolic basis. It has been found that this type of proximal motor neuropathy is more likely to be associated with a distal sensory neuropathy than is the asymmetric form with a more rapid onset (Subramony and Wilbourn, 1982). The symmetric proximal syndrome of insidious onset must be uncommon. It has not been observed despite extensive experience of patients with diabetic neuropathy (P. J. Watkins, personal communication).

The older literature contains reports of distal symmetric motor polyneuropathies occurring in patients with diabetes (Girard *et al.*, 1957; Boudin *et al.*, 1958; Azerad *et al.*, 1961; Bonduelle *et al.*, 1966; Fabregoule *et al.*, 1957). These had a subacute or chronic course. The reports often lacked nerve conduction studies and the precise nature of these cases is therefore uncertain. Some could well have represented coincidental associations. Others perhaps had chronic inflammatory demyelinating polyneuropathy (CIDP) superimposed upon diabetic neuropathy as a secondary immune event, as is known to occur in patients with hereditary motor and sensory neuropathy (Dyck *et al.*, 1982). Cornblath *et al.* (1987), in reporting four diabetic patients with CIDP, raised this issue; a number have been encountered by the authors of this review. Other patients are also occasionally seen with a chronic distal predominantly motor polyneuropathy that electrophysiologically and on nerve biopsy is an axonopathy and for which no cause other than diabetes is evident. The explanation is uncertain.

REFERENCES

Aguayo, A. J., Nair, P. V. and Bray, G. M. (1971). Peripheral nerve abnormalities in the Riley–Day syndrome: findings in a sural nerve biopsy. *Arch. Neurol.*, **24**, 106–116

Alvarez, F., Landrieu, P., Laget, P. *et al.* (1983). Nervous and ocular disorders in children with cholestasis and vitamin A and E deficiencies. *Hepatology*, **3**, 410–414

Archer, A. G., Watkins, P. J., Thomas, P. K. *et al.* (1983). The natural history of acute painful neuropathy in diabetes mellitus. *J. Neurol. Neurosurg. Psychiatry*, **46**, 491–499

Asbury, A. K. (1973). Renaut bodies – a forgotten endoneurial structure. *J. Neuropathol. Exp. Neurol.*, **32**, 334–342

Asbury, A. K. (1977). Proximal diabetic neuropathy. *Ann. Neurol.*, **2**, 179–187

Axelrod, F. B., Iyer, K. and Fish, I. (1981). Progressive sensory loss in familial dysautonomia. *Pediatrics*, **67**, 517–522

Azerad, E., Boudin, G., Pepin, B. and Lubetski, G. (1961). Sur une forme particulière amyotrophique de neuropathie diabétique. *Presse Méd.*, **69**, 1419–1428

Azizi, E., Zaidman, J. L., Eschar, J. and Szeinberg, A. (1978). Abetalipoproteinaemia treated with parenteral and oral vitamin A and E, and with medium chain triglycerides. *Acta Paediatr. Scand.*, **67**, 797–801

Azulay, J.-P., Blin, O., Bille, F. *et al.* (1992). High-dose intravenous human immunoglobulins are effective in the treatment of lower motor neuron syndromes associated with elevated serum anti-GM1 antibody titers: a double-blind, placebo-controlled study. *Neurology*, **42** (suppl 3), 334

Bailey, C. C. and Root, H. F. (1947). Neuropathic foot lesions in diabetes mellitus. *N. Engl. J. Med.*, **236**, 387–404

Bakchine, S., Mas, J. L., Rottembourg, R. *et al.* (1987). Polyneuropathy as the first sign of primary Sjögren's syndrome. Treatment by plasmatic exchanges. *Rev. Neurol. (Paris)*, **143**, 839–840

Ben Hamida, C., Doerflinger, N., Belel, S. *et al.* (1993). Localization of Friedreich ataxia phenotype with selective vitamin E deficiency to chromosome 8q by homozygosity mapping. *Nature Genetics*, **5**, 195–200

Blumenfeld, A., Slaugenhaupt, S. A., Axelrod, F. B. *et al.* (1993). Localization of the gene for familial dysautonomia on chromosome 9 and definition of DNA markers for genetic diagnosis. *Nature Genetics*, **4**, 160–164

Bonduelle, M., Deuil, R. and Yazbek, A. (1966). Les radiculonévrites subaiguës régressives des diabétiques. *Diabète*, **14**, 21–33

Boudin, G., Pepin, B., Borguignon, A. and Auffret, M. (1958). Neuropathie périphérique diabétique avec particularités sémiologiques. *Bull. Mém. Soc. Méd. Hôpitaux de Paris*, **74**, 789–798

Boulton, A. J. M., Hardisty, C. A., Betts, R. P. *et al.* (1983). Dynamic foot pressures and other studies as diagnostic and management aids in diabetic neuropathy. *Diabetes Care*, **6**, 26–33

Boulton, A. J. M., Angus, E., Ayyar, D. R. and Weiss, R. (1984). Diabetic thoracic polyradiculopathy presenting as an abdominal swelling. *Br. Med. J.*, **289**, 798–799

Boulton, A. J. M., Kubrusly, D. B., Bowker, J. H. *et al.* (1986). Impaired vibratory foot perception and diabetic foot ulceration. *Diabetic Medicine*, **3**, 335–337

Brown, J. W. and Podosin, R. (1966). A syndrome of the neural crest. *Arch. Neurol.*, **15**, 294–299.

Brown, M. J., Martin, J. R. and Asbury, A. K. (1976). Painful diabetic neuropathies. A morphometric study. *Arch. Neurol.*, **33**, 164–171

Bruns, L. (1890). Über neuritische Lähmungen beim Diabetes mellitus. *Berliner klinische Wochenschrift*, **27**, 509–525

Burck, V., Goebel, H. H., Kuhlendahl, H. D. *et al.* (1981). Neuromyopathy and vitamin E deficiency in man. *Neuropediatrics*, **12**, 267–278

Burman, J. F., Mollin, D. L., Sourial, N. A. and Sladden, R. A. (1979). Inherited lack of transcobalamin III in serum and megaloblastic anaemia: a further patient. *J. Haematol.*, **43**, 27–38

Carmel, R., Watkins, D., Goodman, S. I. and Rosenblatt, D. S. (1988). Hereditary defect of cobalamin metabolism (cblG mutation) presenting as a neurologic disorder in adulthood. *N. Engl. J. Med.*, **318**, 1738–1741

Cavanagh, N. P., Eames, R. A., Galvin, R. J. *et al.* (1979). Hereditary sensory neuropathy with spastic paraplegia. *Brain*, **102**, 79–94

Cavanagh, P. R., Young, M. J., Adams, J. E. and Boulton, A. J. M. (1994). Radiographic abnormalities in diabetic feet. In *The Foot in Diabetes*, 2nd edn. (A. J. M. Boulton, H. Connor and P. R. Cavanagh, eds) pp. 165–176, Chichester: Wiley

Chalk, C. H., Lennon, V. A., Stevens, J. C. and Windebank, A. J. (1993). Seronegativity for type 1 antineuronal nuclear antibodies ("anti-Hu") in subacute sensory neuronopathy patients without cancer. *Neurology*, **43**, 2209–2211

Chamberlain, S., Shaw, V., Rowland, A. *et al.* (1988). The mutation causing Friedreich's ataxia maps to human chromosome 9p22-cm. *Nature*, **334**, 248–250

Chanarin, I. and Perry, J. (1968). Metabolism of 5-methyltetrahydrofolate in pernicious anaemia. *Br. J. Haematol.*, **14**, 297–301

Chanarin, I., Deacon, R., Lumb, M. and Perry, J. (1992). Cobalamin and folate: recent developments. *J. Clin. Pathol.*, **45**, 277–283

Chaudhry, V., Corse, A. M., Cornblath, D. R. *et al.* (1993a). Multifocal motor neuropathy: response to human immune globulin. *Ann. Neurol.*, **33**, 237–242

Chaudhry, V., Corse, A. M., Cornblath, D. R. *et al.* (1993b). Multifocal motor neuropathy: electrodiagnostic features. (Unpublished)

Christensen, N. J. and Ørskov, H. (1969). Vibratory perception during ischaemia in uraemic patients and in subjects with mild carbohydrate intolerance. *J. Neurol. Neurosurg. Psychiatry*, **32**, 519–524

Clarke, C. A. and Sneddon, I. B. (1946). Nutritional neuropathy in prisoners-of-war and internees from Hong Kong. *Lancet*, **i**, 734–739

Coe, C. J. (1989). Guillain–Barré syndrome in Korean children. *Yonsei Medical Journal*, **30**, 81–87

Cornblath, D. R., Drachman, D. B. and Griffin, J. W. (1987). Demyelinating motor neuropathy in patients with diabetic polyneuropathy. *Ann. Neurol.*, **22**, 126

Cornblath, D. R. and McArthur, J. C. (1988). Predominantly sensory neuropathy in patients with AIDS and AIDS-related complex. *Neurology*, **38**, 794–796

Cornford, M. E., Ho, H. W. and Vinters, H. V. (1992). Correlation of neuromuscular pathology in acquired immune deficiency syndrome patients with cytomegalovirus infection and zidovudine treatment. *Acta Neuropathol.*, **84**, 516–529

Cundy, T. F., Edmonds, M. E. and Watkins, P. J. (1985). Osteopenia and metatarsal fractures in diabetic neuropathy. *Diabetic Medicine*, **2**, 461–468

Darnell, R. B. and DeAngelis, L. M. (1993). Regression of small-cell lung carcinoma in patients with paraneoplastic neuronal antibodies. *Lancet*, **341**, 21–22

Deacon, R., Chanarin, I., Perry, J. and Lumb, M. (1991). The effect of folate analogues on thymidine utilization by human and rat marrow cells and the effect on the deoxyuridine suppression test. *Postgrad. Med. J.*, **57**, 611–616

Deacon, R., Purkiss, P., Green, R. *et al.* (1986). Vitamin B_{12} neuropathy is not due to failure to methylate myelin basic protein. *J. Neurol. Sci.*, **72**, 113–117

Deacon, R., Bottiglieri, T., Chanarin, I. *et al.* (1990a). Methylthioadenosine serves as a single carbon source to the folate coenzyme pool in rat bone marrow cells. *Biochim. Biophys. Acta*, **1034**, 342–346

Deacon, J., Perry, J., Lumb, M. and Chanarin, I. (1990b). Cobalamin inactivation induces formyltetrahydrofolate synthetase. *FEBS Lett.*, **263**, 303–304

Denny-Brown, D. E. (1947). Neurological conditions resulting from prolonged and severe dietary restriction. *Medicine (Baltimore)*, **26**, 41–47

Denny-Brown, D. (1948). Primary sensory neuropathy with muscular changes associated with carcinoma. *J. Neurol. Neurosurg. Psychiatry*, **11**, 73–87

Denny-Brown, D. (1951). Hereditary sensory radicular neuropathy. *J. Neurol. Neurosurg. Psychiatry*, **14**, 237–252

Dinn, J. J., McCann, S., Wilson, P. *et al.* (1978). Animal model for subacute combined degeneration. *Lancet*, **2**, 1154

Dolman, C. L. (1963). The morbid anatomy of diabetic neuropathy. *Neurology*, **13**, 135–142

Donaghy, M., Hakin, R. N., Bamford, J. M. *et al.* (1987). Hereditary sensory neuropathy with neurotrophic keratitis: description of an autosomomal recessive disorder with a selective reduction of small myelinated nerve fibres and a discussion of the classification of the hereditary sensory neuropathies. *Brain*, **110**, 563–584

Dyck, P. J., Lambert, E. H. and Nichols, P.C. (1971). Quantitative measurements of sensation related to compound action potential and number and sizes of myelinated fibers of sural nerve in health, Friedrich's ataxia, hereditary sensory neuropathy, and tabes dorsalis. In *Handbook of Electroencephalography and Clinical Neurophysiology* (W. A. Cobb, ed.) **9**, 83–103. Amsterdam: Elsevier

Dyck, P. J. (1993). Neuronal atrophy and degeneration predominantly affecting peripheral sensory and autonomic neurons. In *Peripheral Neuropathy*, 3rd edn (P. J. Dyck, P. K. Thomas, J. W. Griffin et al., eds), pp. 1065–1093, Philadelphia: W. B. Saunders

Dyck, P. J. and Lais, A. C. (1973). Evidence for segmental demyelination secondary to axonal degeneration in Friedreich's ataxia. In *Clinical Studies in Myology* (B. A. Kakulas, ed), pp. 253–263, Amsterdam: Excerpta Medica

Dyck, P. J. and Bastron, J. (1983). 'Burning feet' as the only manifestation of dominantly inherited neuropathy. *Mayo Clin. Proc.*, **58**, 426–432

Dyck, P. J., Low, P. A., Bartelson, J. D. *et al.* (1982). Prednisolone responsive hereditary motor and sensory neuropathy. *Mayo Clin. Proc.*, **57**, 239–245

Dyck, P. J., Mellinger, J. F., Reagan, T. J. *et al.* (1983). Not 'indifference to pain' but varieties of hereditary sensory and autonomic neuropathy. *Brain*, **106**, 373–390

Dyck, P. J., Zimmerman, B. R., Vilen, T. H. *et al.* (1988). Nerve glucose, fructose, sorbitol, myo-inositol and fiber degeneration and regeneration in diabetic neuropathy. *N. Engl. J. Med.*, **319**, 542–548

Edmonds, M. E. (1987). Experience in a multi-disciplinary foot clinic. In *The Foot in Diabetes*, 1st edn. (H. Connor, A. J. M. Boulton and J. D. Ward, eds), pp. 121–133, Chichester: Wiley

Edmonds, M. E. and Foster, A. V. M. (1994). Classification and management of neuropathic and neuroischaemic ulcers. In *The Foot in Diabetes*, 2nd edn. (A. J. M. Boulton, H. Connor and P. R. Cavanagh, eds), pp. 109–120, Chichester: Wiley

Edmonds, M. E., Archer, A. G. and Watkins, P. J. (1983). Ephedrine: a new treatment for diabetic neuropathic oedema. *Lancet*, **1**, 548–557

Edmonds, M. E., Blundell, M. P., Morris, M. E. *et al.* (1986). Improved survival of the diabetic foot: the role of a specialised foot clinic. *Q. J. Med.*, **60**, 763–772

Ellenberg, M. (1974). Diabetic neuropathic cachexia. *Diabetes*, **23**, 418–423

Enders, U., Karch, H., Toyka, K. V. *et al.* (1993). The spectrum of immune responses to *Campylobacter jejuni* and glycoconjugates in Guillain–Barré syndrome and in other neuroimmunological disorders. *Ann. Neurol.*, **34**, 136–144.

Fabregoule, M., Eisenbeth, R. and Dutel, M. (1957). Neuropathie diffuse et régressive à type de polynévrite motrice d'origine diabétique. *Algérie Médecine*, **61**, 365–379

Feldman, E. L., Bromberg, M. B., Albers, J. W. and Pestronk, A. (1991). Immunosuppressive treatment in multifocal neuropathy. *Ann. Neurol.*, **30**, 397–401

Fine, E. J. and Hallett, M. (1980). Neurophysiological study of subacute combined degeneration. *J. Neurol. Sci.*, **45**, 331–336

Fisher, C. M. (1955). Residual neuropathological changes in Canadians held prisoners-of-war by the Japanese. *Canadian Services Med. J.*, **11**, 157–166

Flavin, M., Ortiz, P. J. and Ochoa, S. (1955). Metabolism of propionic acid in animal tissue. *Nature*, **176**, 823–826.

Font, J., Valls, J., Cervera, R. *et al.* (1990). Pure sensory neuropathy in patients with primary Sjögren's syndrome: clinical, immunological, and electromyographic findings. *Ann. Rheum. Dis.*, **49**, 775–778

Fox, R. I., Robinson, C. A., Curd, J. E. *et al.* (1986). Sjögren's syndrome. Proposed criteria for classification. *Arthritis Rheum.*, **29**, 577–585

Fujimura, H., LaCroix, C. and Said, G. (1991). Vulnerability of nerve fibres to ischaemia. A quantitative light and electron microscopic study. *Brain*, **114**, 1929–1942

Fuller, G. N., Jacobs, J. M. and Guiloff, R. J. (1989). Association of painful peripheral neuropathy in AIDS with cytomegalovirus infection. *Lancet*, **2**, 937–941

Fuller, G. N., Jacobs, J. M. and Guiloff, R. J. (1993). Nature and incidence of peripheral nerve syndromes in HIV infection. *J. Neurol. Neurosurg. Psychiatry*, **56**, 372–381.

Gabbay, K. H. (1973). Role of sorbitol pathway in neuropathy. In *Vascular and Neurological Changes in Early Diabetes* (R. A. Camerini-Davalos and H. S. Cole, eds), pp. 417–424, New York: Academic Press

Gabelli, C. (1992). The lipoprotein metabolism of apolipoprotein B mutants. *Curr. Opin. Lipids*, **3**, 208–214

Garland, H. (1955). Diabetic amyotrophy. *Br. Med. J.*, **2**, 1287–1291

Girard, M., Schott, B., Guillermet, J. and Alex, R. (1957). Polyradiculonévrite sensitivomotrice avec dissociation albuminocytologique au cours d'un diabète avec dénutrition. *Lyon Médecine*, **197**, 159–171

Glass, J. D., Griffin, J. W., Seiler, D. *et al.* (1994). Asynchronous degeneration of motor and sensory fibers during Wallerian degeneration. *Ann. Neurol.*, **36**, 287

Goebel, H. H., Veit, S. and Dyck, P. J. (1980). Confirmation of virtual unmyelinated fiber absence in hereditary sensory neuropathy type IV. *J. Neuropathol. Exp. Neurol.*, **39**, 670–675

Goldstein, J. M., Azizi, S. A., Booss, J. and Vollmer, T. L. (1993). Human immunodeficiency virus-associated motor axonal polyradiculoneuropathy. *Arch. Neurol.*, **50**, 1316–1319

Graus, F., Elkon, K. B., Cordon-Cardo, C. and Posner, J. B. (1986). Sensory neuronopathy and small cell lung cancer: an antineuronal antibody that also reacts with the tumor. *Am. J. Med.*, **80**, 45–52

Graus, F., Pou, A., Kanterwicz, E. and Anderson, N. E. (1988). Sensory neuronopathy and Sjögren's syndrome: clinical and immunologic study of two patients. *Neurology*, **38**, 1637–1639

Greenbaum, D., Richardson, P. C., Salmon, M. V. and Urich, H. (1964). Pathological observations on six cases of diabetic neuropathy. *Brain*, **87**, 201–214

Greenfield, J. G., Shy, G. M., Alvord, E. C. and Berg, J. L. (1957). *An Atlas of Muscle Pathology in Neuromuscular Diseases*. Edinburgh: E & S Livingstone

Gregersen, G. (1967). Diabetic neuropathy: influence of age, sex, metabolic control, and duration of diabetes on motor conduction velocity. *Neurology (Minneapolis)*, **17**, 972–980

Griffin, J. W. and Ho, T. W. (1993). The Guillain–Barré syndrome at 75: the *Campylobacter* connection (editorial). *Ann. Neurol.*, **34**, 125–127

Griffin, J. W., Cornblath, D. R., Alexander, E. *et al.* (1990). Ataxic sensory neuropathy and dorsal root ganglionitis associated with Sjögren's syndrome. *Ann. Neurol.*, **27**, 304–315

Griffin, J. W., Li, C. Y., Ho, T. W. *et al.* (1995a). Neuropathology of the "axonal" Guillain–Barré syndrome after *Campylobacter jejuni* infection. *Ann. Neurol.* (in press)

Griffin, J. W., Li, C. Y., Ho, T. W. *et al.* (1995b). Guillain–Barré syndrome in northern China: the spectrum of neuropathic changes in clinically defined cases. *Brain* (in press)

Guggenheim, M. A., Jackson, V., Lilly, J. and Silverman, A. (1983). Vitamin E deficiency and neurologic disease in children with cholecystasis: a progressive study. *J. Pediatr.*, **102**, 577–585

Guy, R. J. C., Clark, C. A., Malcolm, P. N. and Watkins, P. J. (1985). Evaluation of thermal and vibration sensation in diabetic neuropathy. *Diabetologia*, **28**, 131–137

Hankey, G. J. and Gubbay, S. S. (1987). Peripheral neuropathy associated with sicca syndrome. *J. Neurol. Neurosurg. Psychiatry*, **50**, 1085

Harding, A. E. (1984). *The Hereditary Ataxias and Related Disorders*. Edinburgh: Churchill Livingstone

Harding, A. E. (1987). Vitamin E and the nervous system. *CRC Crit. Rev. Neurobiol.*, **3**, 89–103

Harding, A. E., Muller, D. P. R., Thomas, P. K. and Willison, H. J. (1982). Spinocerebellar degeneration secondary to chronic intestinal malabsorption: a vitamin E deficiency syndrome. *Ann. Neurol.*, **12**, 419–424

Harding, A. E., Matthews, S., Jones, S. *et al.* (1985). Spinocerebellar degeneration with a selective defect of vitamin E absorption. *N. Engl. J. Med.*, **313**, 32–35

Hardman, D. A., Pullinger, C. R., Hamilton, R. L. *et al.* (1991). Molecular and metabolic basis for the metabolic disorder normotriglyceridemic abetalipoproteinemia. *J. Clin. Invest.*, **88**, 1722–1729

Heller, I. H. and Robb, P. (1955). Hereditary sensory neuropathy. *Neurology*, **5**, 15–20

Hicks, E. P. (1922). Hereditary perforating ulcer of the foot. *Lancet*, **1**, 319–321

Ho, T. W., Mishu, B., Li, C. Y. *et al.* (1995). Guillain–Barré syndrome in northern China: relationship to *Campylobacter jejuni* infection and anti-glycolipid antibodies. *Brain* (in press)

Horwich, M. S., Cho, L., Porro, R. S. and Posner, J. B. (1977). Subacute sensory neuropathy: a remote effect of carcinoma. *Ann. Neurol.*, **2**, 7–19

Hull, R. G., Morgan, S. H., Harding, A. E. and Hughes, G. R. V. (1984). Sjögren's syndrome presenting as a severe sensory neuropathy including involvement of the trigeminal nerve. *Br. J. Rheumatol.*, **23**, 301–303

Inoue, K., Hirano, A. and Hassin, J. (1979). Friedreich's ataxia selectively involves the large neurons of the dorsal root ganglia. *Ann. Neurol.*, **6**, 150

Jedrzejowska, H. and Milczarek, H. (1976). Recessive hereditary sensory neuropathy. *J. Neurol. Sci.*, **29**, 371–387

Jestico, J. V., Urry, P. A. and Efphimiou, J. (1985). An hereditary sensory and autonomic neuropathy transmitted as an X-linked recessive trait. *J. Neurol. Neurosurg. Psychiatry*, **48**, 1259–1264

Jitpimolmard, S., Small, J., King, R. H. M. *et al.* (1993). The sensory neuropathy of Friedreich's ataxia: an autopsy study in a case with prolonged survival. *Acta Neuropathol. (Berlin)*, **86**, 29–35

Judzewitsch, R. G., Jaspan, J. B., Polonsky, K. S. *et al.* (1983). Aldose reductase inhibition improves nerve conduction velocity in diabetic patients. *N. Engl. J. Med.*, **308**, 119–125

Jughenn, H., Krücke, W. and Wadulla, H. (1949). Zur Frage der familiären Syringomyelie: klinische-anatomisch Untersuchungen über familiäre neuro-vasculäre Dystrophie der Extremitäten. *Archiv. für Psychiatrie Nervenkrankreiten*, **182**, 153–159

Kaji, R., Shibasaki, H. and Kimura, J. (1992). Multifocal demyelinating motor neuropathy: cranial nerve involvement and immunoglobulin therapy. *Neurology*, **42**, 506–509

Kaji, R., Oka, N., Tsuji, T. *et al.* (1993). Pathological findings at the site of conduction block in multifocal motor neuropathy. *Ann. Neurol.*, **33**, 152–158

Kaplan, J. G., Rosenberg, R., Reinitz, E. *et al.* (1990). Invited review: peripheral neuropathy in Sjögren's syndrome. *Muscle Nerve*, **13**, 570–579

Kennett, R. P. and Harding, A. E. (1986). Peripheral neuropathy associated with the sicca syndrome. *J. Neurol. Neurosurg. Psychiatry*, **49**, 90–92

Khalifeh, R. R. and Zellweger, H. (1963). Hereditary sensory neuropathy with spinal cord disease. *Neurology*, **13**, 405–411

Knazan, M., Bohlega, S., Berry, K. and Eisen, A. (1990). Acute sensory neuronopathy with preserved SEPs and long-latency reflexes. *Muscle Nerve*, **13**, 381–384

Koenig, R. H. and Spiro, A. J. (1970). Hereditary spastic paraparesis with sensory neuropathy. *Dev. Med. Child Neurol.*, **12**, 576–581

Kondo, K. and Horikawa, Y. (1974). Genetic heterogeneity of hereditary sensory neuropathy. *Arch. Neurol.*, **30**, 336–343

Kosik, K. S., Mullins, T. F., Bradley, W. G. *et al.* (1980). Coma and axonal degeneration in vitamin B$_{12}$ deficiency. *Arch. Neurol.*, **37**, 590–592

Krarup, C., Stewart, J. D., Sumner, A. J. *et al.* (1990). A syndrome of asymmetrical limb weakness and motor conduction block. *Neurology*, **40**, 118–127

Krendel, D. A., Gilchrist, J. M., Johnson, O. A. and Boessen, E. H. (1987). Isolated deficiencies of vitamin E with progressive neurologic deterioration. *Neurology*, **37**, 538–540

Kumazawa, K., Sobue, G., Yamamoto, K. *et al.* (1993). Autonomic dysfunction in sensory ataxic neuropathy with Sjögren's syndrome (in Japanese). *Rinsho Shinkeigaku*, **33**, 1059–1065

Laloux, P., Brucher, J. M., Guerit, J. M. *et al.* (1988). Subacute sensory neuronopathy associated with Sjögren's sicca syndrome. *J. Neurol.*, **235**, 352–354

Lambert, E. H. and Dyck, P. J. (1975). Compound action potentials of sural nerve in vitro in peripheral neuropathy. In *Peripheral Neuropathy* (P. J. Dyck, P. K. Thomas and E. H. Lambert, eds), pp. 427–441, Philadelphia: W. B. Saunders

Landor, J. V. and Pallister, R. A. (1935). Avitaminosis B$_2$. *Trans. R. Soc. Trop. Med. Hyg.*, **29**, 121–125

Landrieu, P., Selva, J., Alvarez, F. *et al.* (1985). Peripheral nerve involvement in children with chronic cholecystasis and vitamin E deficiency. *Neuropediatrics*, **16**, 194–197

Landrieu, P., Said, G. and Allaire, C. (1990). Dominantly transmitted congenital indifference to pain. *Ann. Neurol.*, **27**, 574–581

Lange, D. J., Blake, D. M., Hirano, M. *et al.* (1990). Multifocal conduction block motor neuropathy: diagnostic value of stimulating nerve roots. *Neurology*, **40** (suppl), 182

Lange, D. J., Trojaborg, W., Latov, N. *et al.* (1992). Multifocal motor neuropathy with conduction block: is it a distinct clinical entity? *Neurology*, **42**, 497–505

LaPlante, P., Vanasse, M., Michaud, J. *et al.* (1988). A progressive neurological syndrome associated with an isolated vitamin E deficiency. *J. Lab. Clin. Invest.*, **111**, 558–559

Layzer, R. (1978). Myeloneuropathy after prolonged exposure to nitrous oxide. *Lancet*, **2**, 1227–1230

Leger, J. M. (1992). Atteinte du system nerveux peripherique au cours de l'infection par le VIH: exploration electromyographique et vitesses de conduction nerveuses. (Involvement of the peripheral nervous system in HIV infection: electromyographic study and nerve conduction velocity) (Review). *Neurophysiologie Clinique*, **22**, 403–416

Lewis, R. A., Sumner, A. J., Brown, M. J. and Asbury, A. K. (1982). Multifocal demyelinating neuropathy with persistent conduction block. *Neurology*, **32**, 958–964

Liang, B. C., Albers, J. W., Sima, A. A. and Niostrant, T. T. (1994). Paraneoplastic pseudo-obstruction, mononeuropathy multiplex, and sensory neuronopathy. *Muscle Nerve*, **17**, 91–96

Lincoff, N. S., Odel, J. G. and Hirano, M. (1993). 'Outbreak' of optic and peripheral neuropathy in Cuba. *JAMA.*, **270**, 511–518

Llewelyn, J. G., Thomas, P. K., Fonseca, V. *et al.* (1986). Acute painful diabetic neuropathy precipitated by strict glycaemic control. *Acta Neuropathol. (Berlin)*, **72**, 157–163

Llewelyn, J. G., Gilbey, S. G., Thomas, P. K. *et al.* (1991). Sural nerve morphometry in diabetic autonomic and painful sensory neuropathy: a clinicopathological study. *Brain*, 114, 867–892

Locke, S., Lawrence, D. G. and Legg, M. A. (1963). Diabetic amyotrophy. *Am. J. Med.*, **34**, 775–780

Low, P. A., Burke, W. J. and McLeod, J. G. (1978). Congenital sensory neuropathy with selective loss of small myelinated nerve fibres. *Ann. Neurol.*, **3**, 179–182

Malinow, K., Yannakakis, G. D., Glusman, S. M. *et al.* (1986). Subacute sensory neuronopathy secondary to dorsal root ganglionitis in Sjögren's syndrome. *Ann. Neurol.*, **20**, 535–537

McCombe, P. A. and McLeod, J. G. (1984). The peripheral neuropathy of vitamin B$_{12}$ deficiency. *J. Neurol. Sci.*, **66**, 117–121

McKhann, G. M., Cornblath, D. R., Griffin, J. W. *et al.* (1993). Acute motor axonal neuropathy: a frequent cause of acute flaccid paralysis in China. *Ann. Neurol.*, **33**, 333–342

McLeod, J. G. (1971). An electrophysiological and pathological study of peripheral nerves in Friedreich's ataxia. *J. Neurol. Sci.*, **12**, 333–349

McLeod, J. G. (1993). Paraneoplastic neuropathies. In *Peripheral Neuropathy* (P. J. Dyck, P. K. Thomas, J. W. Griffin, P. A. Low and J. F. Poduslo, eds), pp. 1583–1590, Philadelphia: W. B. Saunders

McLeod, J. G. and Evans, W. A. (1981). Peripheral neuropathy in spinocerebellar degenerations. *Muscle Nerve*, **4**, 51–61

McLoughlin, J. L. and Cantrill, R. C. (1986). Nitrous oxide induced vitamin B$_{12}$ deficiency: measurement of methylation reactions in the fruit bat (*Rousethus aegypticus*). *Int. J. Biochem.*, **18**, 199–202

Mellgren, S. I., Conn, D. L., Stevens, J. C. and Dyck, P. J. (1989). Peripheral neuropathy in primary Sjögren syndrome. *Neurology*, **39**, 390–394

Métivier, V. M. (1941). Eye disease due to vitamin deficiency in Trinidad. *Am. J. Ophthalmol.*, **24**, 1265–1272

Miller, R. G., Nielsen, S. L. and Sumner, A. J. (1976). Hereditary sensory neuropathy and tonic pupils. *Neurology*, **26**, 931–939

Mott, F. W. (1907). A case of Friedreich's disease with autopsy. *Arch. Neurol. (London)*, **3**, 180–200

Muller, D. P. R., Harries, J. T. and Lloyd, J. K. (1970). Vitamin E therapy in a-beta-lipoproteinaemia. *Arch. Dis. Child.*, **45**, 715–722

Murray, T. J. (1973). Congenital sensory neuropathy. *Brain*, **96**, 387–394,

Nelson, J. S., Fitch, C. D., Fischer, V. W. *et al.* (1981). Progressive neuropathologic lesions in vitamin E deficient rhesus monkeys. *J. Neuropathol. Exp. Neurol.*, **40**, 166–186

Nemoto, H., Fujioka, T., Okada, S. (1992). A case of carcinomatous autonomic and sensory neuropathy (in Japanese). *Rinsho Shinkeigaku*, **32**, 543–546.

Neville, H. E., Ringel, S. P., Guggenheim, M. A. *et al.* (1983). Ultrastructural and histochemical abnormalities of skeletal muscle in patients with chronic vitamin E deficiency. *Neurology*, **33**, 483–488

Nishiyama, K., Kurisaki, H., Masuda, N. *et al.* (1993). Carcinomatous neuropathy associated with hepatic cell carcinoma: an autopsy case report. *Neuromuscular Disorders*, **3**, 227–229

Nobile-Orazio, E., Baldini, L., Barbieri, S. *et al.* (1988). Treatment of patients with neuropathy and anti-MAG IgM M-proteins. *Ann. Neurol.*, **24**, 93–97

Nobile-Orazio, E., Meucci, N., Barbieri, S. *et al.* (1993). High-dose intravenous immunoglobulin therapy in multifocal motor neuropathy. *Neurology*, **43**, 537–544

Nordborg, C., Conradi, N., Sourander, P. and Westerberg, B. (1981). A new type of non-progressive sensory neuropathy in children with atypical dysautonomia. *Acta Neuropathol. (Berlin)*, **55**, 135–141

Nukada, H., Pollock, M. and Haas, L. F. (1982). The clinical spectrum and morphology of type II hereditary sensory neuropathy. *Brain*, **105**, 647–666

Ogryzlo, M. A. (1946). A familial peripheral neuropathy of unknown etiology resembling Morvan's disease. *Can. Med. Assoc. J..*, **54**, 547–553

Ohta, M., Ellefson, R. D., Lambert, E. H. and Dyck, P. J. (1973). Hereditary sensory neuropathy type II. Clinical, electrophysiologic, histologic and biochemical studies of a Quebec kinship. *Arch. Neurol. (Chicago)*, **29**, 23–37

Ouvrier, R. A., McLeod, J. G. and Conchin, T. E. (1982). Friedreich's ataxia. Early detection and progression of peripheral nerve abnormalities. *J. Neurol. Sci.*, **55**, 137–145

Ojala, J. M., Matikaien, E. and Groop, L. (1985). Body sway in diabetic neuropathy. *J. Neurol.*, **232** (suppl. 188), 188.

Panegyres, P. K., Reading, M. C. and Esiri, M. M. (1993). The inflammatory reaction of paraneoplastic ganglionitis and encephalitis: an immunohistochemical study. *J. Neurol.*, **240**, 93–97

Parry, G. J. and Floberg, J. (1989). Diabetic truncal neuropathy presenting as an abdominal hernia. *Neurology*, **9**, 1488–1490

Pearson, J. and Pytel, B. (1978). Quantitative studies of sympathetic ganglia and spinal cord intermediolateral gray columns in familial dysautonomia. *J. Neurol. Sci.*, **39**, 47–59

Pearson, J. Budzilovich, G. and Finegold, M. J. (1971). Sensory, motor and autonomic dysfunction: the nervous system in familial dysautonomia. *Neurology (Minneapolis)*, **21**, 486–493

Peraita, M. (1946). Deficiency neuropathies observed in Madrid during the civil war (1936–39). *Br. Med. J.*, **2**, 784–793

Perry, J., Chanarin, I., Deacon, R. and Lumb, M. (1983). Chronic cobalamin inactivation impairs folate polyglutamate synthesis in the rat. *J. Clin. Invest.*, **71**, 1183–1190

Pestronk, A., Cornblath, D. R., Ilyas, A. A. *et al.* (1988). A treatable multifocal motor neuropathy with antibodies to GM1 ganglioside. *Ann. Neurol.*, **24**, 73–78

Pestronk, A., Chaudhry, V., Feldman, E. L. *et al.* (1990). Lower motor neuron syndromes defined by patterns of weakness, nerve conduction abnormalities, and high titers of antiglycolipid antibodies. *Ann. Neurol.*, **27**, 316–326

Pinsky, L. and Di George, A. M. (1966). Congenital familial sensory neuropathy with anhidrosis. *J. Pediatr.*, **68**, 1–13

Pollock, M. and Kies, B. (1990). Benign hereditary cerebellar ataxia with extensive thermoanalgesia. *Brain*, **113**, 857–865

Raff, M., Sangalang, V. and Asbury, A. K. (1968). Ischemic mononeuropathy multiplex associated with diabetes mellitus. *Arch. Neurol. (Chicago)*, **18**, 487–495

Rance, N., McArthur, J. C., Cornblath, D. R. *et al.* (1988). Gracile tract degeneration in patients with sensory neuropathy and AIDS. *Neurology*, **38**, 265–271

Rith-Najarian, S. J., Stolusky, T. and Ghodes, D. M. (1992). Identifying diabetic patients at high risk for lower-extremity amputation in a primary health care setting. *Diabetes Care*, **15**, 1386–1389

Rizzutto, N., Monaco, S., Moretto, G. *et al.* (1981). Friedreich's ataxia. A light and electron microscopic study of peripheral nerve biopsies. *Acta Neuropathol. (Berlin)*, (Suppl. 7), 344–347

Robert, M. E., Geraghty, J. J., III, Miles, S. A. *et al.* (1989). Severe neuropathy in a patient with acquired immune deficiency syndrome (AIDS). Evidence for widespread cytomegalovirus infection of peripheral nerve and human immunodeficiency virus-like immunoreactivity of anterior horn cells. *Acta Neuropathol.*, **79**, 255–261

Rothwell, J. C., Traub, M. M., Day, B. L. *et al.* (1982). Manual motor performance in a deafferented man. *Brain*, **105**, 515–542

Ryle, C. and Donaghy, M. (1995). Glycation of peripheral nerve proteins in diabetes mellitus. *J. Neurol. Sci.* **129**, 62–68

Sadiqu, S. A., Thomas, F. P., Kilidireas, K. *et al.* (1990). The spectrum of neurologic disease associated with anti-GM$_1$ antibodies. *Neurology*, **40**, 1067–1072

Said, G., Slama, G. and Selva, J. (1983). Progressive centripetal degeneration of axons in small fibre type diabetic polyneuropathy. A clinical and pathological study. *Brain*, **106**, 791–807

Said, G., Marion, M.-H., Selva, J. and Jamet, C. (1986). Hypotrophic and dying-back nerve fibres in Friedreich's ataxia. *Neurology*, **36**, 1292–1299

Said, G., Goulon-Goeau, C., Slama, G. and Tchobroutsky, G. (1992). Severe early-onset polyneuropathy in insulin-dependent diabetes mellitus. *N. Engl. J. Med.*, **326**, 1257–1263

Said, G., Goulon-Goeau, C., LaCroix, C. and Moulonguet, A. (1994). Nerve biopsy findings in different patterns of proximal diabetic neuropathy. *Ann. Neurol.*, **35**, 559–569

Sanes, J. N., Mauritz, K.-H., Dalakas, M. C. and Evarts, E. V. (1985). Motor control in humans with large-fiber sensory neuropathy. *Hum. Neurobiol.*, **4**, 101–114.

Santoro, M., Thomas, F. P., Fink, M. E. *et al.* (1990). IgM deposits at nodes of Ranvier in a patient with amyotrophic lateral sclerosis, anti-GM$_1$ antibodies, and multifocal motor conduction block. *Ann. Neurol.*, **28**, 373–377

Scaravilli, F., Sinclair, E., Arango, J.-C. *et al.* (1992). The pathology of the posterior root ganglia in AIDS and its relationship to the pallor of the gracile tract. *Acta Neuropathol.*, **84**, 163–170

Schneider, W., Neidermeier, W. and Graff, P. (1993a). The paradox between resistance to hypoxia and liability to hypoxic damage in hyperglycaemic peripheral nerves. Evidence for glycolysis involvement. *Diabetes*, **42**, 981–987

Schneider, W., Quasthoff, S., Mitrovic, N. and Graff, P. (1993b). Hyperglycaemic hypoxia alters after potential and fast K$^+$ conductance of rat axons by cytoplasmic acidification. *J. Physiol. (London)*, **465**, 679–697

Scott, H. H. (1918). An investigation into an acute outbreak of 'central neuritis'. *Ann. Trop. Med. Parasitol.*, **12**, 109–115

Scott, J. M., Dinn, J. J., Wilson, P. and Weir, D. G. (1981). Pathogeneis of subacute combined degeneration. A result of methyl group deficiency. *Lancet*, **2**, 334–337

Selby, P. L., Young, M. J. and Boulton, A. J. M. (1994). Biphosphonates: a new treatment for diabetic Charcot neuroarthropathy. *Diabetic Medicine*, **11**, 28–31

Seneviratne, K. N. and Peiris, O. A. (1968). The effect of ischaemia on the excitability of sensory nerves in diabetes mellitus. *J. Neurol. Neurosurg. Psychiatry*, **31**, 348–353

Sima, A. A. F., Bril, V., Nathaniel, V. *et al.* (1988). Regeneration and repair of myelinated fibres in sural nerve biopsies from patients with diabetic neuropathy treated with sorbinil, an investigational aldose reductase inhibitor. *N. Engl. J. Med.*, **319**, 548–555

Small, J. R., Thomas, P. K. and Schapira, A. H. V. (1993). Dorsal root ganglion proteins in Friedreich's ataxia. *Neurosci. Lett.*, **163**, 182–184

Smith, B. E., Windebank, A. J. and Dyck, P. J. (1993). Nonmalignant inflammatory sensory polyganglionopathy. In *Peripheral Neuropathy*, Vol. 2 (P. J. Dyck, P. K. Thomas, J. W. Griffin, P. A. Low and J. F. Poduslo, eds), pp. 1525–1531, Philadelphia: W. B. Saunders

So, Y. T., Holtzman, D. M., Abrams, D. I. and Olney, R. K. (1988). Peripheral neuropathy associated with acquired immunodeficiency syndrome: prevalence and clinical features from a population-based survey. *Arch. Neurol.*, **45**, 945–948

Sokol, R. J., Guggenheim, M. A., Iannacone, S. T. *et al.* (1985). Improved neurologic function after long-term correction of vitamin E deficiency in children with chronic cholestasis. *N. Engl. J. Med.*, **313**, 1580–1588

Sokol, R. J., Kayden, H. J., Bettis, D. B. *et al.* (1988). Isolated vitamin E deficiency in the absence of fat malabsorption – familial and sporadic cases: characterization and investigation of causes. *J. Lab. Clin. Med.*, **111**, 548–559

Sosenko, J. M., Kato, M., Soto, R. and Bild, D. E. (1990). Comparison of quantitative sensory test measurements and their association with foot ulceration in diabetic patients. *Diabetes Care*, **13**, 1057–1061

Southam, E., Thomas, P. K., King, R. H. M. *et al.* (1991). Experimental vitamin E deficiency in rats. Morphological and functional evidence of abnormal axonal transport secondary to free radical damage. *Brain*, **114**, 915–936

Spencer, P. S. and Schaumburg, H. H. (1976). Central-peripheral distal axonopathy – the pathology of dying-back polyneuropathies. *Prog. Neuropathol.*, **3**, 253–295

Spillane, J. D. (1947). *Nutritional Disorders of the Nervous System*. Edinburgh: E. and S. Livingstone

Spillane, J. D. and Scott, G. I. (1945). Obscure neuropathy in the Middle East. *Lancet*, **2**, 261–266

Steele, J. M., Young, R. J. Lloyd, G. G. and Clarke, B. F. (1987). Clinically apparent eating disorders in young diabetic women: associations with painful neuropathy and other complications. *Br. Med. J.*, **294**, 859–866

Sterman, A. B., Schaumburg, H. H. and Asbury, A. K. (1980). The acute sensory neuropathy syndrome: a distinct clinical entity. *Ann. Neurol.*, **7**, 354–358

Strachan, H. (1888, cited by Victor, 1975). Malarial multiple peripheral neuritis. *Sajou's Annual of the Universal Medical Sciences*, **1**, 139

Strachan, H. (1897). On a form of multiple neuritis prevalent in the West Indies. *Practitioner*, **59**, 477–481

Stumpf, D. A., Sokol, R., Bettis, D. *et al.* (1987). Friedrich's disease: V. Variant form with vitamin E deficiency and normal fat absorption. *Neurology*, **37**, 68–74

Subramony, S. H. and Wilbourn, A. J. (1982). Diabetic proximal neuropathy. Clinical and electromyographic studies. *J. Neurol. Sci.*, **53**, 293–304

Sugimura, K. and Dyck, P. J. (1982). Multifocal fiber loss in proximal sciatic nerve in symmetric distal diabetic neuropathy. *J. Neurol. Sci.*, **53**, 501–509

Sun, S. F. and Streib, E. W. (1981). Diabetic thoracoabdominal neuropathy: clinical and electrodiagnostic features. *Ann. Neurol.*, **9**, 75–79

Swanson, A. G. (1963). Congenital insensitivity to pain with anhidrosis. *Arch. Neurol.*, **8**, 299–302

Swanson, A. G., Buchan, G. C. and Alvord, E. C. Jr. (1965). Anatomic changes in congenital insensitivity to pain. Absence of small primary sensory neurons in ganglia, roots and Lissauer's tract. *Arch. Neurol. (Chicago)*, **12**, 12–18

Thévenard, A. (1942). L'acropathie ulcéro-mutilante familiale. *Rev. Neurol. (Paris)*, **74**, 193–201

Thomas, F. P., Adapon, H. P., Goldberg, G. P. *et al.* (1989). Localization of neural epitopes that bind to IgM monoclonal autoantibodies (M-proteins) from two patients with motor neuron disease. *J. Neuroimmunol.*, **21**, 31–39

Thomas, F. P., Trojaborg, W., Nagy, C. *et al.* (1990). Experimental autoimmune neuropathy in rabbits immunized with Gal(beta1-3)Gal NAc or GM1, with partial conduction block and IgG and IgM deposits at nodes of Ranvier. *J. Neurol. Sci.*, **98** (suppl), 69

Thomas, P. K. (1992). The Guillain–Barré syndrome: no longer a simple concept. *J. Neurol.*, **239**, 361–362

Thomas, P. K. (1994). Growth factors and diabetic neuropathy. *Diab. Med.*, **11**, 732–739

Thomas, P. K. and Ormerod, I. E. C. (1993). Hereditary neuralgic amyotrophy associated with a relapsing multifocal sensory neuropathy. *J. Neurol. Neurosurg. Psychiatry* **56**, 107–109

Thomas, P. K. and Tomlinson, D. R. (1993). Diabetic and hypoglycemic neuropathy. In *Peripheral Neuropathy*, 3rd edn. (P. J. Dyck, P. K. Thomas, J. W. Griffin, P. A. Low and J. F. Poduslo, eds), pp. 1219–1250, Philadelphia: W. B. Saunders

Thomas, P. K., Hoffbrand, A. V. and Smith, I. S. (1982). Neurological involvement in hereditary transcobalamin II deficiency. *J. Neurol. Neurosurg. Psychiatry*, **45**, 72–77

Thomas, P. K., Cooper, J. M., King, R. H. M. *et al.* (1993). Myopathy in vitamin E deficient rats: muscle fibre necrosis associated with disturbances of mitochondrial function. *J. Anat.*, **183**, 451–461

Thomas, P. K., Plant, G., Baxter, P. J. and Santiago Luis, R. (1994). An epidemic of optic neuropathy and painful sensory neuropathy in Cuba. *J. Neurol. Neurosurg. Psychiatry*, **57**, 1288

Thompson, F., Veves, A., Ashe, H. *et al.* (1991). A team approach to diabetic foot care. *The Foot*, **1**, 75–82

Timperley, W. R., Boulton, A. J., Davies-Jones, G. A. *et al.* (1985). Small vessel disease in progressive neuropathy associated with good metabolic control. *J. Clin. Pathol.*, **38**, 1030–1039

Towfighi, J. (1981). Effects of chronic vitamin E deficiency on the nervous system of the rat. *Acta Neuropathol.*, **54**, 261–267

Trapp, B. D., Andrews, S. B., Wong, A. *et al.* (1989). Co-localization of the myelin-associated glycoprotein and the microfilament components f-actin and spectrin in Schwann cells of myelinated fibers. *J. Neurocytol.*, **18**, 47–60

Tuck, R. R., Schmelzer, J. D. and Low, P. A. (1984). Endoneurial blood flow and oxygen tension in the sciatic nerve of rats with experimental diabetic neuropathy. *Brain*, **107**, 935–950

Valldeoriola, F., Vega, F., Rene, R. *et al.* (1992). Neurologic syndromes associated with anti-Hu antibody. Study of 24 patients (in Spanish). *Medicina Clinica (Barcelona)*, **99**, 361–364

Van Epps, C. and Kerr, H. D. (1940). Familial lumbosacral syringomyelia. *Radiology*, **35**, 160–168

Veves, A., Murray, H. J., Young, M. J. and Boulton, A. J. M. (1992). The risk of foot ulceration in diabetic patients with high foot pressure: a prospective study. *Diabetologia*, **35**, 660–663

Victor, M. (1974). Polyneuropathy due to nutritional deficiency and alcoholism. In *Peripheral Neuropathy* (P. J. Dyck, P. K. Thomas and E. H. Lambert, eds), pp. 1030–1066, Philadelphia: W. B. Saunders

Viera-Makings, E., Metz, J., Van Der Westhuyzen, J. *et al.* (1990). Cobalamin neuropathy. Is S-adenosylhomocysteine toxicity a factor? *Biochem. J.*, **266**, 707–711

Vivaqua, R. J., Myerson, R. M., Prescott, D. J. and Rabinowitz, J. L. (1966). Abnormal propionic-methyl malonic succinic acid metabolism in vitamin B_{12} deficiency and its possible relationship to the neurologic syndrome of pernicious anaemia. *Am. J. Med. Sci.*, **251**, 507–515

Vriesendorp, F. J., Mishu, B., Blaser, M. and Koski, C. L. (1993). Serum antibodies to GM1, peripheral nerve myelin, and *Campylobacter jejuni* in patients with Guillain–Barré syndrome and controls: correlation and prognosis. *Ann. Neurol.*, **34**, 130–135

Wadia, N., Irani, P., Mehta, L. and Purohit, A. (1978). Evidence of peripheral neuropathy in a variety of heredo-familial olivo-ponto-cerebellar degeneration frequently seen in India. In *Spinocerebellar Degenerations* (I. Sobue, ed.), pp. 239–250, Tokyo: University of Tokyo Press

Ward, J. D., Barnes, C. G., Fisher, D. J. *et al.* (1971). Improvement in nerve conduction following treatment in newly-diagnosed diabetics. *Lancet*, **1**, 428–431

Watkins, P. J. (1990). Natural history of the diabetic neuropathies. *Q. J. Med.*, **77**, 1209–1218

Weir, D. G., Keating, S. and Molloy, A. (1988). Methylation deficiency causes vitamin B_{12}-associated neuropathy in the pig. *J. Neurochem.*, **51**, 1949–1952

Willis, T. (1685). *The London Practice of Pysick*. New York: The Classics of Neurology & Neurosurgery Library

Windebank, A. J., Blexrud, M. D., Dyck, P. J. *et al.* (1990). The syndrome of acute sensory neuropathy: clinical features and electrophysiologic and pathologic changes. *Neurology*, **40**, 584–591

Wright, R. A. and Dyck, P. J. (1995). Hereditary sensory neuropathy with sensorineural hearing loss and early-onset dementia. *Neurology*, in press

Xu, Y., Sladky, J. T. and Brown, M. J. (1989). Dose-dependent expression of neuronopathy after experimental pryridoxine intoxication. *Neurology*, **39**, 1077–1083

Yokota, T., Wada, Y., Furukaura, T. *et al*, (1987). Adult-onset spinocerebellar syndrome with idiopathic vitamin E deficiency. *Ann Neurol.*, **22**, 84–87

Yoshioka, A., Ueda, Y., Sakai, K. *et al.* (1992). Immunohistochemical studies of paraneoplastic subacute sensory neuropathy – an analysis of antineuronal antibody and infiltrated lymphocytes (in Japanese). *Rinsho Shinkeigaku*, **32**, 397–404

Young, M. J., Manes, C. and Boulton, A. J. M. (1992). Vibration perception threshold predicts foot ulceration. *Diabetic Medicine*, **9** (suppl 2), 542

Young, S. G., Bihain, B., Flynn, L. M. *et al.* (1994). Asymptomatic homozygous hypobetalipoproteinemia associated with apolipoprotein B 45.2. *Hum. Mol. Genet.*, **3**, 741–744

Yuki, N., Yoshino, H., Sato, S. and Miyatake, T. (1990). Acute axonal polyneuropathy associated with anti-GM_1 antibodies following *Campylobacter jejuni* enteritis. *Neurology*, **40**, 1900–1902

Yuki, N., Yoshino, H., Sato, S. *et al.* (1992). Severe acute axonal form of Guillain–Barré syndrome associated with IgG anti-GD_{1a} antibodies. *Muscle Nerve*, **15**, 899–903

Zaheer, W., Friedland, M. L., Cooper, E. B. *et al.* (1993). Spontaneous regression of small cell carcinoma of lung associated with severe neuropathy. *Cancer Invest. (New York)*, **11**, 306–309

Zhao, B., Yang, T., Huang, H. and Liu, X. (1981). Acute polyradiculitis (Guillain–Barré syndrome): an epidemiological study of 156 cases observed in Beijing. *Ann. Neurol.*, **9** (suppl), 146–148

Zoghbi, H. Y., Frontali, M., Orr, H. T. *et al.* (1993). Linkage studies in dominantly inherited ataxias. In *Inherited Ataxias* (A. E. Harding and T. Denfel, eds), *Adv. Neurol.*, **61**, 133–137

5
Autonomic neuropathy: aspects of diagnosis and management
C. J. Mathias

INTRODUCTION

The autonomic nervous system has two major efferent divisions, the craniosacral parasympathetic and the thoracolumbar sympathetic. It is, however, dependent upon a variety of afferent pathways, which are activated by pressure, cutaneous, muscle and visceral receptors. These pathways, through cerebral and/or spinal connections, influence the autonomic outflow. Virtually every organ in the body is supplied by one or both autonomic pathways which play key roles in both local and integrative function.

Involvement of peripheral autonomic pathways occurs in a wide variety of disorders. In some the autonomic nervous system only may be affected. The dysfunction may be highly specific as in the isolated deficiency of dopamine betahydroxylase (DBH) with failure to synthesize noradrenaline and adrenaline (Mathias and Bannister, 1992a); it may involve only one efferent pathway as in pure cholinergic dysautonomia (Thomashetsky *et al.*, 1972); or it may encompass the entire autonomic nervous system (without other neurological involvement) as in pure autonomic failure (Bannister and Mathias, 1992). An autonomic neuropathy may complicate neurological disorders as in the Guillain–Barré syndrome, endocrine diseases such as diabetes mellitus and various medical conditions, ranging from renal failure to human immunodeficiency virus (HIV) infection (McLeod, 1992).

In this chapter, aspects of the diagnosis and management of the autonomic neuropathies will be reviewed. A classification is provided, which will concentrate predominantly on peripheral disorders. This will be followed by a description of the major abnormalities resulting from autonomic dysfunction, and key aspects of investigation and management. Further details on individual disorders are available in major textbooks on autonomic disorders.

CLASSIFICATION OF AUTONOMIC NEUROPATHIES

Autonomic neuropathies may be either localized or generalized. In some of the localized disorders there may be few symptoms directly attributable to autonomic involvement itself, but the signs provide an important clue to the underlying

Table 5.1 Examples of conditions that result in localized autonomic dysfunction

---

Horner's syndrome
Reflex sympathetic dystrophy
Gustatory sweating (Frey's syndrome)
Crocodile tears (Bogorad's syndrome)
Chagas' disease (*Trypanosomiasis cruzii*)
Hirschsprung's disease (congenital megacolon)

Surgery
    Sympathectomy – regional
    Vagotomy and gastric drainage procedures resulting in dumping syndrome
    Organ transplantation – heart

In Chagas' disease, which is initially a systemic infection, there is targeting of the heart, oesophagus and colon. A localized disorder, such as gustatory sweating may result from regional surgery (to the parotid gland) or complicate a systemic disorder such as diabetes mellitus.

diagnosis (Table 5.1). An example is Horner's syndrome which can lead to detection of Pancoast's tumour at the apex of the lung, or diagnosis of a dissecting aneurysm of the internal carotid artery. Severe local symptoms may occur in reflex sympathetic dystrophy (also known as Sudeck's osteodystrophy or causalgia), where the relationship between the clinical manifestations, pain pathways, sympathoneural activity and neuropeptides is not clear (see also Chapter 3).

The autonomic neuropathies can be divided into primary, where the aetiology is not known, and secondary, where there is a clear association with disease, and/or where the site of the lesion is known (Table 5.2). Within the primary autonomic disorders the acute/subacute dysautonomias mainly involve peripheral pathways, unlike the chronic autonomic failure syndromes. In the latter group, pure autonomic failure (PAF, previously called idiopathic orthostatic hypotension) is a peripheral disorder; separation from the Shy–Drager syndrome (often synonymous with multiple system atrophy), which is predominantly a central disorder, can be difficult in the early stages. The presence or development of additional neurological manifestations is a feature of the Shy–Drager syndrome (Figure 5.1).

The secondary autonomic neuropathies outlined in Table 5.2 are classified under different groups. In addition, there are two other groups which are caused by, or may cause peripheral autonomic dysfunction which are separately classified. Neurally mediated syncope includes common faints (vasovagal syncope), and syncope associated with carotid sinus hypersensitivity, glossopharyngeal neuralgia and swallowing. Syncope in these situations results from excessive or abnormal autonomic activity, which between episodes appears to be normal. In conditions such as vasovagal syncope, the relative roles of peripheral, central or efferent components in causing the fall in blood pressure is unclear. Drugs are a common cause of peripheral autonomic dysfunction (Table 5.3) and may do this in a variety of ways.

CLINICAL AND INVESTIGATIVE APPROACH IN SUSPECTED AUTONOMIC NEUROPATHY

The clinical manifestations of an autonomic neuropathy vary widely, and may thus mimic other disorders. The history and clinical examination, therefore, is of particular importance in determining which investigative path to take. A history

Table 5.2 Classification of autonomic neuropathies

Primary
Aetiology unknown
  Acute/subacute dysautonomias
    Pure pandysautonomia
    Pure cholinergic dysautonomia
    With neurological features
  Chronic
    Pure autonomic failure

Congenital   Nerve growth factor deficiency

Secondary
Hereditary
  Autosomal dominant
    Familial amyloid neuropathy
    Porphyria
  Autosomal recessive
    Familial dysautonomia/Riley–Day syndrome
    Dopamine β-hydroxylase deficiency
  X-linked recessive
    Fabry's disease

Metabolic
  Chronic renal failure
  Chronic liver disease
  Vitamin B_{12} deficiency
  Alcohol

Toxins
  Botulism

Inflammatory
  Guillain–Barré syndrome

Infections
  Bacterial   Leprosy
  Viral   HIV infection
  Parasitic   Chagas' disease

Malignancy
  Paraneoplastic to include adenocarcinomas – lung, pancreas and
  Lambert–Eaton syndrome

Connective tissue disorders
  Rheumatoid arthritis
  Systemic lupus erythematosus
  Mixed connective tissue disease

Surgery
  Regional sympathectomy – upper limb, splanchnic
  Vagotomy and drainage procedures – dumping syndrome
  Organ transplantation – heart

Neurally mediated syncope
  Vasovagal syncope
  Swallow syncope
  With glossopharyngeal neuralgia

Drugs
  (see Table 5.3)

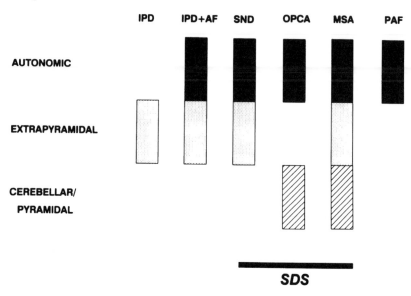

Figure 5.1 Schematic representation indicating the major clinical features in primary auto-nomic failure (AF). In pure autonomic failure (PAF), there are no other neurological signs, unlike the other groups: IPD, idiopathic Parkinson's disease; SND, striatonigral degenera-tion; OPCA, olivopontocerebellar atrophy; MSA, multiple system atrophy. The Shy–Drager syndrome includes the SND, OPCA and MSA forms. (Adapted from Mathias and Williams, 1994.)

of symptoms of cerebral ischaemia, including syncope, associated with head-up postural change, favours postural hypotension which will need appropriate inves-tigation. In carotid sinus hypersensitivity, the history may be crucial in deciding on specific testing, such as carotid sinus massage, as routine autonomic function testing between attacks is usually normal. Patients may present with one or a variety of symptoms, as outlined in Table 5.4. A history of consanguinity (as in familial dysautonomias, such as the Riley–Day syndrome), or a family history (as in familial amyloid polyneuropathy) is of importance. A detailed drug his-tory is particularly valuable; drugs such as L-dopa may enhance or unmask postural hypotension, or may cause an autonomic neuropathy, as with perhexi-lene mealeate. The clinical examination and basic bedside tests may provide clues to the diagnosis. The presence of a peripheral neuropathy, postural hypo-tension and proteinuria, when present with glycosuria will indicate diabetes mellitus, but without glycosuria will warrant exclusion of systemic amyloidosis.

In investigating a possible autonomic neuropathy it is initially necessary to deter-mine if autonomic function is normal or abnormal. Autonomic screening tests are mainly directed towards cardiovascular assessment and form a useful first step. As they are usually normal between attacks in neurally mediated syncope, a detailed history is needed for specific targeting. In autonomic neuropathies affecting systems other than the circulation, such as the urinary bladder or bowel, additional testing will be needed (Table 5.5). If the tests indicate that autonomic function is abnormal, it is then important to determine the degree of dysfunction, the site of the lesion, and

Table 5.3 Drugs, chemicals, heavy metals and toxins which cause or may contribute to peripheral autonomic dysfunction*

Decreasing sympathetic activity
  Sympathetic neuron (guanethidine, bethanadine)
  α-adrenoceptor blockade (phenoxybenzamine, prazosin)
  β-adrenoceptor blockade (propranolol, timolol)

Increasing sympathetic activity
  Releasing noradrenaline (tyramine)
  Monoamine oxidase inhibitors (tranylcypromine)
  β-adrenoceptor stimulants (isoprenaline)

Decreasing parasympathetic activity
  Antidysrhythmics (disopyramide)
  Anticholinergics (atropine, probanthine)
  Toxins (botulinum)

Increasing parasympathetic activity
  Cholinomimetics (carbachol, bethanechol, pilocarpine, mushroom poisoning)
  Anticholinesterases
    Reversible inhibitors (pyridostigmine, neostigmine)
    Organophosphorus inhibitors (parathion)

Miscellaneous
  Alcohol, thiamine (vitamin B_1) deficiency
  Vincristine
  Perhexilene maleate
  Thallium, arsenic, mercury
  Cyclosporin

---

*Adapted from Mathias (1991).

whether the disorder is of the primary or secondary variety. This may entail a range of additional tests (from neuroimaging and electrophysiological   studies to sural nerve biopsy and genetic typing) designed to exclude or confirm the underlying disorder. These are helpful for predicting outcome and prognosis, which vary in the different disorders. They are necessary in evolving appropriate management strategies, which should encompass complications resulting from the autonomic deficits and also the other systems affected by the primary disorder.

The clinical manifestations, investigations and management of abnormalities affecting major systems in autonomic neuropathies will now be considered. Although this will deal mainly with peripheral disorders, there will be reference to central disorders from which they need to be distinguished. High spinal cord lesions cause substantial peripheral dysfunction, and will also be briefly discussed.

Cardiovascular

A major problem is postural hypotension. Supine hypertension, lability of blood pressure with paroxysmal hypertension, bradycardia and tachycardia may occur as a result of autonomic dysfunction.

Table 5.4 Some clinical manifestations of autonomic dysfunction

---

Cardiovascular
  Postural hypotension
  Supine hypertension
  Lability of blood pressure
  Paroxysmal hypertension
  Tachycardia
  Bradycardia

Sudomotor
  Hypo- or anhidrosis
  Hypohidrosis
  Localized sweating abnormalities – gustatory sweating

Alimentary
  Xerostomia
  Dysphagia
  Gastric stasis
  Dumping syndromes
  Constipation
  Diarrhoea

Urinary
  Nocturia
  Frequency, urgency, retention, incontinence

Sexual
  Erectile failure
  Ejaculatory failure
  Retrograde ejaculation

Eye
  Pupillary abnormalities
  Ptosis
  Alacrima
  Excessive lacrimation

Hypotension

Postural hypotension is one of the cardinal features of autonomic failure. It is arbitrarily defined as a fall in systolic blood pressure of 20 mmHg or more, with or without symptoms. The symptoms accompanying postural hypotension vary considerably, as indicated in Table 5.6. Some are readily recognized, such as those resulting from cerebral ischaemia (Table 5.7). Others recently added to the symptom list include suboccipital, neck and shoulder pain (in the 'coathanger' region) which is common in primary autonomic failure with severe postural hypotension (Bleasdale-Barr and Mathias, 1994). There may be a dissociation between symptoms of postural hypotension and the blood pressure fall. In some instances this may be due to an increased ability of the cerebral circulation to cope with a low pressure. In others, such as in patients with familial amyloid neuropathy in whom there may be few symptoms, the reasons are unclear and include a gradual onset and their younger age (Mathias *et al.*, 1994). A large number of factors can influence postural hypotension

Table 5.5 Outline of investigations in autonomic failure*

Cardiovascular physiological
    Head-up tilt (45°); standing; Valsalva manoeuvre
    Pressor stimuli – isometric exercise, cutaneous cooling, mental arithmetic
    Heart rate responses – deep breathing, hyperventilation, standing, head-up tilt, 30:15 ratio
    Carotid sinus massage
    Liquid meal challenge
    Exercise testing

Biochemical
    Plasma noradrenaline – supine and standing; urinary catecholamines; plasma renin activity and
       aldosterone

Pharmacological
    Noradrenaline – α-adrenoceptors – vascular
    Isoprenaline – β-adrenoceptors – vascular and cardiac
    Tyramine – pressor and noradrenaline response
    Edrophonium – noradrenaline response
    Clonidine – growth hormone response
    Atropine – heart rate response

Sweating
    Central regulation – increase core temperature by 1°C
    Sweat gland response to intradermal acetyl choline

Gastrointestinal
    Barium studies, videocinefluoroscopy, endoscopy, gastric-emptying studies

Renal function and urinary tract
    Day and night urine volumes and sodium/potassium excretion
    Urodynamic studies, intravenous urography, ultrasound examination, urethral sphincter
    electromyography

Sexual function
    Penile plethysmography
    Intracavernosal papaverine

Respiratory
    Laryngoscopy
    Sleep studies to assess apnoea/oxygen desaturation

Eye
    Schirmer's test
    Pupillary function – pharmacological and physiological

---

*From Mathias and Bannister (1992b).

Table 5.6   Some of the symptoms resulting from postural hypotension

---

Non-specific – weakness, lethargy
Cerebral ischaemia
Paracervical and suboccipital ('coathanger') ache
Chest discomfort – angina pectoris
Lower back/buttock ache
Spinal cord ischaemia
Calf claudication

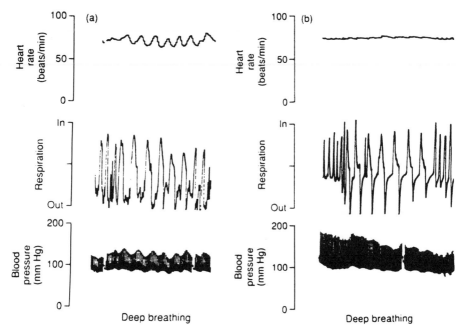

Figure 5.2 The effect of deep breathing on heart rate and blood pressure in (a) a normal subject and (b) a patient with autonomic failure. There is no sinus arrhythmia in the patient, despite a fall in blood pressure. Respiratory changes are indicated in the middle panel. (From Mathias and Bannister, 1992b.)

Table 5.7   Some of the key symptoms resulting from cerebral ischaemia

Dizziness
Visual disturbances
  Blurred vision
  Tunnel vision
  Scotoma
  Greying out
  Blacking out
  Colour defects
Loss of consciousness

(Table 5.8). A postural fall in blood pressure of less than 20 mmHg, but with an appropriate history, warrants investigation.

The investigation of postural hypotension provides the basis for determining the integrity of various autonomic reflexes and the function of efferent sympathetic and parasympathetic pathways. An outline is provided in Table 5.5. Technological advances enable these tests to be performed non-invasively, with measurement of beat-by-beat blood pressure and heart rate. A key component is determining postural hypotension in response to passive change with head up tilt, and/or with standing. The Valsalva manoeuvre provides a measure of overall baroreceptor function. The various pressor tests are dependent upon peripheral or central activation,

Table 5.8   Factors influencing postural hypotension

Speed of positional change
Time of day (worse in morning)
Prolonged recumbency
Warm environment (hot weather, central heating, hot bath)
Raising intrathoracic pressure – micturition, defaecation or coughing
Food and alcohol ingestion
Physical exertion
Physical manoeuvres and positions (bending forward, abdominal compression, leg crossing, squatting
  activating calf muscle pump)*
Drugs with vasoactive properties (including dopaminergic agents)

*These manoeuvres usually reduce the postural fall in blood pressure, unlike the others.

the common pathway being the sympathetic efferent outflow. The heart rate responses to postural change, the Valsalva manoeuvre, deep breathing (Figure 5.2), and hyperventilation provide an indication of cardiac parasympathetic activity.

Additional tests to determine the responses to food ingestion and exercise, while supine and during head-up postural change, may be needed (Mathias *et al.*, 1991; Smith *et al.*, 1993) (Figures 5.3 and 5.4). Twenty-four hour ambulatory non-invasive blood pressure monitoring (Figure 5.5) is of value in determining the blood pressure and heart rate responses to a variety of factors. These include assessing postural responses at different times of the day (as hypotension is often worse in the morning), and after food ingestion and exercise, two key factors which exacerbate postural hypotension.

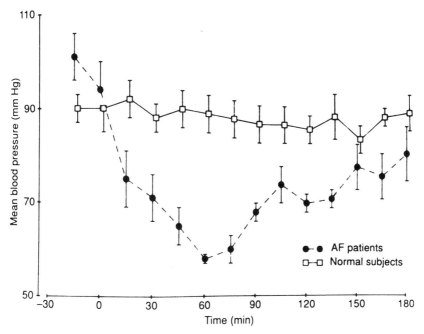

Figure 5.3 Percentage change in mean blood pressure in a group of patients with chronic autonomic failure (- - -, ●) and in normal subjects (—, □) before and after food ingestion at times 0. The bars indicate means ± SEM. (From Mathias *et al.*, 1989a.)

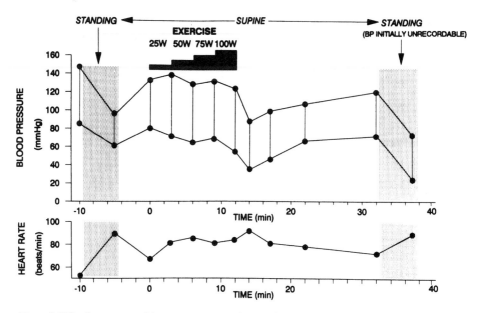

Figure 5.4 Blood pressure and heart rate response in a patient with primary autonomic failure before exercise, during exercise (supine) and post exercise. Standing after exercises causes a marked increase in postural hypotension. (From Smith *et al.*, 1993).

Plasma noradrenaline levels are useful in confirming a neurogenic cause for postural hypotension. Either minimal or no change in plasma noradrenaline levels with head-up postural change, provides biochemical evidence of sympathetic failure (Figure 5.6). Non-neurogenic causes of postural hypotension (Table 5.9) may need to be considered.

Plasma catecholamine measurement may differentiate the central Shy–Drager syndrome from peripheral disorders such as PAF; they also may diagnose DBH deficiency (Figure 5.6). Basal levels in the Shy–Drager syndromes are often similar to normal levels, while in PAF levels are considerably lower than normal. In DBH deficiency, plasma noradrenaline and adrenaline are undetectable, while plasma dopamine is abnormally elevated (Robertson *et al.*, 1986; Man In't Veld *et al.*, 1987; Mathias *et al.*, 1990). In the nerve growth factor (NGF) deficiency syndrome, which includes absence of DBH, there are similar biochemical changes to isolated DBH deficiency except that plasma dopamine levels are low, suggesting tyrosine hydroxylase deficiency (Mathias *et al.*, 1990).

Special tests may be needed to confirm some of the rarer catecholamine disorders. In DBH deficiency, plasma DBH activity is undetectable. Electron microscopy and immunohistochemical studies of skin and axillary gland biopsies are normal, except for absent DBH immunoreactivity (Mathias *et al.*, 1990). Low tissue nerve growth factor levels provide an explanation for why there is depletion of sensory neuropeptides (substance P and CGRP), in addition to absent tyrosine hydroxylase and DBH in NGF deficiency (Anand *et al.*, 1991).

Pharmacological testing may be needed in certain situations. An example is cholinergic muscarinic blockade with atropine to define cardiac parasympathetic involvement. Physiological testing of these pathways often provides the answers, but is dependent on subject cooperation. Atropine testing is useful when subjects are

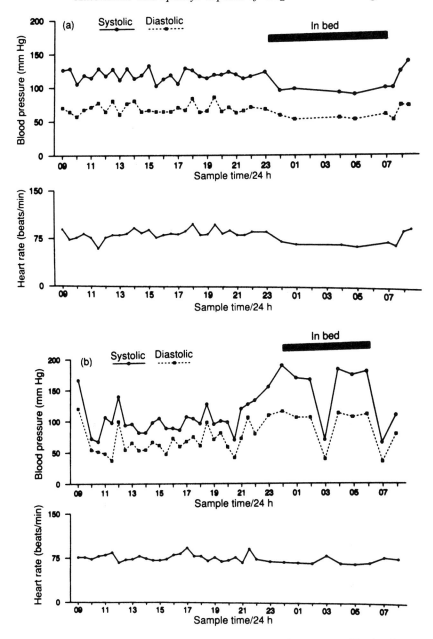

Figure 5.5 Twenty-four-hour non-invasive ambulatory blood pressure profile, showing systolic (—●—) and diastolic (- -■- -) blood pressure and heart rate at intervals through the day and night. (a) The changes in a normal subject with no postural fall in blood pressure; there was a fall in blood pressure at night while asleep with a rise in blood pressure on wakening. (b) The marked fluctuations in blood pressure in a patient with pure autonomic failure. The marked falls in blood pressure are usually the result of postural changes, either sitting or standing. Supine blood pressure, particularly at night is elevated. Getting up to micturate causes a marked fall in blood pressure (at 03:00 h). There is a reversal of the diurnal changes in blood pressure. There are relatively small changes in heart rate, considering the marked changes in blood pressure. (From Mathias and Bannister, 1992b).

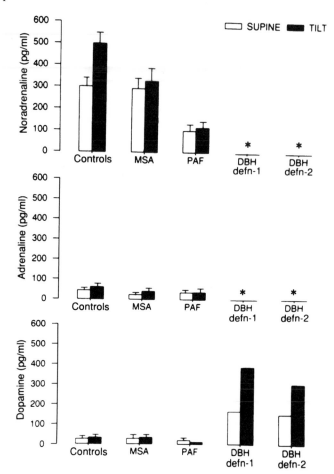

Figure 5.6 Plasma noradrenaline, adrenaline, and dopamine levels (measured by high-pressure liquid chromatography) in normal subjects (controls), patients with multiple system atrophy (MSA), pure autonomic failure (PAF), and two individual patients with dopamine β-hydroxylase (DBH defn 1 and 2) deficiency while supine and after head-up tilt to 45° for 10 min. The asterisk indicates levels below the detection limits for the assay, which are less than 5 pg/ml for noradrenaline and adrenaline and less than 20 pg/ml for dopamine. Bars indicate ± SEM. (From Mathias and Bannister, 1992b).

unconscious, or on a ventilator. Adrenoreceptor agonists, such as noradrenaline, may be needed to determine the presence of cardiovascular supersensitivity or subsensitivity; the former is present in PAF and the latter if there is amyloid infiltration of heart and blood vessels. The clonidine–growth hormone test is a promising means of separating central from peripheral autonomic failure syndromes, which can be especially difficult in the early stages (Thomaides *et al.*, 1992) (Figure 5.7). Growth hormone levels rise in normal subjects and PAF patients with peripheral involvement, but not in those with central impairment accompanying the Shy–Drager

Table 5.9   Non-neurogenic causes of postural hypotension

Low intravascular volume	
Blood/plasma loss	Haemorrhage, burns, haemodialysis
Fluid/electrolyte	Inadequate intake – anorexia nervosa, fluid loss, vomiting
	Diarrhoea – including losses from ileostomy
	Renal/endocrine – salt-losing nephropathy, adrenal insufficiency (Addison's disease), diabetes insipidus, diuretics
Vasodilatation	Drugs – glyceryl trinitrate
	Alcohol
	Heat, hyperpyrexia
	Hyperbradykinism
	Extensive varicose veins
Cardiac impairment	
Myocardial	Myocarditis
Impaired ventricular filling	Artrial myxoma, constrictive pericarditis
Impaired output	Aortic stenosis

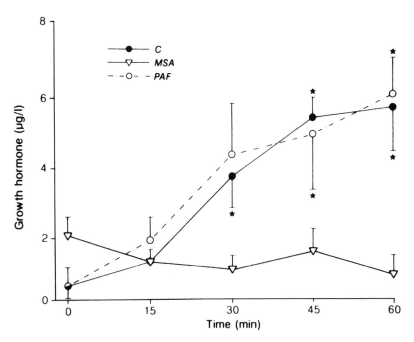

Figure 5.7 Plasma growth hormone concentrations before (0) and 15, 30 45 and 60 min after clonidine in normal subjects (controls, C) and patients with Shy–Drager syndrome/multisystem atrophy (MSA) or pure autonomic failure (PAF). The error bars indicate SEM. *P < 0.05. (From Thomaides *et al.*, 1992.)

syndrome. In amyloidosis, deposition of amyloid in the adrenal gland may cause adrenocortical deficiency which will need to be excluded by a synacthen test.

The management of postural hypotension includes a combination of non-pharmacological and pharmacological approaches (Mathias and Bannister, 1992c) which ideally should be tailored individually (Table 5.10). Some of the former are directly related to the various factors, listed in Table 5.8, which influence postural hypotension. Advice about physical counter-measures which increase muscle activity (such as crossing the legs or tensing calf muscles) often helps to reduce symptoms (Wieling *et al.*, 1992). Head-up tilt at night, if tolerated, can improve postural hypotension and reduce supine hypertension, if present. Smaller and more frequent meals should be taken. Salt intake should be increased. Physical methods may either not work adequately or, as is the case with G-suits, be effective only when in operation. They

Table 5.10 Non-pharmacological and pharmacological approaches to management of postural hypotension

---

Non-pharmacological
  Avoid
    Sudden head-up postural change, especially in the morning
    Straining during micturition and defaecation
    High environmental temperature
    Severe exertion
    Large meals, especially with carbohydrate and fat
    Alcohol
    Drugs with vasodepressor properties
  Use
    Head-up tilt nocturnally
    Small frequent meals
    High salt intake
  Physical counter-measures
    Elastic stockings
    Abdominal binders
    Anti-gravity suits

Pharmacological
  Reducing salt loss/plasma volume expansion
    Mineralocorticoids (fludrocortisone)
  Vasoconstriction – sympathomimetics
    Direct
      Resistance vessels (midodrine, phenylephrine)
      Capitance vessels (dihydroergotamine)
    Indirect   (ephedrine, tyramine, monoamine oxidase inhibitors, yohimbine)
  Preventing vasodilatation
    Prostaglandin synthetase inhibitors (indomethacin, flurbiprofen)
    Dopamine receptor blockade (metoclopropamide, domperidone)
    Beta-2 adrenoceptor blockade (propranolol)
  Preventing postprandial hypotension
    Adenosine receptor blockade (caffeine)
    Peptide release inhibitors (somatostatin analogue, octreotide)
  Increasing cardiac output (pindolol, xamoterol)
  Increasing red cell mass and oxygen capacity (erythropoetin)
  Reducing nocturnal polyuria
    V2 receptor agonists (desmopressin)

---

usually make the subject more susceptible to symptoms when not in use. Supplementation of non-pharmacological approaches with drugs is often needed (Mathias and Bannister, 1992c). The drugs are directed towards increasing plasma volume (fludrocortisone), causing vasoconstriction (the sympathomimetic agents ephedrine and midodrine) and preventing vasodilatation (the peptide release inhibitor octreotide). In DBH deficiency, specific targeting with the drug L-dihydroxyphenylserine (L-dops), bypasses the enzyme deficiency, results in the formation of noradrenaline and is highly successful in reducing symptoms and signs of postural hypotension (Mathias and Bannister, 1992a). L-dops has been used successfully in familial amyloid polyneuropathy.

Hypertension

Supine hypertension often accompanies severe postural hypotension. It can be a problem at night, especially in subjects on pressor agents. It may result from a variety of factors which include fluid shifts from the extravascular to the intravascular, and peripheral to central, compartments while lying flat, the inability of baroreflexes to control blood pressure, and the additional effects of pressor supersensitivity to therapeutic agents. Supine hypertension is best managed by head-up-tilt and reduction of the evening dose of pressor agents. Occasionally, antihypertensive agents may be needed at night.

Marked lability of blood pressure, including severe hypertension, may occur in the Guillain–Barré syndrome. The mechanisms include an afferent baroreceptor lesion contributing to uncontrolled sympathetic discharge (Fagius and Wallin, 1983). In high spinal cord lesions, paroxysmal hypertension may occur as part of autonomic dysreflexia, which is a response to afferent stimulation involving the skin, viscera or skeletal muscles. Stimulation initiates a spinal reflex with an increase in sympathetic efferent activity, not inhibited by cerebral pathways, as would occur normally (Mathias and Frankel, 1992). Other factors, including adrenoreceptor supersensitivity may contribute. In the Guillain-Barré syndrome hypertension control may need α-adrenoreceptor blocking drugs; β-adrenoreceptor blockers often are also needed because of tachycardia. The management of paroxysmal hypertension in high spinal cord lesions is dependent upon the initiating cause, which should be rectified. Sympathetic efferent outflow may be reduced by a variety of measures (Table 5.11).

Table 5.11 Some of the drugs used in the management of autonomic dysreflexia in high spinal cord lesions classified according to their major site of action on the reflex arc and target organs

Afferent		
Spinal cord		Topical lignocaine
		Clonidine*
		Reserpine*
		Spinal anaesthetics
Efferent	Sympathetic ganglia	Hexamethonium
	Sympathetic nerve terminals	Guanethidine
	α-adrenoreceptors	Phenoxybenzamine
Target organs	Blood vessels	Glyceryl trinitrate
		Nifedipine
	Sweat glands	Propantheline

*These drugs may have multiple effects.

Tachycardia

This may be a problem in disorders such as the Guillain–Barré syndrome, and may necessitate the use of β-adrenoreceptor blockers. A high heart rate (over 100 beats/ min), which remains unchanged ('fixed') in response to various stimuli, may occur in diabetes mellitus and amyloidosis, and is indicative of cardiac parasympathetic failure. This often precedes sympathetic impairment.

Bradycardia

A resting bradycardia is unusual in autonomic neuropathies, especially if there is both sympathetic and parasympathetic failure. In DBH deficiency, with cardiac parasympathetic sparing, the basal heart rate may be low.

Bradycardia in response to specific stimuli, however, occurs in carotid sinus hypersensitivity and swallow syncope. It is a key feature of vasovagal syncope. Carotid sinus massage may induce an attack if there is hypersensitivity, which is now recognized as a factor in the elderly with otherwise unexplained syncope. In carotid sinus hypersensitivity there is often a cardioinhibitory component, caused by increased vagal activity; atropine or cardiac pacing prevents the bradycardia, but may not prevent the fall in blood pressure. The vasodepressor component appears to be due to withdrawal of sympathetic activity; the precise reasons for withdrawal remain unclear (Smith *et al.*, 1992). Similar changes may occur during syncope caused by swallowing and accompanying glossopharyngeal neuralgia (Figure 5.8) (Wallin *et al.*, 1984). The vasodepressor component may not occur with the subject supine and may only occur during head-up tilt or standing, when there is maximal need for

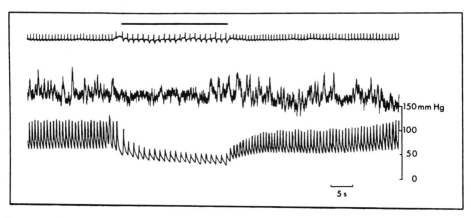

Figure 5.8 The electrocardiogram (upper trace), muscle sympathetic activity (as mean voltage neurograms middle trace) and intra-arterial blood pressure (lower trace), before, during and after an attack of glossopharyngeal neuralgia associated with syncope. Attacks occurred when the patient coughed or yawned, but at times were observed without a triggering event. The horizontal bar indicates when the cardiac pacemaker was activated; despite this the blood pressure fell and sympathetic bursts were considerably reduced. Termination of syncope occurred spontaneously, with an increase in sympathetic activity, restoration of endogenous heart rate and a gradual return of blood pressure to original levels. (From Wallin *et al.*, 1984.)

sympathoneural activation to maintain blood pressure (Mathias *et al.*, 1992). Testing in carotid sinus hypersensitivity and swallow syncope, therefore, ideally should include responses also while tilted. In vasovagal syncope a variety of methods to induced syncope have been used; these include prolonged head-up tilt, isoprenaline infusion and combined tilt and lower body negative pressure (El-Badawi and Hainsworth, 1994). Whether any of these stimuli are related to the initiating cause is uncertain.

Demand cardiac pacemakers may be of value in syncope associated with a prominent cardioinhibitory component. The management of the vasodepressor component in carotid sinus hypersensitivity and in vasovagal syncope remains unsatisfactory and a variety of vasopressor agents, of doubtful benefit, have been used. In carotid sinus hypersensitivity, denervation of the relevant carotid sinus may be an effective means of preventing syncope, especially in the unilateral form. Glossopharyngeal nerve section may be needed in glossopharyngeal neuralgia. Severe bradycardia and cardiac arrest may occur in high cervical spinal cord lesions needing artificial ventilation, especially during tracheal suction-induced hypoxia. Afferent stimuli from the trachea increase vagal activity, which is enhanced because of hypoxia, lack of opposing sympathetic activity and the inability to respire. The management consists of adequate oxygenation; prophylactic atropine or a demand cardiac pacemaker are used if necessary (Mathias and Frankel, 1992).

Sudomotor system

Hypo/anhidrosis

The eccrine sweat glands are supplied by sympathetic cholinergic fibres and may be severely affected in generalized autonomic neuropathies, such as pure autonomic failure. In hot climates, this causes heat intolerance, which in combination with cutaneous vasodilatation may result in severe hypotension and collapse. Segmental areas of anhidrosis may accompany the Holmes–Adie syndrome, as described in Ross' syndrome (Ross, 1958; Weller *et al.*, 1992). Sweating is preserved in DBH and NGF deficiency syndromes, which spare cholinergic function. The thermoregulatory control of sudomotor function can be tested by determining the sweat responses (using quinazarin dye) to a 1°C elevation in body temperature (Low and Fealey, 1992). Regional abnormalities of sweating can be further determined with locally iontophoresed acetyl choline, as in the quantitative sudomotor axon reflex test. The acetyl choline spot test or quinazarin tape test are useful to assess impairment in smaller areas, as occurs in leprosy.

There is no specific treatment for anhidrosis. Avoiding warm environmental temperatures and the use of cold drinks and adequate hydration is needed.

Hyperhidrosis

Occasionally hyperhidrosis may be the initial symptom in an autonomic neuropathy, with later progression to anhidrosis. The hyperhidrosis may be compensatory, because of impaired sweating in other parts, although it may reflect a form of supersensitivity in partially denervated areas.

In palmar or more generalized hyperhidrosis there may be no specific cause found, assuming thyrotoxicosis and rare disorders such as phaeochromocytoma have been excluded. In some of these cases it may be difficult to determine if psychological abnormalities, including stress/anxiety cause hyperhidrosis. There is increasing use of minimally invasive procedures such as endoscopic transthoracic sympathectomy, which is highly successful in reducing sweating over the palms and arms. The operation, however, can be complicated by excessive sweating over the trunk and lower limbs (Masters and Rennie, 1992); this is presumably a form of compensatory hyperhidrosis, although the reasons for this are unclear.

The management of hyperhidrosis includes the use of local antiperspirants, and systemic agents to reduce sweating. Anticholinergic drugs such as propantheline may be effective, but have side effects which include a dry mouth and blurred vision. Centrally acting sympatholytic agents, such as clonidine, are sometimes beneficial. As indicated above, surgical sympathectomy may be effective, but there may be troublesome complications.

Localized paroxysmal sweating can be a particular problem. An example is gustatory sweating with abnormally profuse sweating over the head, face and neck. This can occur after bland food and sometimes even be caused by the thought of food. It results from aberrant connections between cholinergic fibres from the vagus and/or efferent (glossopharyngeal) supply to the salivary glands, with sympathetic cholinergic efferent pathways supplying facial sweat glands (Thomas and Mathias, 1993). It may occur in the recovery phase after an acute autonomic neuropathy, as a complication in diabetes mellitus, following surgery to the parotid gland (Frey's syndrome) or after operations at the root of the neck which involve the vagus nerve and upper sympathetic outflow. The management includes the use of anticholinergic agents such as propantheline. Surgical section of the sympathetic supply, auriculotemporal nerve, or tympanic branch of the glossopharyngeal nerve may be needed in extreme cases.

Alimentary tract

The salivary glands and gut are richly supplied by the autonomic nervous system, and involvement at different levels may occur in the various autonomic neuropathies.

Hyposalivation or xerostomia is a prominent feature in acute cholinergic dysautonomia and causes difficulty in chewing and swallowing food. The functional ability of salivary glands can be tested with the cholinomimetic bethanecol, which should induce salivation. In chronic neuropathies, xerostomia may result from gland involvement and salivary gland biopsy may show inflammatory changes in Sjögren's syndrome or amyloid infiltration in amyloidosis. Artificial saliva is of benefit.

In acute cholinergic dysautonomia, a prominent feature may be dysphagia due to dilatation and stasis of the lower third of oesophagus. This does not occur in PAF. In Chagas' disease, the oesophagus and colon are targeted, with involvement of the intrinsic plexuses (Auerbach's and Meissner's); this results in megaoesophagus and megacolon (Fernandez et al., 1992). Investigation may include radiological studies and also manometry, especially to determine cholinergic postsynaptic receptor sensitivity in response to cholinomimetic agents such as bethanecol.

There are two major dumping syndromes, which result from a combination of surgical vagotomy and a drainage procedure, such as a gastrojejunostomy (Roberts *et al.*, 1954; Le Quesne *et al.*, 1960). In the early dumping syndrome, systemic manifestations include dizziness, tachycardia and excessive perspiration within a short period after ingestion of food, especially with a high carbohydrate content. The presence of an hyperosmotic load in the jejunum results in fluid absorption, reduction in intravascular volume and a compensatory sympathetic response which accounts for the manifestations. In the late dumping syndrome, which is associated with excessive insulin release, a variety of features secondary to hypoglycaemia may occur. Management includes small meals with a low refined carbohydrate content. Abnormal release of enteric peptides may contribute to the syndrome and some are helped by the somatostatin analogue octreotide, which inhibits peptide release (Long *et al.*, 1985). In diabetes mellitus, gastric stasis (gastroparesis diabeticorum) may be a troublesome problem; it appears to be secondary to vagal or enteric neural damage (Guy *et al.*, 1984) and may respond to macrolides such as erythromycin which act on motilin receptors to increase gastric motility (Janssens *et al.*, 1990).

In the early stages after high spinal cord injury there is often increased vagal activity which may be secondary to absent spinal and thus peripheral sympathetic activity. This may contribute to the high incidence of peptic ulceration and upper gastrointestinal bleeding, which can be prevented by the prophylactic use of H2 antagonists and allied agents.

Constipation is common in many of the chronic autonomic neuropathies, such as PAF and amyloidosis. Occasionally diarrhoea may occur. Symptomatic management of constipation should follow standard guidelines. Diarrhoea, sometimes nocturnal, may be extremely troublesome in autonomic neuropathy complicating diabetes mellitus. It may be associated with a combination of factors which include pancreatic exocrine deficiency, deranged motility secondary to abnormalities in enteric peptide release and bacterial overgrowth. The management includes a trial of antibiotics (such as tetracycline or metronidazole), the somatostatin analogue octreotide, and the opiates loperamide and codeine phosphate.

An exaggerated gastrocolic reflex and diarrhoea may occur when there is isolated sympathetic failure, presumably because of a relative increase in parasympathetic activity (Cortelli *et al.*, 1992). Unexplained diarrhoea in HIV infection may be associated with increased parasympathetic activity and may respond to anticholinergic agents (Coker *et al.*, 1992).

Urinary system

Nocturia is common when postural hypotension is a prominent feature of an autonomic neuropathy, as in PAF and amyloidosis. It is mainly related to recumbency rather than to abnormal circadian rhythms (Kooner *et al.*, 1987). It is probably the result of relocation of fluid from the periphery into the central compartment. Other factors may include excessive atrial natriuretic peptide release and the inability of sympathetically denervated tubules to re-absorb sodium. The combination of nocturia and impaired urinary bladder function, can cause considerable disability. Measurement of day and night urine output is a useful way to assess the problem and determine the response to therapy. Desmopressin, a vasopressin analogue with predominantly V2 agonist effects on the renal tubules is effective in reducing overnight urine secretion (Mathias *et al.*, 1986). Care should be taken to ensure that hyponatraemia does not occur.

In the cholinergic dysautonomias, urinary bladder atony often occurs because of paralysis of the detrusor muscle. In PAF there is less urinary bladder involvement than in central autonomic syndromes such as the Shy–Drager syndrome, where frequency and urge incontinence is common; in this situation the lesion appears to be mainly in Onufs' nucleus within sacral neurons, and can be detected by urethral sphincter electromyography, which shows a characteristic pattern of denervation and reinnervation (Kirby *et al.*, 1986). A variety of abnormalities may occur in diabetes mellitus (Beck *et al.*, 1994).

The investigations include urodynamic studies, and if necessary urethral and/or anal sphincter electromyography to exclude sacral neuronal involvement. Management depends upon the disability. In detrusor instability and overactivity, anticholinergics such as oxybutynin are of value, while in sphincter overactivity, α-adrenoreceptor blockers are helpful. Intermittent self-catheterization, an indwelling urethral or suprapubic catheter, or other urological procedures may be needed.

Sexual function

In males, both erectile and ejaculatory failure may occur. Erection is dependent largely on the parasympathetic nerve supply in addition to other substances, such as the autocoid nitric oxide. Ejaculation appears dependent on sympathetic pathways. Retrograde ejaculation may occur if there is an abnormal urethral sphincter and following sphincterotomy. In PAF there is both erectile and ejaculatory failure. In DBH deficiency, however, erection is preserved but ejaculation is difficult to achieve; the replacement drug, L-dops, which elevates noradrenaline levels, improves ejaculatory ability (Man In't Veld *et al.*, 1987). A number of additional factors, which include psychogenic and local vascular factors, could contribute to erectile and ejaculatory failure, especially in diabetes mellitus.

A variety of approaches can be used in management (Beck *et al.*, 1994). Penile prostheses may help in erectile failure, if mechanical aids such as a suction pump have failed. The intracavernosal injection of substances such as papaverine and prostaglandins have a limited role.

In females, sexual and reproductive function does not appear to be directly affected.

The eye

A variety of pupillary abnormalities may occur, but there are few, if any, symptoms. In Horner's syndrome miosis is accompanied by mild ptosis, facial vasodilatation and lack of sweating. In the Holmes–Adie syndrome there is a dilated, myotonic pupil with tendon areflexia. Symptoms may arise when cholinergic blockade (as part of a cholinergic dysautonomia or after drugs such as atropine) cause dilated pupils and ciliary muscle paresis. The former diminishes the ability to cope with bright light and the latter causes blurred vision. Intraocular pressure may rise, especially in those prone to glaucoma.

Pupillary abnormalities may be investigated using pharmacological or physiological tests (Smith, 1992). The former utilize local ocular instillation of drugs and are designed to determine supersensitivity or subsensitivity. The physiological tests assess the functional ability of the pupil in different circumstances. These help determine the pathway involved and the site of the lesion. Specific treatment of pupillary abnormalities usually is not needed. In severe cholinergic dysautonomia cholinomimetic drops (such as pilocarpine) reduce light sensitivity and blurring of vision.

Alacrima is a feature of acute cholingeric dysautonomias. Hypolacrima may occur in some chronic autonomic neuropathies. In amyloidosis, gland infiltration may be contributory. The lack of tears results in dry eyes with irritation and infection. Lacrimal gland secretion can be assessed with Schirmer's test. Artificial tears, such as hypromellose drops, are necessary to prevent ocular complications.

Excessive lacrimal secretion during chewing food and stimuli which cause salivation occurs in the syndrome of crocodile tears (paroxysmal lacrimation, Bogorad's syndrome). It results from aberrant connections between the cholinergic nerve supply to the salivary and lacrimal glands. It can follow surgery or injury to the nerve supply to the parotid gland and occasionally complicates a lower motor neuron facial palsy with lesions proximal to the geniculate ganglion where the various nerves travel together (Thomas and Mathias, 1993). Management consists of division of the glossopharyngeal nerve supply to the parotid gland, although part removal of the lacrimal gland may help.

ACKNOWLEDGEMENTS

I would like to acknowledge the support of the Wellcome Trust and the assistance of Mrs Corinne Docherty.

REFERENCES

Anand, P., Rudge, P., Mathias, C. J. *et al.* (1991). New autonomic and sensory neuropathy with loss of adrenergic sympathetic function and sensory neuropeptides. *Lancet*, **337**, 1253–1254

Bannister, R. and Mathias, C. J. (1992). Clinical features and investigations of primary autonomic failure syndromes. In *Autonomic Failure. A Textbook of Clinical Disorders of the Autonomic Nervous System*, 3rd edn (R. Bannister and C. J. Mathias, eds), pp. 531–547, Oxford: Oxford University Press

Beck, R. O., Fowler, C. J. and Mathias, C. J. (1994). Genitourinary dysfunction in disorders of the autonomic nervous system. In *Handbook of Neuro-Urology* (D. Rushton, ed.), pp. 281–301, New York: Marcel-Dekker

Bleasdale-Barr, K. and Mathias, C. J. (1994). Suboccipital (coathanger) and other muscular pains – frequency in autonomic failure and other neurological problems, in association with postural hypotension. *Clin. Autonom. Res.*, **4**, 82

Coker, R. J., Horner, P., Bleasdale-Barr, K. *et al.* (1992). Increased gut parasympathetic activity and chronic diarrhoea in a patient with the acquired immunodeficiency syndrome. *Clin. Autonom. Res.*, **2**, 295–298

Cortelli, P., Parchi, P., Contin, M. *et al.* (1992). Isolated failure of noradrenergic transmission in a case with orthostatic hypotension and hyperactivity of gastrocolic reflex. *Clin. Autonom. Res.*, **2**, 177–182

El-Badawi, K. M. and Hainsworth, R. (1994). Combined head-up tilt and low body suction: a test of orthostatic tolerance. *Clin. Autonom. Res.*, **4**, 41–48

Fagius, J. G. and Wallin, B. G. (1983). Microneurographic evidence of excessive sympathetic outflow in the Guillain–Barré syndrome. *Brain*, **106**, 589–600

Fernandez, A., Hontebeyrie, M. and Said, G. (1992). Autonomic neuropathy and immunological abnormalities in Chagas' disease. *Clin. Autonom. Res.*, **2**, 409–414

Guy, R. J. C., Dawson, J. L., Garret, J. R. *et al.* (1984). Diabetic gastroparesis from autonomic neuropathy: surgical considerations and changes in vagus nerve morphology. *J. Neurol. Neurosurg. Psychiatry*, **47**, 686–691

Janssens, J., Pectens, T. L., Van-Trappen, G. *et al.* (1990). Improvement of gastric emptying in diabetic gastroparesis by erythromycin. *N. Engl. J. Med.*, **322**, 1028–1031

Kirby, R. S., Fowler, C. J., Gosling, J. *et al.* (1986). Urethro-vesical dysfunction in progressive autonomic failure with multiple system atrophy. *J. Neurol. Neurosurg. Psychiatry*, **49**, 554–562

Kooner, J. S., Da Costa, D. F., Frankel, H. L. *et al.* (1987). Recumbency induces hypertension, diuresis and natriuresis in autonomic failure following renal angioplasty in a patient with one functioning kidney. *Br. Med. J.*, **295**, 527–528

Le Quesne, L. P., Hobsley, M. and Hand, B. A. (1960). The dumping syndrome. *Br. Med. J.*, **1**, 141–151

Long, R. G., Adrian, T. E. and Bloom, S. R. (1985). Somatosatin and the dumping syndrome. *Br. Med. J.*, **290**, 886–888

Low, P. A. and Fealey R. D. (1992). Testing of sweating. In *Autonomic Failure. A Textbook of Clinical Disorders of the Autonomic Nervous System*, 3rd edn (R. Bannister and C. J. Mathias, eds), pp. 413–420, Oxford: Oxford University Press

Man In't Veld, A. J., Boosma, F., Van Den Meiraeker, A. H. *et al.* (1987). Congenital dopamine beta-hydroxylase deficiency. *Lancet*, **2**, 1172–1175

Masters, A. and Rennie, J. A. (1992). Endoscopic transthoracic sympathectomy for idiopathic upper limb hyperhidrosis. *Clin. Autonom. Res.*, **2**, 349–353

Mathias, C. J. (1991). Disorders of the autonomic nervous system. In *Neurology in Clinical Practice*, Vol. II (W. G. Bradley, R. B. Daroff, G. M. Fenichel and C. D. Marsden, eds), pp. 1661–1685, Stoneham, Massachusetts: Butterworths

Mathias, C. J. and Bannister, R. (1992a). Dopamine–beta-hydroxylase deficiency and other genetically determined autonomic disorders. In *Autonomic Failure. A Textbook of Clinical Disorders of the Autonomic Nervous System*, 3rd edn (R. Bannister and C. J. Mathias, eds), pp. 837–879, Oxford: Oxford University Press

Mathias, C. J. and Bannister, R. (1992b). Investigation of autonomic disorders. In *Autonomic Failure. A Textbook of Clinical Disorders of the Autonomic Nervous System*, 3rd edn (R. Bannister and C. J. Mathias, eds), pp. 255–290, Oxford: Oxford University Press

Mathias, C. J. and Bannister, R. (1992c). The management of postural hypotension. In *Autonomic Failure. A Textbook of Clinical Disorders of the Autonomic Nervous System*, 3rd edn (R. Bannister and C. J. Mathias, eds), pp. 622–644, Oxford: Oxford University Press

Mathias, C. J. and Frankel H. L. (1992). The cardiovascular system in tetraplegia and paraplegia. In *Handbook of Clinical Neurology, Vol 61, Spinal Cord Trauma*. (P. J. Vinken, G. W. Bruyn and H. L. Klawans, eds; H. L. Frankel, vol. ed.), pp. 435–456, Amsterdam: Elsevier

Mathias, C. J. and Williams, A. C. (1994). The Shy–Drager syndrome (and multiple system atrophy). In *Neurodegenerative Disorders* (D. Calne, ed.), pp. 743–767, Philadelphia: W. B. Saunders

Mathias, C. J., Armstrong, E., Browse, N. *et al.* (1992). Value of non-invasive continuous blood pressure monitoring in the detection of carotid sinus hypersensitivity. *Clin. Autonom. Res.*, **2**, 157–159

Mathias, C. J., Bannister, R., Cortelli, P. *et al.* (1990). Clinical autonomic and therapeutic observations in two siblings with postural hypotension and sympathetic failure due to an inability to synthesise noradrenaline from dopamine because of a deficiency of dopamine beta hydroxylase. *Q. J. Med.*, **278**, 617–633

Mathias, C. J., Bleasdale-Barr, K., Smith, G. *et al.* (1994). Dissociation between autonomic symptoms and signs in familial amyloid polyneuropathy – the need for cardiovascular autonomic assessment. *J. Neurol.*, **241** (suppl 1), S35–S37

Mathias, C. J., Da Costa, D. F., Fosbraey, P. *et al.* (1989). Cardiovascular, biochemical and hormonal changes during food induced hypotension in chronic autonomic failure. *J. Neurol. Sci.*, **94**, 255–269

Mathias, C. J., Fosbraey, P. Da Costa, D. F., *et al.* (1989). Desmopressin reduces nocturnal polyuria, reverses overnight weight loss and improves morning postural hypotension in autonomic failure. *Br. Med. J.*, **293**, 353–354

Mathias, C. J., Holly, E., Armstrong, E. *et al.* (1991). The influence of food on postural hypotension in three groups with chronic autonomic failure; clinical and therapeutic implications. *J. Neurol. Neurosurg. Psychiatry*, **54**, 726–730

McLeod, J. G. (1992). Autonomic dysfunction in peripheral nerve disease. In *Autonomic Failure. A Textbook of Clinical Disorders of the Autonomic Nervous System*, 3rd edn (R. Bannister and C. J. Mathias, eds), pp. 659–681, Oxford: Oxford University Press

Roberts, K. E., Randall, H. T. and Farr, H. W. (1954). Cardiovascular and blood volume alterations resulting from intrajejunal administration of hypertonic solutions to gastrectomised patients: The relationship of these changes to the dumping syndrome. *Ann. Surg.*, **140**, 631–640

Robertson, D., Goldberg, M. R., Onrot, J. *et al.* (1986). Isolated failure of autonomic noradrenergic transmission; evidence for impaired beta-hydroxylation of dopamine. *N. Engl. J. Med.*, **314**, 1494–1497

Ross, A. T. (1958). Progressive selection sudomotor denervation. A case co-existing with Adie's syndrome. *Neurology*, **8**, 809–817

Smith, S. A. (1992). Pupil function: tests and disorders. In *Autonomic Failure. A Textbook of Clinical Disorders of the Nervous System*, 3rd edn (R. Bannister and C. J. Mathias, eds), pp. 421–441, Oxford: Oxford University Press

Smith, G. D. P., Bannister, R. and Mathias, C. J. (1993). Post-exercise dizziness as the sole presenting symptom in autonomic failure. *Br. Heart J.*, **69**, 359–361

Smith, M. L., Ellenbogen, K. A. and Eckberg, L. D. (1992). Sympathoinhibition and hypotension in carotid sinus hypersensitivity. *Clin. Autonom. Res.*, **2**, 389–392

Thomaides, T., Chaudhuri, K. R., Maule, S. *et al.* (1992). The growth hormone response to clonidine in central and peripheral primary autonomic failure. *Lancet*, **340**, 263–266

Thomas, P. K. and Mathias, C. J. (1993). Diseases of the ninth, tenth, eleventh and twelfth cranial nerves. In *Peripheral Neuropathy*, 3rd edn (P. J. Dyck, P. K. Thomas, J. W. Griffin, P. A. Low and J. F. Podulso, eds), pp. 869–885, Philadelphia: W. B. Saunders

Thomashetksy, A. J., Horwitz, S. J. and Feingold, M. H. (1972). Acute autonomic neuropathy. *Neurology (Minneapolis)*, **22**, 251–255

Wallin, B. G., Westerberg, C. E. and Sundlof, G. (1984). Syncope induced by glossopharyngeal neuralgia: sympathetic outflow to muscle. *Neurology*, **34**, 522–524

Weller, M., Wilhelm, H., Sommer, M. *et al.* (1992). Tonic pupil, areflexia, and segmental anhidrosis: two additional cases of Ross syndrome and review of the literature. *J. Neurol.*, **239**, 231–234

Wieling, W., Van Lieshout, J. J. and Van Leeuwen, A. M. (1992). Physical manoeuvres that reduce postural hypotension in autonomic failure. *Clin. Autonom. Res.*, **2**, 57–66

6
Molecular genetics of inherited neuropathies

A. E. Harding and M. M. Reilly

INTRODUCTION

The purpose of this chapter is to review advances in inherited neuropathies (Table 6.1), emphasizing disorders in which molecular genetic techniques have made an impact on clinical practice. This is particularly the case in leukodystrophies, familial amyloidoses, hereditary motor and sensory neuropathies and related disorders, and X-linked bulbospinal neuronopathy. An overview of the clinical and genetic features of inherited neuropathies in general was provided in the first volume of this series on peripheral neuropathies (Harding and Thomas, 1984)

LEUKODYSTROPHIES

Metachromatic leukodystrophy (MLD)

The clinical features of this heterogeneous disorder were reviewed previously (Harding and Thomas, 1984). It is characterized by the accumulation of cerebroside sulphate due to deficiency of the enzyme aryl sulphatase A (ASA). Three clinical forms can be identified, depending on age of onset (infantile, juvenile and adult), and severity is correlated with enzyme activity. Peripheral nerve involvement is universal in the infantile form, but variable in the others. As expected, molecular genetic studies have shown heterogeneity at a mutational level, with reports of at least eight different mutations of the ASA gene and some correlation between genotype and phenotype (Aubourg, 1993).

A problem arising in the diagnosis of MLD is the existence of ASA pseudodeficiency. About 1–2% of the population are homozygous for an ASA allele which produces low activities of ASA in most assays used in clinical practice, but does not cause disease. Such individuals are inevitably identified in the investigation of patients with neurodegenerative disorders, and it cannot be assumed that the diagnosis of MLD is secure unless storage of sulphatides can be demonstrated in tissue biopsies (brain or nerve) or by the presence of metachromatic granules in renal epithelial cells obtained from urine. The mutation responsible for ASA

Table 6.1 Classification of inherited neuropathies

I.   NEUROPATHIES ASSOCIATED WITH SPECIFIC METABOLIC DEFECTS
Disturbances of lipid metabolism
    Leukodystrophies
        Metachromatic
        Globoid cell (Krabbe)
        Adrenoleukomyeloneuropathy
    Lipoprotein deficiencies
        Alphalipoprotein deficiency (Tangier disease)
        Abetalipoproteinaemia (Bassen–Kornzweig disease)
    Phytanic acid storage diseases
        Classical Refsum disease
        Infantile Refsum disease
    Alpha-galactosidase deficiency (Fabry disease)
    Cholestanolosis
    Spingomyelin lipidoses

Inherited amyloidoses
    Transthyretin-related
    Apolipoprotein A1-related
    Gelsolin-related

Porphyrias
    Acute intermittent
    Variegate
    Hereditary coproporphyria
    ALA dehydratase deficiency

Disorders with defective DNA repair
    Xeroderma pigmentosum
    Ataxia telangiectasia
    Cockayne syndrome

Neuropathies associated with defects of PMP-22
    Hereditary motor and sensory neuropathy type Ia
        With duplication of PMP-22
        With point mutation(s) of PMP-22
    Hereditary liability to pressure palsies
        Deletion of PMP-22
        Point mutation(s) of PMP-22

Neuropathies associated with defects of P_0
    Hereditary motor and sensory neuropathy type Ib:
        With point mutation(s) of P_0

Neuropathies associated with defects of connexin-32
    X-linked hereditary motor and sensory neuropathy
        With point mutation(s) of connexin-32

Neuropathy associated with CAG expansion in androgen receptor gene
    X-linked bulbospinal neuronopathy

Neuropathies associated with defects of the mitochondrial respiratory chain and/or mitochondrial DNA

Table 6.1 Classification of inherited neuropathies (*continued*)

II.   NEUROPATHIES OF UNKNOWN CAUSATION
Hereditary motor neuronopathies (spinal muscular atrophy)

Hereditary motor and sensory neuropathies
  Type I (hypertrophic Charcot–Marie–Tooth disease)
    Autosomal dominant
      (Localization not known)
    Autosomal recessive
      Locus on 8q
      Others (localization not known)
  Type II (neuronal Charcot–Marie–Tooth disease)
    Autosomal dominant
      IIa (chromosome 1p)
      Others (localization not known)
    Autosomal recessive
    Severe childhood form (autosomal recessive)
  Type III (Dejerine–Sottas disease, congential hypomyelinating neuropathy; some autosomal
    recessive and heterogeneous, some due to fresh dominant mutation of PMP-22 or P_0)
  Complex forms (with optic atrophy, pigmentary retinopathy, deafness, etc.)

Hereditary sensory and autonomic neuropathies
  Autosomal dominant
    Autosomal dominant sensory neuropathy
    Sensory neuropathy with spastic paraplegia
  Autosomal recessive
    Autosomal recessive sensory neuropathy
      Congenital non-progressive
      Progressive
    Congential sensory neuropathy with anhidrosis
    Familial dysautonomia (Riley–Day syndrome)
    Sensory neuropathy with spastic paraplegia
    Sensory neuropathy with predominant loss of small myelinated fibres
    Others, less well defined
  X-linked sensory neuropathy

Miscellaneous, including
  Brachial plexus neuropathy
  Giant axonal neuropathy
  Neuroacanthocytosis
  Chediak–Higashi disease
  Neuropathy in hereditary ataxias

---

pseudodeficiency alters a polyadenylation signal of the gene (Gieselmann *et al.*, 1989), and this can easily be detected by DNA analysis. The absence of this mutation in both alleles would make pseudodeficiency unlikely, but pseudodeficiency may occur in combination with functional deficiency mutations.

Adrenoleukodystrophy (ALD)

An axonal peripheral neuropathy occurs in the adrenoleukomyeloneuropathy phenotype of ALD, usually in combination with spastic paraplegia and/or ataxia (Thomas, 1993). This disorder is of X-linked inheritance and is associated with impaired β-oxidation of very long-chain fatty acids, particularly hexacanoic acid (C26:0), a process which normally takes place in peroxisomes. The ALD gene maps to chromosome Xq28 and was identified by positional cloning; it encodes a protein, termed ALD protein, which is homologous to a known peroxisomal membrane protein, peroxisomal membrane protein-70 (Mosser *et al.*, 1993). ALD has not yet been fully investigated at a mutational level, but there is already evidence of substantial heterogeneity, with the description of both deletions and point mutations (Cartier *et al.*, 1993; Mosser *et al.*, 1993). It is therefore not clear how straightforward or useful mutation analysis will be in ALD.

FAMILIAL AMYLOIDOSES

The familial amyloid polyneuropathies (FAP) are a heterogeneous group of autosomal dominant disorders first described by Andrade in northern Portugal (Andrade, 1952). Pathologically, FAP shares the common feature of all amyloidoses, deposition of a fibrillar protein with an abundant β-pleated structure in the extracellular space. Amyloid also contains a non-fibrillar glycoprotein, the P component, and a variety of mucopolysaccharides and other plasma and tissue proteins. Many different proteins can form amyloid and it is the individual constituent protein of each type of amyloid which defines the disease (Benson, 1989). In FAP the most common protein deposited as amyloid is transthyretin (TTR, formerly known as pre-albumin) but FAP can also occur secondary to apolipoprotein A-1 or gelsolin deposition.

Costa and colleagues (1978) first showed that the fibril protein in the Portuguese type of FAP was immunologically related to TTR. The three-dimensional structure of plasma transthyretin is known. It is a tetramer (55 kDa) composed of four identical monomer subunits, and shows an extensive β-pleated structure which presumably explains its propensity to form amyloid. Over 90% of TTR is produced in the liver, the remainder being synthesized in the choroid plexus and the retina. The mature protein has two known functions. It is responsible for about 20% of plasma thyroxine binding, and also binds with retinol binding protein, although the site of binding is not known (Hamilton *et al.*, 1993).

TTR is the product of a gene mapping to chromosome 18q11.2-q12.1, which contains four exons coding for a 127-amino acid mature protein and an 18-residue signal peptide. The first exon codes for the signal peptide and the first three amino acids of the protein. No mutations have been reported in this exon. Numerous mutations have been described in the other three exons (Benson, 1991; Saraiva, 1991). Those associated with FAP (as opposed to harmless polymorphisms or others causing non-neurological dysfunction) are listed in Table 6.2.

Classification of FAP

FAP used to be classified into four types on the basis of clinical presentation (Harding and Thomas, 1984): predominantly involving the lower limbs (FAP I) described mainly in Portuguese, Japanese and Swedish families; initially upper limb involvement (FAP II) originally described in Indiana/Swiss and German/Maryland kindreds; causing lower-limb neuropathy with nephropathy and gastric ulcers (FAP III), originally reported in an Iowa kinship; and the Finnish type of cranial neuropathy with corneal lattice dystrophy (FAP IV). This clinical

Table 6.2 Transthyretin (TTR) mutations associated with familial amyloid polyneuropathies

Exon	Amino acid substitution	Ethnic origin	Predominant clinical features
2	Arg 10	Hungarian	N, late onset
	Met 30	Portuguese	N, A
	Ala 30	German	N
	Leu 30	Japanese	N
	Ile 33	Jewish	N, vitreous
	Leu 33	Polish/American	N, A, C
	Pro 36	Greek	N, C, vitreous, renal
	Gly 42	Japanese	N, A
	Arg 47	Japanese	N, A
3	Ala 49	Italian	N, C, vitreous
	Arg 50	Japanese	ULN, A
	Ile 50	Japanese	N
	Pro 55	Dutch/German	N, C
	His 58	German/Maryland	N, CTS, C
	Arg 58	Japanese	ULN, A, vitreous
	Ala 60	Irish/Appalachian	N, A, C, late onset
	Lys 61	Japanese	N, A
	Leu 64	Italian	N, CTS
	His 69	American	N, vitreous
	Asn 70	German	N, CTS, vitreous
	Ala 71	French	N
	Tyr 77	Illinois/German	N
	Ser 84	Swiss/Indiana	N, CTS, vitreous
	Asn 84	Italian	N, vitreous
	Gln 89	Italian	N, CTS, C
	Asn 90	Italian	N, C, vitreous
	Gly 97	Japanese	N, late onset
4	Cys 114	Japanese	N

N, neuropathy, generally involving lower limbs first; ULN, symptoms presenting in upper limbs; C, cardiomyopathy; A, severe and early autonomic dysfunction; CTS, carpal tunnel syndrome.

classification has largely been replaced by a classification based on mutations in the amyloidogenic proteins in FAP. The ever increasing number of pathogenic mutations described, especially in the TTR gene (Table 6.2), has highlighted the overlapping clinical syndromes between the different types of FAP, although in an individual patient ethnic origin or clinical features may suggest a particular mutation.

The clinical and genetic features of the more common types of FAP, particularly the Portuguese type associated with a mutation in the TTR gene causing a substitution of methionine for valine at amino acid 30 of the TTR protein, will be reviewed here.

TTR-related FAP

FAP met 30 (Portuguese)

FAP met 30 is most common in patients of Portuguese origin (Saraiva, 1991) but has also been described in patients from Sweden (Drugge *et al.*, 1993), Japan (Nakazato *et al.*, 1987), Cyprus and Greece (Holt *et al.*, 1989), other Mediterranean countries, France and England (Bhatia *et al.*, 1993). There is marked variation, with some consistency in each major cluster of the disease, in relation both to age of onset (ranging from 17 to 78 years; Coelho *et al.*, 1994) and the nature of the initial presentation. Portuguese patients tend to present in the third or fourth decades of life, whereas Swedish patients with the same mutation tend to present in their late fifties. Swedish patients also differ from Portuguese patients in frequently having vitreous opacities.

The typical presenting symptom is painful dysaesthesias in the lower legs, followed by progressive numbness and sensory loss. There is early lack of pain and temperature sensation due to greater small fibre involvement but eventually all sensory modalties are impaired. Painless injury to the feet complicated by ulcers, cellulitis, osteomyelitis and Charcot joints may occur. Motor involvement develops later in the course of the disease, causing wasting and weakness. There is progressive loss of reflexes. The arms are affected months to years after onset in the legs. Carpal tunnel syndrome can occur in this type of FAP, but it is rarely the presenting feature. Most patients have early autonomic involvement, causing orthostatic hypotension, alternating constipation and diarrhoea, gastric atony, impotence, urinary hesitancy and dry skin.

Neurophysiologically there is evidence of a predominantly sensory axonal neuropathy in established cases. Sensory nerve action potentials may be of normal amplitude early in the course of the disease, again reflecting mainly small fibre involvement. Nerve biopsy with immunohistochemistry is useful in confirming the diagnosis of TTR-related amyloidosis, but occasionally no amyloid deposits are detected because of their patchy nature. Biopsy of other tissues, for example rectal mucosa, can also be useful in detecting amyloid. In patients where there is a strong suspicion of FAP, DNA analysis is the first investigation of choice (see later).

Other systems which may be involved in FAP met 30 include the heart (causing a restrictive cardiomyopathy), the vitreous and the kidneys. In Portuguese patients death, from systemic involvement and sepsis, occurs typically about 15 years after onset. The disease tends to be less rapidly progressive if onset is later. It was originally thought that all patients with FAP met 30, including those in Japan and Sweden, were Portuguese in origin and had a common founder. However, studies of DNA polymorphisms in the non-coding part of the TTR gene have shown at least three different haplotypes associated with this mutation in Japanese, Portuguese and other European populations (Yoshioka *et al.*, 1989; Reilly *et al.*, 1995a), suggesting that is has occurred several times independently. A high frequency of mutation at this position may be explained by the fact that it occurs in a C_pG dinucleotide sequence which is susceptible to mutation (Yoshioka *et al.*, 1989).

Other TTR variants with a similar phenotype

A similar clinical picture to that seen in FAP met 30 is observed in patients with other variants of TTR including leucine 33 (Nakazato *et al.*, 1984; Ii *et al.*, 1991), tyrosine 77 (Wallace *et al.*, 1986), asparagine 90 (Skare *et al.*, 1989), cysteine 114 (Ueno *et al.*, 1990a), glycine 42 (Ueno *et al.*, 1990b), arginine 47 (Murakami *et al.*, 1992), alanine 49 (Almeida *et al.*, 1992), and alanine 71 (Benson II *et al.*, 1993). Several of these have been described in only one family.

FAPs ser 84, his 58, and others with a similar phenotype

These disorders were originally described in a large kindred in Indiana of Swiss origin (ser 84) (Dwulet and Benson, 1986) and an extended pedigree comprising 11 families in Maryland of German origin (his 58) (Nichols *et al.*, 1989). The presentation is with carpal tunnel syndrome, most commonly starting in the early forties. Later the neuropathy, mainly sensory, extends more generally in the upper limbs and then involves the legs. Autonomic failure is common and a restrictive cardiomyopathy can also occur. More recently, patients presenting either with carpal tunnel syndrome or a more generalized neuropathy which starts in the upper limbs have been found to have TTR mutations at arginine 50 (Ueno *et al.*, 1990b), arginine 58 (Saeki *et al.*, 1991), leucine 64 (Ii *et al.*, 1991), asparagine 70 (Izumoto *et al.*, 1992) and glutamine 89 (Almeida *et al.*, 1992).

FAP ala 60 (Irish/Appalachian), and others with a similar phenotype

This type of FAP was first reported in a family living in the Appalachian region of the USA (Benson *et al.*, 1987) but it has since become apparent that the mutation originated in North-West Ireland. A cluster of families from Donegal (North-West Ireland) has the same mutation (Staunton *et al.*, 1987, 1991; Reilly *et al.*, 1995b). Onset is late, usually in the sixth or seventh decade, and both motor involvement and large-fibre sensory loss are more prominent than in FAP met 30. Cardiomyopathy is often severe and may be the presenting feature (Staunton *et al.*, 1987). A similar phenotype was reported with the arginine 10 and lysine 61 mutations (Uemichi *et al.*, 1992, Shiomi *et al.*, 1993). A further TTR mutation (glycine 97) causes a late-onset neuropathy and cardiomyopathy without autonomic dysfunction (Yasuda *et al.*, 1994).

Pathogenesis

The various TTR point mutations described in FAP usually exist in the heterozygous state and are inherited as an autosomal dominant trait. Homozygosity for TTR met 30 is associated with a similar phenotype to that seen in heterozygotes (Holmgren *et al.*, 1992). Transmission from an affected mother confers earlier onset in affected offspring than in those of affected fathers (Drugge *et al.*, 1993). There is good evidence for reduced penetrance in TTR-related FAP, particularly well documented with the met 30 mutation but also observed in others, for example ala 60 and glu 89 (Holt *et al.*, 1989; Almeida *et al.*, 1992; Coelho *et al.*, 1994; Reilly *et al.*, 1995b). These observations, together with the late onset of these disorders, suggest that there are other factors involved in disease pathogenesis and expression besides the amyloidogenic potential of TTR itself. This has been investigated using transgenic mice expressing the human TTR met 30 mutation. In these mice amyloid deposition started at 6 months in the gastrointestinal tract, cardiovascular system and kidneys. By 24 months the pattern of amyloid deposition was the same as that seen in autopsy cases of human FAP except for its absence in the peripheral and autonomic nervous system and the choroid plexus (Yi *et al.*, 1991). Transgenic mice carrying the autologous TTR regulatory sequences have amyloid deposits in the choroid plexus and the meninges but not in the peripheral nerves (Saraiva, 1991). Another type of transgenic mouse, carrying the human mutant TTR gene and the human serum amyloid P (SAP) gene (SAP is found associated with all types of amyloid), exhibited the same clinical course and pattern of tissue amyloid deposition as mice with only the mutant TTR gene (Tashiro *et al.*, 1991). This suggests that SAP is not important for the initiation or progression of amyloid deposition. Further studies on transgenic mice may be useful in understanding mechanisms of amyloid fibril formation.

Apolipoprotein A-1-related FAP

One type of FAP, seen in an Iowa kindred described by Van Allen (1969), has been shown to be associated with deposition of a variant apolipoprotein A-1 in which an arginine for glycine substitution occurs at position 26 (Nichols *et al.*, 1990). The phenotype is similar to that of FAP met 30.

Gelsolin-related FAP

This disease, first described in a Finnish kindred by Meretoja (1969), usually presents in the fourth decade of life with a corneal lattice dystrophy. This is followed by a progressive cranial neuropathy, initially involving the upper facial muscles. Other cranial nerves may become affected, especially the trigeminal, hyopoglossal and vestibulocochlear nerves (Kiuru *et al.*, 1992). The facial skin is at first thickened but with time becomes thin and lax. A mild sensory neuropathy, with autonomic involvement, develops later in the limbs.

The fibril protein in this disease is an abnormal fragment of a plasma protein, gelsolin, in which there is most commonly a substitution of asparagine for aspartic acid at residue 187 (position 15 of the amyloid protein; Levy *et al.*, 1990). As well as being described in more than 200 Finnish families, this disorder has been reported in patients of Dutch (de la Chapelle *et al.*, 1992), Japanese (Sunada *et al.*, 1993) and Irish–American origins (Gorevic *et al.*, 1991). Two further families with this syndrome have been reported, one Danish (Boysen *et al.*, 1979) and one Czech, with a different gelsolin mutation involving the same codon, changing aspartic acid to tyrosine instead of asparagine at residue 187 (de la Chapelle *et al.*, 1992).

DNA diagnosis of FAP

This largely concerns TTR mutations as apolipoprotein A-1 and gelsolin-related amyloidosis are very rare in most populations. For diagnostic purposes, many point mutations (including the most common, met 30, ala 60 and tyr 77) change cleavage sites for restriction endonucleases and are therefore easily detected by amplification of the relevant sequence using the polymerase chain reaction (PCR) and subsequent restriction (Figure 6.1). For those mutations that do not change restriction sites, either allele-specific PCR or mismatch PCR can be used (Nichols *et al.*, 1989; Uemichi *et al.*, 1992). In patients with a family history of FAP and a documented mutation, diagnostic analysis is straightforward. It is more complex in patients with biopsy-proven or possible amyloid neuropathy, with or without affected relatives, unless there are clues from ethnic origin, for example they are Portuguese or Irish in which case it is logical to look for the met 30 or ala 60

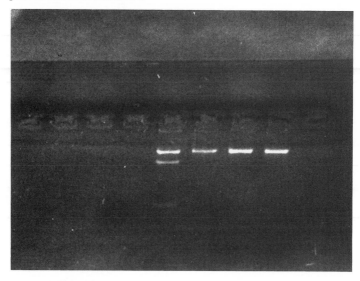

Figure 6.1 Diagnosis of the Portuguese type of familial amyloid neuropathy using the PCR and digestion with *Nsi*I, for which the mutation introduces a new restriction site. 414 bp of exon 2 of the transthyretin gene have been amplified; in the sample on the left there are two additional fragments (295 and 119 bp in length, the latter less clearly seen) in addition to the normal 414 bp product which is seen alone in three normal individuals on the right. (From Davis *et al.*, 1993, with permission).

mutations. If there are no such clues, the policy in the DNA laboratory at the National Hospital is to screen for the most common mutations seen in our patient base, i.e. met 30, ala 60 and tyr 77. If these are not present and the patient has either: (1) immunohistochemically proven TTR-related and amyloidosis or (2) a suggestive clinical picture (a predominantly small-fibre neuropathy with autonomic dysfunction) and a positive family history, we sequence the TTR gene directly. This is more efficient than performing multiple restriction analyses for rare known mutations, and also allows detection of unknown mutations. It is possible to screen exons for mutations before sequencing by several techniques including single-strand conformation polymorphism analysis (Uemichi *et al.*, 1992), but this is not known to be 100% sensitive.

In families with known mutations detection of these can also be used for pre-symptomatic and prenatal testing. Both require pre- and post-test genetic counselling, using the same principles as in Huntington's disease (World Federation of Neurology Research Group on Huntington's Disease, 1993). The main problem in presymptomatic testing relates to the reduced penetrance seen in most types of FAP which is about 80% in FAP met 30, but not quantified in relation to most of the other mutations.

Treatment

Until recently treatment of FAP was limited to rehabilitative measures and symptomatic therapies, for example for orthostatic hypotension and carpal tunnel syndrome. There is still no proven effective treatment for FAP. Plasma exchange has been shown to lower variant TTR concentrations, but has not been shown to affect disease progression. Another recently suggested potential treatment is extracorporeal immunoadsorption on immobilized anti-transthyretin antibodies but this has yet to be subjected to clinical trials (Regnault *et al.*, 1992). Liver transplantation has been performed in patients with FAP met 30 based on the rationale that over 90% of TTR is produced in the liver. The biochemical effect of transplantation is good as demonstrated by a dramatic reduction in variant TTR plasma and scintigraphic evidence of reduced amyloid deposits postoperatively. Clinically, improvement has been noted in gastrointestinal function and postural hypotension; the neuropathy may stop progressing (Holmgren *et al.*, 1993; Skinner *et al.*, 1994). These results are encouraging but liver transplantation is a major procedure and is hazardous in patients with advanced autonomic failure; we are aware of one such patient who died in the early postoperative procedure as a result of intractable hypotension. The ideal time to perform this procedure has not as yet been determined, but is probably at a relatively early stage of the disease.

HEREDITARY MOTOR AND SENSORY NEUROPATHIES

The hereditary motor and sensory neuropathies (HMSN) are a heterogeneous group of disorders which can be classified on the basis of their clinical, genetic, neurophysiological and pathological features. They will increasingly be classified on the basis of which mutant gene and protein causes the disease (see Table 6.1).

Clinical and pathological features

HMSN I (also called Charcot–Marie–Tooth disease type 1) is characterized by slowly progressive distal weakness and wasting, predominantly affecting the anterior tibial and peroneal muscles. Foot deformity, areflexia and distal sensory loss are common, and upper limb ataxia or tremor and peripheral nerve hypertrophy occur in about one-third of patients. The last reflects the underlying pathology of a hypertrophic demyelinating peripheral neuropathy. Autosomal dominant HMSN I is the commonest type of inherited neuropathy, with a prevalence of about 1 in 5000 in the UK. The disorder varies in severity and about 20% of patients are seriously handicapped. HMSN II has similar clinical features, but these are associated with a chronic axonal, as opposed to demyelinating, neuropathy. Both disorders are usually dominantly inherited, although autosomal recessive forms have been described (Harding and Thomas, 1980a).

The existence of X-linked HMSN was disputed (Harding and Thomas, 1980b) until recently, but it is probably one of the more common types of HMSN, with a prevalence perhaps approaching that of HMSN II. Males tend to be more severely affected than females, who may have a mild symptomatic neuropathy or be asymptomatic (Rozear *et al.*, 1987; Hahn *et al.*, 1990). The neurophysiological features in males may resemble those of HMSN I, whereas those in females suggest an axonal degeneration (Nicholson and Nash, 1993). Sporadic cases of HMSN present particular problems in terms of diagnosis and genetic counselling, as it is still not clear how many represent new mutations as opposed to an autosomal recessive form of disease.

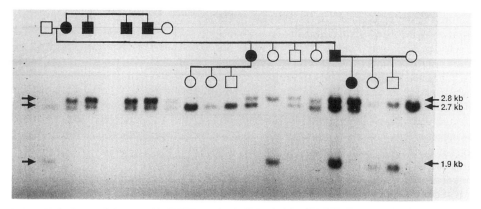

Figure 6.2 Pedigree of family with HMSN type Ia, with *Msp*I restriction digests hybridized to probe VAW409R3 (which maps within the 17p11.2 duplication) from each individual immediately under their pedigree symbol. Normal subjects (open symbols) show only one fragment (homozygotes) or two of equal intensity (heterozygotes). Individual II.5 is affected (filled symbols) and exhibits three fragments, demonstrating the presence of the duplication. The other affected subjects show two bands, but one is more intense than the other, indicating three copies of this locus. (From Hallam *et al.*, 1992, with permission.)

HMSN III, or Dejerine–Sottas disease, is generally defined as a severe demyelinating/hypomyelinating neuropathy with extremely slow motor nerve conduction velocities and delayed motor development which is thought to be autosomal recessive (Dyck *et al.*, 1993). However, there is substantial pathological and genetic heterogeneity in this syndrome. Some severely affected patients with dominant HMSN I have the same clinical phenotype, and the distinction between autosomal recessive HMSN I and HMSN III may be impossible without nerve biopsy; many authors consider evidence of hypomyelination to be an essential component of HMSN III. Gabreëls-Festen and Gabreëls (1993) have reviewed this difficult area and divided recessive and sporadic forms of demyelinating HMSN into five groups: two types of autosomal recessive HMSN I with either basal lamina onion bulbs or focally folded myelin, and three types of HMSN III, with amyelination, basal lamina onion bulbs or classical onion bulbs. As will be discussed later, an increasing proportion of patients with the clinical syndrome of HMSN III have been shown to have *de novo* mutations of genes which are involved in the pathogenesis of dominant HMSN I.

Molecular genetics of HMSN

HMSN I

Genetic linkage studies have shown that autosomal dominant HMSN I is genetically heterogeneous, involving at least three gene loci. The first locus identified is on chromosome 1 (HMSN Ib) (Lebo *et al.*, 1991), although this type of HMSN appears to be rare. It was subsequently shown that the peripheral myelin P_0 gene maps to chromosome 1 (Hayasaka *et al.*, 1991), and mutations of this gene have been identified in four families previously known to have a chromosome 1 locus (Hayasaka *et al.*, 1993a,b; Kulkens *et al.*, 1993; Su *et al.*, 1993). In addition, *de novo* P_0 mutations have been reported in two patients with the clinical phenotype of HMSN III (Hayasaka *et al.*, 1993c). With one possible exception, the mutations reported to date are in exons 2 or 3 of the P_0 gene, which code for the extracellular and trans-membranous domains of the protein. The functional effects of these are as yet unknown. One area of confusion is that two different mutations have been reported in the same family by different groups (Hayasaka *et al.*, 1993a; Su *et al.*, 1993), the latter suggesting a splice junction mutation rather than one in coding sequence.

Most families with autosomal dominant HMSN I have a disease locus on chromosome 17 (HMSN Ia), within band 17p11.2 (Vance *et al.*, 1991). In 1991 two groups reported independently the discovery of a large DNA duplication within 17p11.2 in individuals with HMSN Ia (Lupski *et al.*, 1991; Raeymaekers *et al.*, 1991). This observation has been confirmed by many other investigators (Brice *et al.*, 1992; Hallam *et al.*, 1992), including in patients from small families unsuitable for linkage studies, and it is clear that most families with HMSN Ia, and probably about 90% of those with dominant HMSN I overall, carry the duplication. It does not occur in normal subjects or in patients with other types of HMSN. The duplication has also been demonstrated in several patients without a history of affected relatives and genetically normal parents (Hoogendijk *et al.*, 1992; Wise *et al.*, 1993). Of interest is the observation of one patient with an IgM kappa paraproteinaemia, and the widely spaced myelin characteristic of this type of paraproteinaemic neuropathy (Gregory *et al.*, 1993). It seems unlikely that these two pathologies are coincidental; there is some evidence that patients with HMSN type I are more susceptible to developing CIDP (Low *et al.*, 1982) and possibly other dysimmune neuropathies.

This mechanism of causing an apparently straightforward mendelian genetic disease in humans, termed segmental trisomy, is currently unique. The duplication is large, involving about 1.5 megabases (mb) of DNA. Evidence to date suggests that the duplicated region is constant in the vast majority of patients (Wise *et al.*, 1993); only one family with a precisely sized, smaller, duplication (~460 kb) has been reported (Valentijn *et al.*, 1993). In families with the 'common' duplication, these appear to have arisen independently and probably by interchromosomal exchange, as different and heterozygous allelic forms are found in different families, and fresh mutation occurs. Physical mapping studies have shown that the duplication is a tandem repeat of 1.5 mb which is flanked by a repeated sequence 17–29 kb in length. *De novo* duplications probably arise from unequal crossing over due to misalignment of these repeats during meiosis (Pentao *et al.*, 1992); these appear to be mainly, if not exclusively, of paternal origin (Palau *et al.*, 1993).

Coincident with description of the HMSN Ia duplication were reports of two point mutations in a newly described myelin gene in the *Trembler* and *Trembler-J* mouse mutants. These had been proposed as models for HMSN I, based on the features of an autosomal dominant demyelinating/hypomyelinating neuropathy, and localization to a region of the mouse genome (chromosome 11) which shows homology to human chromosome 17. The point mutations substitute aspartic acid for glycine and proline for leucine in *Trembler* and *Trembler-J* respectively, in a peripheral myelin protein (PMP-22) (Suter *et al.*, 1992a,b).

Several groups then showed that PMP-22 is within the HMSN Ia duplication (Matsunami *et al.*, 1992; Patel *et al.*, 1992; Timmerman *et al.*, 1992; Valentijn *et al.*, 1992a). It thus seems very likely that a dosage effect related to this gene in patients with HMSN Ia causes the neuropathy. Further evidence for this comes from the offspring of two parents with HMSN I and the duplication; this individual had four copies of 17p11.2 and was particularly severely affected (Lupski *et al.*, 1992). The important role of PMP-22 in HMSN Ia was confirmed by studies of a Dutch family in which linkage to the relevant region of chromosome 17 could be demonstrated but the duplication was not detected. Affected members of this kindred carried the same mutation of PMP-22 seen in *Trembler-J* (Valentijn *et al.*, 1992b). Further dominant pedigrees with different point mutations of PMP-22 were reported by Nelis and colleagues (1994) and Roa and co-workers (1993a). In the latter family the index case had a very severe neuropathy, described as Dejerine–Sottas syndrome by the authors, although his mother was also affected.

De novo mutations of PMP-22 have been reported in two patients with HMSN, one with a severe phenotype reminiscent of HMSN III and the other with more typical HMSN I which was transmitted to offspring (Roa *et al.*, 1993a,b). A most unusual family was reported by Roa and colleagues (1993c), in which several members had hereditary liability to pressure palsies and the associated deletion of chromosome 17p11.2 (see later). One patient had the phenotype of HMSN I; in addition to the deletion, she carried a point mutation of PMP-22 in her only copy of this gene. One of her sons had inherited this mutation and was clinically and neurophysiologically normal. The authors suggested that these observations provided evidence for pathogenicity of recessive PMP-22 mutations in HMSN I.

The PMP-22 gene is homologous to a gene isolated earlier from mouse fibroblasts termed growth arrest specific 3. The sequence of the rat, murine and human PMP-22 genes predicts a 18-kDa protein with four putative membrane-spanning domains (Suter *et al.*, 1993). One highly conserved sequence of the gene is a glycosylation site, indicating that there is post-translational modification, in agreement with the apparent molecular weight of 22 kDa on SDS gels. PMP-22 expression is strongly down-regulated distal to nerve injury, recovering after regeneration of axons, suggesting that axons regulate expression of this gene in Schwann cells (Welcher *et al.*, 1991). With one exception (Nelis *et al.*, 1994), the dominant mutations described to date in HMSN I have altered amino acids which are deep in the putative membrane-spanning domains of the protein. The apparently recessive nature of the mutation reported by Roa *et al.*, (1993c) may be explained by the fact that it lies either at one end of the third domain, or immediately beyond it. However, Nelis and colleagues (1994) reported a dominant mutation in the first nucleotide of the last intron of PMP-22. This alters the consensus 5′ splice site, which could have serious consequences on RNA processing.

There is now a real opportunity to investigate the molecular pathogenesis of HMSN Ia, particularly as an animal model is already available. The pathological changes hint that the development of these hinges on disturbances in axon-Schwann cell relationships. We need to establish how either over-expression of PMP-22, as in the 17p duplication, or point mutations or deletions of this gene lead to different phenotypes of demyelination, hypomyelination and dysmyelination.

In some families with dominant HMSN I, linkage to both chromosome 1 and chromosome 17 loci has been excluded (Chance *et al.*, 1990), indicating that yet further genes may be involved in producing this phenotype, perhaps other peripheral myelin protein genes.

One autosomal recessive form of HMSN I has been mapped to chromosome 8q in Tunisian families (Ben Othmane *et al.*, 1993a). Patients in these families had an early onset neuropathy with severe distal weakness, and an average median motor nerve conduction velocity of 29 m/s. Nerve biopsies showed loss of myelinated fibres and hypomyelination. Autosomal recessive HMSN I is clearly genetically heterogeneous as other Tunisian families with this syndrome did not show linkage to chromosome 8.

Other types of HMSN

Evidence for linkage to chromosome 1p markers has been reported in three of six families with autosomal dominant HMSN II, suggesting that this disorder is also genetically heterogeneous (Ben Othmane *et al.*, 1993b).

The locus for X-linked HMSN (HMSN X) maps to the proximal long arm of the X chromosome (Xq13.1; Bergoffen *et al.*, 1993a). The gene for the gap junction protein connexin 32 also maps to this region, leading to its consideration as a candidate gene for HMSN X. Bergoffen and colleagues (1993b) identified seven different mutations of this gene in eight families with HMSN X. Two other groups confirmed these findings in a further 13 families, demonstrating another 11 mutations of connexin 32 (Fairweather *et al.*, 1994; Ionasescu *et al.*, 1994). However, these studies did not identify mutations of the connexin 32 coding sequence in seven families, even though linkage data were compatible with a locus in this region. It is possible that splice site or promotor region mutations are responsible for HMSN X in these kindreds.

Defects of connexin 32 are somewhat unexpected in HMSN (Spray, 1994), as gap junctions have not been detected in human peripheral nerve by freeze-fracture electron microscopy (Gabriel *et al.*, 1986). Furthermore, connexin 32 is widely expressed in other tissues not affected in HMSN X, including liver and brain (Bergoffen *et al.*, 1993b). These observations suggest that connexin 32 may serve a different function in peripheral nerve.

Immunohistochemical studies showed that connexin 32 was present at nodes of Ranvier and Schmidt–Lanterman incisures, perhaps indicating that the protein forms intracellular gap junctions between the folds of Schwann cell cytoplasm (Bergoffen *et al.*, 1993b). It is of interest that temporary gap junctions were reported in chicken sciatic nerve during degeneration and subsequent regeneration (Tetzlaff, 1982). Like PMP-22, connexin 32 has four transmembranous domains, but identified mutations are not confined to these, involving extracellular loops and cytoplasmic domains as well (Bergoffen *et al.*, 1993b; Fairweather *et al.*, 1994; Ionasescu *et al.*, 1994).

Clinical applications

From the clinical point of view, it is clear that DNA analysis for the 17p duplication is useful in diagnosis. It is particularly helpful in sporadic cases and serves to distinguish HMSN Ia from other demyelinating neuropathies, particularly chronic inflammatory demyelinating polyneuropathy (CIDP). It is not indicated in patients with possible HMSN II. The methods for duplication detection which are suitable for clinical use are not particularly rapid or technically straightforward. Pulsed field gel electrophoresis, which consistently detects a pathologically large fragment, and densitometric/Phosphor-Imaging dosage analysis of Southern blots with appropriate controls (Hensels *et al.*, 1993; Wise *et al.*, 1993) provide reliable results.

In patients with dominantly inherited HMSN I (from pedigrees showing male-to-male transmission), if the duplication is not present then point mutations of PMP-22, or P_0 are possible. Screening for these is still largely a research procedure. If there is no male-to-male transmission it is worth considering whether inheritance could be X-linked. This suspicion would be supported by males being consistently more severely affected within the family, and accompanying discordance of nerve conduction data ('demyelinating' in males and 'axonal' in females) (Nicholson and Nash, 1993). It is probable that many of the so called 'intermediate' families which provoked controversy in relation to the division of HMSN into types I and II (e.g. Davis *et al.*, 1978) are, in fact, examples of HMSN X. It is important to establish whether inheritance is dominant or X-linked for genetic counselling purposes. Screening for connexin 32 mutations is, at present, again a research procedure.

In isolated cases of HMSN I, or possible cases of HMSN III, detection of the duplication confirms the diagnosis of HMSN Ia, with a resulting 50% risk of transmission to offspring. If the duplication is absent, it is worth considering a diagnosis of CIDP. Some patients with CIDP have onset in childhood or adolescence, with an indolent course and resulting skeletal deformity. Non-uniform slowing of nerve conduction velocities, sometimes with evidence of conduction block, suggests an inflammatory rather than a genetic neuropathy. A nerve biopsy should be performed in such patients, particularly if the cerebrospinal fluid (CSF) protein concentration is high, to detect possible inflammatory changes or specific pathological features of some recessive types of HMSN such as focally folded myelin sheaths (Gabreëls-Festen and Gabreëls, 1993).

It is clear that the phenotype of HMSN III (early onset, motor delay, motor nerve conduction velocities < 10 m/s) has a genetically heterogeneous basis and it cannot be assumed that inheritance is autosomal recessive in patients without affected sibs. It may well turn out that the majority of these represent *de novo* mutations of either PMP-22 or P_0. Although screening for these is not an established clinical test, most research groups in this field would be interested to analyse DNA from suitable patients in this category.

In families with known genetic defects, of which the duplication of 17p11.2 is clearly the most frequent, it is possible to use the DNA analysis for presymptomatic and prenatal screening. In family members at risk, DNA analysis is a suitable alternative to nerve conduction studies. This is entirely appropriate in requesting adults who are aware of the implications of a positive result in relation to reproduction, employment and health insurance. The question of testing children is less straightforward. The fact that children in HMSN families have been investigated by nerve conduction studies for three decades does not mean that this issue should not be considered carefully. The main argument for testing children, a coherent one, is to identify affected individuals who will need to be followed carefully to detect early skeletal deformities which can be prevented with appropriate orthotic and orthopaedic measures. This probably outweighs the argument that individuals at risk of genetic disorders (particularly late onset ones) should make their own decision about testing when they have reached the age of majority. There is little point in performing such screening before the age of 2 or 3 years. If parents do not wish to know their children's genetic status, all their children should be examined annually for the reason given above after the age of 3 or 4 years.

Personal experience with many HMSN Ia families suggests that requests for prenatal diagnosis will be relatively infrequent. Couples' views on this issue will inevitably be coloured by their experience of the disease, either in themselves or their relatives. Many couples feel that termination of an affected fetus is not justified by the (usually) relatively mild disability of HMSN Ia. It is of course impossible to distinguish by DNA analysis for the 17p duplication whether the individual will be severely or mildly affected. However, some couples cannot countenance having an affected child, with about a 20% probability of being significantly disabled by early adult life, and will opt for prenatal diagnosis with termination of an affected fetus. DNA is ideally analysed from chorionic villus samples obtained at about 10 weeks' gestation. Testing should not be undertaken unless the couple concerned is committed to terminating affected pregnancies. There is nothing to be gained in knowing fetal genetic status for any other reason, and potentially much to be lost. Chorionic villus sampling has about a 2% risk of causing miscarriage.

HEREDITARY LIABILITY TO PRESSURE PALSIES

The model of duplication generation referred to above in HMSN Ia, unequal crossing over, requires the production of a chromosome in which the duplicated region is deleted. This has been shown to be associated with an entirely different phenotype, hereditary neuropathy with liability to pressure palsies (HNPP) or tomaculous neuropathy (Chance *et al.*, 1993, 1994). Deletion of 17p11.2 was observed in affected members of three families with this disease, and *de novo* deletion was documented in one pedigree. This observation accords with data suggesting that PMP-22 is important in axon–myelin interactions.

Tyson and colleagues (1995) investigated 41 patients with multifocal neuropathies for this deletion of chromosome 17p11.2. The deletion was detected in 18 patients, including 10 from eight out of nine families in whom HNPP had been considered likely on clinical, neurophysiological and/or pathological grounds. Some patients with a deletion had unusual clinical features for HNPP (Windebank, 1993), including one with a progressive scapuloperoneal syndrome and one progressive asymmetric proximal upper limb weakness. Overall, five (38%) of the 13 index patients with the deletion had no affected relatives, and less than half had evidence of a generalized neuropathy on examination. Nerve conduction studies in 14/19 patients studied showed a fairly uniform pattern of moderate prolongation of distal sensory and motor latencies and slowing of conduction velocities, and variation reduction of sensory or muscle action potential amplitudes. The patients investigated who did not have a deletion of 17p11.2 were heterogeneous and included cases with recurrent neuralgic amyotrophy, two or more peripheral nerve lesions at common sites of entrapment, or a patchy axonal neuropathy of unknown aetiology. In one a diagnosis of HNPP remained most likely; it is possible that this patient has a point mutation of PMP-22. Nicholson and co-workers (1994) have reported a two base-pair deletion in the seventh codon of PMP-22, which must effectively cause a functional deletion of the gene, in one family with HNPP.

DNA analysis for the deletion of 17p11.2 is clearly useful in establishing the diagnosis of HNPP, which should be considered regardless of family history or clinical evidence of a generalized neuropathy, and in patients with multifocal neuropathies which do not conform to the classical clinical picture of HNPP. DNA analysis is less invasive than nerve conduction studies or nerve biopsy, and will be particularly valuable in defining (with appropriate counselling and informed consent) which family members are at risk of pressure palsies and determining advice about lifestyle, including the necessity to take additional precautions to protect peripheral nerves during operative procedures and childbirth.

X-LINKED BULBOSPINAL NEURONOPATHY

X-linked bulbospinal neuronopathy (XLBSN), also called Kennedy's disease, causes progressive generalized neurogenic muscle weakness in males, usually with onset between the ages of 25 and 50 years. Muscle cramps may precede the onset of weakness by several years. The prognosis is variable, and partly dependent on age at onset, but the disease does not usually limit life expectancy. Bulbar symptoms, especially dysphagia, tend to occur relatively late. Fasciculation is particularly prominent, and is striking in the lower face and tongue. This disorder is often classified as a spinal muscular atrophy but this is inaccurate as there is involvement of sensory neurons. Associated features include areflexia, neurophysiological evidence of a sensory axonal neuropathy, occasionally with mild sensory loss in the legs, tremor, gynaecomastia, infertility and diabetes mellitus (Harding *et al.*, 1982). The gene locus was mapped to the proximal long arm of the X chromosome in 1986 (Fischbeck *et al.*, 1986). Subsequently La Spada and colleagues (1991) provided evidence that the causative genetic defect is an abnormally long CAG repeat in the androgen receptor gene which leads to an increase in size of a polygutamine tract in the receptor. The normal CAG repeat ranges from 16 to 26 copies, but patients with XLBSN have between 40 and 62 (La Spada *et al.*, 1992). The functional significance of this is as yet unknown; abnormal androgen receptor binding of dihydrotestosterone is observed in some families but not others (Warner *et al.*, 1992), and there is no correlation between the length of the CAG repeat and clinical evidence of androgen insensitivity

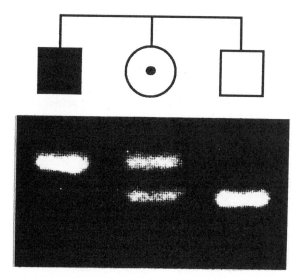

Figure 6.3 Pedigree of a patient with XLBSN (left), his carrier sister (middle) and normal brother (right). PCR products obtained by amplifying the relevant part of the androgen receptor gene are shown below each subject. The affected male has a larger fragment, containing the CAG expansion, than his unaffected brother. Their sister exhibits two fragments, one normal and one containing the expansion.

(La Spada *et al.*, 1992). There is a correlation between length of the repeat and neurological severity (Doyu *et al.*, 1992; La Spada *et al.*, 1992), and androgen receptors are expressed in motor neurons (Warner *et al.*, 1992). There is meiotic instability of the length of the CAG repeat, particularly in male meioses. Both contractions and expansions may occur, but without an obvious relationship to severity within families (Bianacalana *et al.*, 1992; La Spada *et al.*, 1992). However, the magnitude of variation in repeat length is small compared with that seen in other disorders associated with unstable trinucleotide repeats such as myotonic dystrophy, the fragile X syndrome, or Huntington's disease.

DNA analysis for the CAG expression in the androgen receptor gene is extremely useful in confirming the diagnosis (Figure 6.3), particularly in the 50% of patients who do not have affected relatives (Harding *et al.*, 1982). Such patients are often misdiagnosed as having amyotrophic lateral sclerosis (ALS). An accurate diagnosis of XLBSN confers a much better prognosis than that of ALS, and there are important genetic implications. All the daughters of an affected male will be carriers, and his sisters are likely to have a 50% chance of being carriers. No example of fresh mutation has been reported in this disease. Androgen receptor gene analysis can also be used for carrier detection and prenatal diagnosis. The analysis is simple, using the PCR to amplify the relevant part of the gene; a larger than normal allele is easily visualized (Figure 6.3).

REFERENCES

Almeida, M. R., Ferlini, A., Forabosco, A. *et al.* (1992). Two transthyretin variants (TTR Ala-49 and TTR Gln-89) in two Sicilian kindreds with hereditary amyloidosis. *Human Mutation*, **1**, 211–215

Andrade, C. (1952). A peculiar form of peripheral neuropathy: familial atypical generalized amyloidosis with special involvement of the peripheral nerves. *Brain*, **75**, 408–427

Aubourg, P. (1993). The leukodystrophies: a window to myelin. *Nature Genet.*, **5**, 105–106

Ben Othmane, K. B., Hentati, F., Lennon, F. *et al.* (1993a). Linkage of a locus (CMT4A) for autosomal recessive Charcot–Marie–Tooth disease to chromosome 8q. *Hum. Mol. Genet.*, **2**, 1625–1628

Ben Othmane, K., Middleton, L. T., Loprest, L. J. *et al.* (1993b). Localization of a gene (CMT2A) for autosomal dominant Charcot–Marie–Tooth disease type 2 to chromosome 1p and evidence of genetic heterogeneity. *Genomics*, **17**, 370–375

Benson, M. D. (1989). Familial amyloid polyneuropathy. *Trends Neurosci.*, **12**, 88–92

Benson, M. D. (1991). Inherited amyloidosis. *J. Med. Genet.*, **28**, 73–78

Benson, M. D., Wallace, M. R., Tejada, E. *et al.* (1987). Hereditary amyloidosis. Description of a new American kindred with late onset cardiomyopathy. Appalachian amyloid. *Arthritis Rheum.*, **30**, 195–200

Benson II, M. D., Turpin, J. C., Lucotte, G. *et al.* (1993). A transthyretin variant (alanine 71) associated with familial amyloidotic polyneuropathy in a French family. *J. Med. Genet.*, **30**, 120–122

Bergoffen, J. A., Trofatter, J., Pericak-Vance, M. A. *et al.* (1993a). Linkage localization of X-linked Charcot–Marie–Tooth disease. *Am. J. Hum. Genet.*, **52**, 312–318

Bergoffen, J., Scherer, S. S., Wang, S. *et al.* (1993b). Connexin mutations in X-linked Charcot–Marie–Tooth disease. *Science*, **262**, 2039–2042

Bhatia, K., Reilly, M., Adams, D. *et al.* (1993). Transthyretin gene mutations in British and French patients with amyloid neuropathy. *J. Neurol. Neurosurg. Psychiatry*, **56**, 694–697

Bianacalana, V., Serville, F., Pommier, J. *et al.* (1992). Moderate instability of the trinucleotide repeat in spinobulbar muscular atrophy. *Hum. Mol. Genet.*, **1**, 255–258

Boysen, G., Galassi, G. and Kamienecka, J. (1979). Familial amyloidosis with cranial neuropathy and corneal lattice dystrophy. *J. Neurol. Neurosurg. Psychiatry*, **42**, 1020–1030

Brice, A., Ravise, N., Stevanin, G., Gugenheim, M., Bouche, P., Penet, C., Agid, Y. and the French CMT Research Group (1992). Duplication within chromosome 17p11.2 in 12 families of French ancestry with Charcot–Marie–Tooth disease type 1a. *J. Med. Genet.*, **29**, 807–812

Cartier, N., Sarde, C.-O., Douar, A.-M. *et al.* (1993). Abnormal messenger RNA expression and a missense mutation in patients with X-linked adrenoleukodystrophy. *Hum. Mol. Genet.*, **2**, 1949–1951

Chance, P. F., Bird, T. D., Thomas, D. B. *et al.* (1990). Genetic linkage and heterogeneity in type I Charcot–Marie–Tooth disease (hereditary motor and sensory neuropathy type I). *Am. J. Hum. Genet.*, **47**, 915–925

Chance, P. F., Alderson, M. K., Leppig, K. A. *et al.* (1993). DNA deletion associated with hereditary neuropathy with liability to pressure palsies. *Cell*, **72**, 143–151

Chance, P. F., Abbas, N., Lensch, M. W. *et al.* (1994). Two autosomal dominant neuropathies result from reciprocal DNA duplication/deletion of a region on chromosome 17. *Hum. Mol. Genet.*, **3**, 223–228

Coelho, T., Sousa, A., Lourenco, E. and Ramalheira, J. (1994). A study of 159 Portuguese patients with familial amyloidotic polyneuropathy (FAP) whose patients were both unaffected. *J. Med. Genet.*, **31**, 293–299.

Costa, P., Figueira, A. S. and Bravo, R. R. (1978). Amyloid fibril protein related to prealbumin in familial amyloidotic polyneuropathy. *Proc. Natl Acad. Sci. USA*, **75**, 4499–4503

Davis, C. J., Bradley, W. G. and Madrid, R. (1978). The peroneal muscular atrophy syndrome: clinical, genetic, electrophysiological and nerve biopsy studies. I. Clinical, genetic and electrophysiological findings and classification. *J. Génét. Hum.*, **26**, 311–349

Davis, M. B., Rosenberg, R. N. and Harding, A. E. (1993). Molecular genetics and neurologic disease: an introduction. In *The Molecular and Genetic Basis of Neurological Disease* (R. N. Rosenberg, S. B Prusiner, S. DiMauro, R. L. Barchi and L. M. Kunkel, eds), Oxford: Butterworth-Heinemann

de la Chapelle, A., Tolvanen, R., Boysen, G. *et al.* (1992). Gelsolin-derived familial amyloidosis caused by asparagine or tyrosine substitution for aspartic acid at residue 187. *Nature Genet.*, **2**, 157–160

Doyu, M., Sobue, G., Mukai, E. *et al.* (1992). Severity of X-linked recessive bulbospinal neuronopathy correlates with size of tandem CAG repeat in androgen receptor gene. *Ann. Neurol.*, **32**, 707–710

Drugge, U., Anderson, R., Chizari, F. *et al.* (1993). Familial amyloidotic polyneuropathy in Sweden: a pedigree analysis. *J. Med. Genet.*, **30**, 388–392

Dwulet, F. E. and Benson, M. D. (1986). Characterisation of a transthyretin (prealbumin) variant associated with familial amyloidotic polyneuropathy Type II (Indiana/Swiss). *J. Clin. Invest.*, **78**, 880–886

Dyck, P. J., Chance, P., Lebo, R. and Carney, J. A. (1993). Hereditary and motor sensory neuropathies. In *Peripheral Neuropathy*, 3rd edn, (P. J. Dyck, P. K. Thomas, J. W. Griffin, P. A. Low and J. F. Poduslo, eds), pp. 1094–1136, Philadelphia: W. B. Saunders

Fairweather, N., Bell, C., Cochrane, S. *et al.* (1994). Mutations in the connexin 32 gene in X-linked domimant Charcot–Marie–Tooth disease (CMT1). *Hum. Mol. Genet.*, **3**, 29–34

Fischbeck, K. H., Ionasecu, V., Ritter, A. W. *et al.* (1986). Localization of the gene for X-linked spinal muscular atrophy. *Neurology*, **56**, 209–213

Gabreëls-Festen, A. and Gabreëls, F. (1993). Hereditary demyelinating motor and sensory neuropathy. *Brain Pathol.*, **3**, 135–146

Gabriel, G., Thomas, P. K., King, R. H. M. *et al.* (1986). Freeze-fracture observations on human peripheral nerve. *J. Anat.,*, **146**, 153–166

Gieselmann, V., Polten, A., Kreysing, J. and von Figura, K. (1989). Aryl sulfatase A pseudodeficiency: loss of a polyadenylation signal and N-glycosylation site. *Proc. Natl Acad. Sci. USA*, **86**, 9436–9440

Gorevic, P. D., Munoz, P. C., Gorgone, G. *et al.* (1991). Amyloidosis due to a mutation of the gelsolin gene in an American family with lattice corneal dystrophy type II. *N. Engl. J. Med.*, **325**, 1780–1785

Gregory, R., Thomas, P. K., King, R. H. M. *et al.* (1993). Coexistence of hereditary motor and sensory neuropathy type Ia and IgM paraproteinemic neuropathy. *Ann. Neurol.*, **33**, 649–652

Hahn, A. F., Brown, W. F., Koopman, W. J. and Feasby, T. E. (1990). X-linked dominant hereditary motor and sensory neuropathy. *Brain*, **113**, 1511–1526

Hallam, P. J., Harding, A. E., Berciano, J. *et al.* (1992). Gene mapping and mutation detection in hereditary motor and sensory neuropathy type I (Charcot–Marie–Tooth disease type 1). *Ann. Neurol.*, **31**, 570–572

Hamilton, J. A., Steinrauf, L. K., Braden, N. C. *et al.* (1993). The X-ray crystal structure refinements of normal human transthyretin and the amyloidogenic val-30→met variant to 1.7-Å resolution. *J. Biol. Chem.*, **268**, 2416–2424

Harding, A. E. and Thomas, P. K. (1980a). The clinical features of hereditary motor and sensory neuropathies types I and II. *Brain*, **103**, 259–280

Harding, A. E. and Thomas, P. K. (1980b). Genetic aspects of hereditary motor and sensory neuropathies (types I and II). *J. Med. Genet.*, **17**, 329–336

Harding, A. E. and Thomas, P. K. (1984). Genetically determined neuropathies. In *Peripheral Nerve Disorders: a Practical Approach*, (A. K. Asbury and R. W. Gilliatt, eds), pp. 205–242, London: Butterworth International Medical Reviews

Harding, A. E., Thomas, P. K., Baraitser, M. *et al.* (1982). X-linked recessive bulbospinal neuronopathy: a report of ten cases. *J. Neurol. Neurosurg. Psychiatry*, **45**, 1012–1019

Hayasaka, K., Nanao, K., Tahara, M. *et al.* (1991). Isolation and sequence determination of cDNA encoding the major structural component of human peripheral myelin. *Biochem. Biophys. Res. Commun.*, **180**, 515–518

Hayasaka, K., Himoro, M., Sato, W. *et al.* (1993a). Charcot–Marie–Tooth neuropathy type 1B is associated with mutations of the myelin P_0 gene. *Nature Genet.*, **5**, 31–34

Hayasaka, K., Takada, G. and Ionasescu, V. V. (1993b). Mutation of the P_0 gene in Charcot–Marie–Tooth neuropathy type 1B. *Hum. Mol. Genet.*, **2**, 1369–1372

Hayasaka, K., Himoro, M., Sawaishi, Y. *et al.* (1993c). De novo mutation of the myelin P0 gene in Dejerine–Sottas disease (hereditary motor and sensory neuropathy type III). *Nature Genet.*, **5**, 266–268

Hensels, G. W., Janssen, E. A. M., Hoogendijk, J. E. *et al.* (1993). Quantitative measurement of duplicated DNA as a diagnostic test for Charcot–Marie–Tooth disease type Ia. *Clin. Chem.*, **39**, 1845–1849

Holmgren, G., Drugge, U., Haettner, E. *et al.* (1992). Four Swedish patients with homozygosity for the TTR Met 30 gene. *Arquivos de Medicina*, **3**, 193–197

Holmgren, G., Ericzon, B.-G., Groth, C.-G. *et al.* (1993). Clinical improvement and amyloid regression after liver transplantation in hereditary transthyretin amyloidosis. *Lancet*, **341**, 1113–1116

Holt, I. J., Harding, A. E., Middleton, L. *et al.* (1989). Molecular genetics of amyloid neuropathy in Europe. *Lancet*, **1**, 524–526

Hoogendijk, J. E., Hensels, G. W., Gabreëls-Festen, A. A. W. M. *et al.* (1992). De-novo mutation in hereditary motor and sensory neuropathy type I. *Lancet*, **339**, 1081–1082

Ii, S., Minnerath, S., Ii, K. *et al.* (1991). Two-tiered DNA-based diagnosis of transthyretin amyloidosis reveals two novel point mutations. *Neurology*, **41**, 893–898

Ionasescu, V., Searby, C. and Ionasescu, R. (1994). Point mutations of the connexin 32 (GJB1) gene in X-linked dominant Charcot–Marie–Tooth neuropathy. *Hum. Mol. Genet.*, **3**, 355–358

Izumoto, S., Younger, D., Hays, A. P. *et al.* (1992). Familial amyloidotic polyneuropathy presenting with carpal tunnel syndrome and a new transthyretin mutation, asparagine 70. *Neurology*, **42**, 2094–2102

Kiuru, S., Seppäläinen, A. M., Haltia, M. *et al.* (1992). Familial amyloidosis of the Finnish type (FAF) – a clinical study of 30 patients. *J. Neurol.*, **239** (suppl 2), S41

Kulkens, T., Bolhuis, P. A., Wolterman, R. A. *et al.* (1993). Deletion of the serine 34 codon from the major peripheral myelin protein P_0 gene in Charcot–Marie–Tooth disease type 1B. *Nature Genet.*, **5**, 35–39.

La Spada, A. R., Wilson, E. M., Lubahn, D. B. *et al.* (1991). Androgen receptor gene mutations in X-linked spinal and bulbar muscular atrophy. *Nature*, **352**, 77–79

La Spada, A. R., Roling, D. B. and Harding, A. E. (1992). Meiotic stability and genotype–phenotype correlation of the trinucleotide repeat in X-linked spinal and bulbar muscular atrophy. *Nature Genet.*, **2**, 301–304

Lebo, R. V., Chance, P. F., Dyck, P. J. *et al.* (1991). Chromosome 1 Charcot–Marie–Tooth disease (CMT1B) locus in the Fcγ receptor gene region. *Hum. Genet.*, **88**, 1–12

Levy, E., Haltia, M. and Frenandez-Madrid, I. (1990). Mutation in gelsolin gene in Finnish Hereditary Amyloidosis. *J. Exp. Med.*, **172**, 1865–1867

Low, P. A., Bartelson, J. D., Daube, J. and Swanson, C. J. (1982). Prednisone responsive hereditary motor and sensory neuropathy. *Mayo Clin. Proc.*, **57**, 239–246

Lupski, J. R., Montes de Oca-Luna, R., Slaugenhaupt, S. *et al.* (1991). DNA duplication associated with Charcot–Marie–Tooth disease type 1A. *Cell*, **66**, 219–232

Matsunami, N., Smith, B., Ballard, L. *et al.* (1992). Peripheral myelin protein-22 gene maps in the duplication in chromosome 17p11.2 associated with Charcot–Marie–Tooth 1A. *Nature Genet.*, **1**, 176–179

Meretoja, J. (1969). Familial systemic paramyloidosis with lattice dystrophy of the cornea, progressive cranial neuropathy, skin changes and various internal symptoms. *Ann. Clin. Res.*, **1**, 314–324

Mosser, J., Douar, A.-M., Sarde, C.-O. *et al.* (1993). Putative X-linked adrenoleukodystrophy gene shares unexpected homology with ABC transporters. *Nature*, **361**, 726–730

Murakami, T., Maeda, S., Yi, S. *et al.* (1992). A novel transthyretin mutation associated with familial amyloidotic polyneuropathy. *Biochem. Biophys. Res. Commun.*, **182**, 520–526

Nakazato, M., Kangawa, K., Minamino, N. *et al.* (1984). Revised analysis of amino acid replacement in a prealbumin variant (SKO-111) associated with familial amyloidotic polyneuropathy of Jewish origin. *Biochem. Biophys. Res. Commun.*, **123**, 921–928

Nakazato, M., Sasaki, H., Furuya, H. *et al.* (1987). Biochemical and genetic characterization of type I familial amyloidotic polyneuropathy. *Ann. Neurol.*, **21**, 596–598

Nelis, E., Timmerman, V., De Jonghe, P. and Van Broeckhoven, C. (1994). Identification of a 5′ splice site mutation in the PMP-22 gene in autosomal dominant Charcot–Marie–Tooth disease type 1. *Hum. Mol. Genet.*, **3**, 515–516

Nichols, W. C., Leipnieks, J. J., McKusick, V. A. and Benson, M. D. (1989). Direct sequencing of the gene for Maryland/German familial amyloidotic polyneuropathy type II and genotyping by allele-specific enzymatic amplification. *Genomics*, **5**, 535–540

Nichols, W. C., Gregg, R. E., Brewer, B. H. and Benson, M. D. (1990). A mutation in apolipoprotein A-1 in the Iowa type of Familial Amyloidotic Polyneuropathy. *Genomics*, **8**, 318–323

Nicholson, G. A. and Nash, J. (1993). Intermediate nerve conduction velocities define X-linked Charcot–Marie–Tooth neuropathy families. *Neurology*, **43**, 2558–2564

Nicholson, G. A., Valentijn, L. J., Cherryson, A. K. *et al.* (1994). A frame shift mutation in the PMP22 gene in hereditary neuropathy with liability to pressure palsies. *Nature Genet.*, **6**, 263–266

Palau, F., Lofgren, A., De Jonghe, P. *et al.* (1993). Origin of the de novo duplication in Charcot–Marie–Tooth disease type 1A: unequal non sister chromatid exchange during spermatogenesis. *Hum. Mol. Genet.*, **2**, 2031–2035

Patel, P. I., Roa, B. B., Welcher, A. A. *et al.* (1992). The gene for the peripheral myelin protein PMP-22 is a candidate for Charcot–Marie–Tooth disease type 1A. *Nature Genet.*, **1**, 159–165

Pentao, L., Wise, C. A., Chinault, A. C. *et al.* (1992). Charcot–Marie–Tooth type 1A duplication appears to arise from recombination at repeat sequences flanking the 1.5 Mb monomer unit. *Nature Genet.*, **2**, 292–300

Raeymaekers, P., Timmerman, V., Nelis, E. *et al.* (1991). Duplication in chromosome 17p11.2 in Charcot–Marie–Tooth neuropathy type 1a (CMT 1a). *Neuromusc. Dis.*, **1**, 93–97

Regnault, V., Costa, P. M. P., Teixeira, A. *et al.* (1992). Specific removal of transthyretin from plasma of patients with familial amyloidotic polyneuropathy: optimization of an immunoadsorption procedure. *Int. J. Artif. Organs*, **15**, 249–255

Reilly, M. M., Adams, D., Davis, M. B. *et al.* (1995a). Haplotype analysis of French, British and other European patients with familial amyloid polyneuropathy (Met 30 and Tyr 77). *J. Neurol.*, in press

Reilly, M. M., Staunton, H. and Harding, A. E. (1995b). Familial amyloid polyneuropathy (TTR ala 60) in northwest Ireland: a clinical genetic and epidemiological study. *J. Neurol. Neurosurg. Psychiatry*, in press

Roa, B. B., Dyck, P. J., Marks, H. G. *et al.* (1993a). Dejerine–Sottas syndrome associated with point mutation in the peripheral myelin protein 22 (PMP22) gene. *Nature Genet.*, **5**, 269–273

Roa, B. B., Garcia, C. A., Suter, U. *et al.* (1993b). Charcot–Marie–Tooth disease type 1A. Association with a spontaneous point mutation in the PMP22 gene. *N. Engl. J. Med.*, **329**, 96–101

Roa, B. B., Garcia, C. A., Pentao, L. *et al.* (1993c). Evidence for a recessive PMP22 point mutation in Charcot–Marie–Tooth disease type 1A. *Nature Genet.*, **5**, 189–194

Rozear, M. P., Pericak-Vance, M. A., Fischbeck, K. *et al.* (1987). Hereditary and motor sensory neuropathy, X-linked: a half century follow-up. *Neurology*, **37**, 1460–1465

Saeki, Y., Ueno, S., Yorifuji, S. *et al.* (1991). New mutant gene (transthyretin Arg 58) in cases with hereditary polyneuropathy detected with non-isotope method of single-strand conformation polymorphism analysis. *Biochem. Biophys. Res. Commun.*, **180**, 380–385

Saraiva, M. J. M. (1991). Recent advances in the molecular pathology of familial amyloidotic polyneuropathy. *Neuromusc. Dis.*, **1**, 3–6

Shiomi, K., Nakazato, M., Matsukura, S. *et al.* (1993). A basic transthyretin variant (glu 61-lys) causes familial amyloidotic polyneuropathy: protein and DNA sequencing and PCR-induced mutation restriction analysis. *Biochem. Biophys. Res. Commun.*, **194**, 1090–1096.

Skare, J. C., Saraiva, M. J. M., Alves, I. L. *et al.* (1989). A new mutation causing familial amyloidotic polyneuropathy. *Biochem. Biophys. Res. Commun.*, **164**, 1240–1246

Skinner, M., Lewis, W. D., Jones, L. A. *et al.* (1994). Liver transplantation as a treatment for familial amyloidotic polyneuropathy. *Ann. Int. Med.*, **120**, 133–134

Spray, D. C. (1994). CMTX1: a gap junction genetic disease. *Lancet*, **343**, 1111–1112

Staunton, H., Dervan, P., Kale, R. *et al.* (1987). Hereditary amyloid polyneuropathy in north west Ireland. *Brain*, **110**, 1231–1245

Staunton, H., Davis, M. B., Guiloff, R. J. *et al.* (1991). Irish (Donegal) amyloidosis associated with the transthyretin ALA 60 (Appalachian) variant. *Brain*, **114**, 2675–2679

Su, Y., Brooks, D. G., Li, L. *et al.* (1993). Myelin protein zero gene mutated in Charcot–Marie–Tooth type 1B patients. *Proc. Natl Acad. Sci. USA*, **90**, 10856–10860

Sunada, Y., Shimizu, T., Nakase, H. *et al.* (1993). Inherited amyloid polyneuropathy type IV (gelsolin variant) in a Japanese family. *Ann. Neurol.*, **33**, 57–62

Suter, U., Welcher, A. A., Ozcelik, T. *et al.* (1992a). Trembler mouse carries a point mutation in a myelin gene. *Nature*, **356**, 241–244

Suter, U., Moskow, J. J., Welcher, A. A. *et al.* (1992b). A leucine-to-proline mutation in the first transmembrane domain of the 22-kDa peripheral myelin protein in the trembler-J mouse. *Proc. Natl Acad Sci. USA*, **89**, 4382–4386

Suter, U., Welcher, A. A. and Snipes, G. J. (1993). Progress in the molecular understanding of hereditary peripheral neuropathies reveals new insights into the biology of the peripheral nervous system. *Trends Neurosci.*, **16**, 50–55

Tashiro, F., Yi, S., Wakasugi, S. *et al.* (1991). Role of serum amyloid P component for systemic amyloidosis in transgenic mice carrying human mutant transthyretin gene. *Gerontology*, **37**, 56–62

Tetzlaff, W. (1982). Tight junction contact events and temporary gap junctions in the sciatic nerve of the chicken during Wallerian degeneration and subsequent regeneration. *J. Neurocytol.*, **11**, 839–858

Thomas, P. K. (1993). Other inherited neuropathies. In *Peripheral Neuropathy*, 3rd edn (P. J. Dyck, P. K. Thomas, J. W. Griffen, P. A. Low and J. F. Poduslo, eds), pp. 1194–1218, Philadelphia: W. B. Saunders

Timmerman, V., Nelis, E., van Hull, W. *et al.* (1992). The peripheral myelin protein gene PMP-22 is contained within the Charcot–Marie–Tooth disease type 1A duplication. *Nature Genet.*, **1**, 171–175

Tyson, J., Malcolm, S., Thomas, P. K. *et al.* (1995). Deletions of chromosome 17p11.2 in multifocal neuropathies. Submitted

Uemichi, T., Murrell, J. R., Zeldenrust, S. and Benson, M. D. (1992). A new mutant transthyretin (Arg 10) associated with familial amyloid polyneuropathy. *J. Med. Genet.*, **29**, 888–891

Ueno, S., Uemichi, T., Yorifuji, S. and Tarui, S. (1990a). A novel variant of transthyretin (Tyr[114] to Cys) deduced from the nucleotide sequences of gene fragments from familial amyloidotic polyneuropathy in Japanese sibling cases. *Biochem. Biophys. Res. Commun.*, **169**, 143–147

Ueno, S., Uemichi, T., Takahaski, N. *et al.* (1990b). Two novel variants of transthyretin identified in Japanese cases with familial amyloidotic polyneuropathy: transthyretin (Glu[42] to Gly) and transthyretin (Ser[50] to Arg). *Biochem. Biophys. Res. Commun.*, **169**, 1117–1121

Valentijn, L. J., Bolhuis, P. A., Zorn, I. *et al.* (1992a). The peripheral myelin gene PMP-22/GAS-3 is duplicated in Charcot–Marie–Tooth disease type 1A. *Nature Genet.*, **1**, 166–170

Valentijn, L. J., Baas, F., Wolterman, R. A. *et al.* (1992b). Identical point mutations of PMP-22 in Trembler-J mouse and Charcot–Marie–Tooth disease type 1A. *Nature Genet.*, **2**, 288–291

Valentijn, L. J., Baas, F., Zorn, I. *et al.* (1993). Alternatively sized duplication in Charcot–Marie–Tooth disease type 1A. *Hum. Mol. Genet.*, **2**, 2143–2146

Van Allen, M. W., Frohlich, J. A. and Davis, J. R. (1969). Inherited predisposition to generalised amyloidosis. Clinical and pathological study of a family with neuropathy, nephropathy and peptic ulcer. *Neurology (Minneapolis)*, **19**, 10–25

Vance, J. M., Barker, D., Yamaoka, L. H. *et al.* (1991). Localisation of Charcot–Marie–Tooth disease type 1a (CMT1a) to chromosome 17p11.2. *Genomics*, **9**, 623–628

Wallace, M. R., Dwulet, F. E., Williams, E. C. *et al.* (1986). Biochemical and molecular genetic characterization of a new variant prealbumin associated with hereditary amyloidosis. *J. Clin. Invest.*, **78**, 6–12

Warner, C. L., Griffin, J. E., Wilson, J. D. *et al.* (1992). X-linked spinomuscular atrophy: a kindred with associated abnormal androgen receptor binding. *Neurology*, **42**, 2181–2184

Welcher, A. A., Suter, U., de Leon, M. *et al.* (1991). A myelin protein is encoded by the homologue of a growth arrest-specific gene. *Proc. Natl Acad. Sci. USA*, **88**, 7195–7199

Windebank, A. J. (1993). Inherited recurrent focal neuropathies. In *Peripheral Neuropathy*, 3rd edn (P. J. Dyck, P. K. Thomas, J. W. Griffin, P. A. Low and J. F. Poduslo, eds), pp. 1137–1148, Philadelphia: W. B. Saunders

Wise, C. A., Garcia, C. A., Davis, S. N. *et al.* (1993). Molecular analyses of unrelated Charcot–Marie–Tooth (CMT) disease patients suggest a high frequency of the CMT1A duplication. *Am. J. Hum. Genet.*, **53**, 853–863

World Federation of Neurology Research Group on Huntington's Disease (1993). Presymptomatic testing for Huntington's disease. A world-wide survey. *J. Med. Genet.*, **30**, 1020–1022

Yasuda, T., Sobue, G., Doyu, M. *et al.* (1994). Familial amyloidotic polyneuropathy with late-onset and well-preserved autonomic function: a Japanese kindred with novel mutant transthyretin (Ala 97 to Gly). *J. Neurol. Sci.*, **121**, 97–102

Yi, S., Takahashi, K., Naito, M. *et al.* (1991). Systemic amyloidosis in mice carrying the human mutant transthyretin (Met 30) gene. Pathologic similarity to human familial amyloidotic polyneurology, type I. *Am. J. Pathol.*, **138**, 403–412

Yoshioka, K., Furuya, H., Sasaki, H. *et al.* (1989). Haplotype analysis of familial amyloidotic polyneuropathy. *Hum. Genet.*, **82**, 9–13

7
Neurofibromatosis types 1 and 2

J. R. Pleasure, P. F. Chance and D. E. Pleasure

INTRODUCTION

Neurofibromatosis type 1 (NF1, von Recklinghausen neurofibromatosis, peripheral neurofibromatosis) is the most common dominantly inherited disorder affecting the peripheral nervous system (PNS), with a prevalence of approximately 1 in 3000. The clinical features of NF1 include Schwann cell tumours and focal skin and iris hyperpigmentation. Neurofibromatosis type 2 (NF2, central neurofibromatosis) is a rare, dominantly inherited disorder characterized by bilateral acoustic nerve Schwann cell tumours. NF1 and NF2 are caused by mutations of tumour suppressor genes on chromosomes 17 and 22 respectively. This chapter will review the clinical and molecular aspects of these two disorders.

CLINICAL FEATURES OF NF1

Clinical diagnosis of NF1 requires the presence of two or more of the following (Stumpf *et al.*, 1988):

(1) Six or more café-au-lait macules, each over 5 mm in greatest diameter (if prepubertal) or over 15 mm (if postpubertal)
(2) Two or more dermal neurofibromas, or at least one plexiform neurofibroma
(3) Axillary or inguinal freckling
(4) Optic glioma
(5) Iris melanomatous hamartomas (Lisch nodules)
(6) Cranial sphenoid bone dysplasia or long bone cortical thinning with or without pseudarthrosis
(7) A first-degree relative with NF1

Recognition of NF1 may be difficult in the neonatal period. At this age, café-au-lait spots are absent in a significant proportion of patients and, if present, may be small and only subtly different from normal skin in colour (Figure 7.1). Dermal neurofibromas are usually not evident. Congenital neurofibromas, if present, are generally plexiform or highly vascular and may compress critical sites such as the

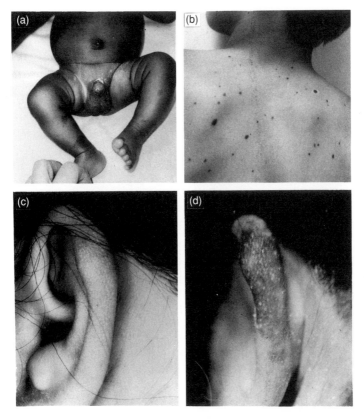

Figure 7.1 Phenotypic features of NF1. (a) Café-au-lait spots on the legs of an infant with NF1. (b) Multiple small café-au-lait spots on the back of an older child with NF1. (c) and (d) A café-au-lait spot on the ear of an adult with NF1, viewed under normal light (c) and under a Woods lamp (d).

airway (Pleasure and Geller, 1967). Dermal and plexiform neurofibromas often increase in number and size during puberty and pregnancy. The plexiform neurofibromas may cause focal nerve compression, for example of the median nerve in the carpal tunnel. There may be generalized overgrowth of a limb or phalanx distal to a plexiform neurofibroma. Orbital plexiform neurofibromas may distort the globe, resulting in buphthalmos and glaucoma. Occasional patients have disseminated plexiform neurofibromas that simulate focal hypertrophic neuropathy. Schwannomas arising from nerve roots may compress the spinal cord. Radiological findings include osteolysis of vertebral bodies with significant kyphosis (Craig and Govender, 1992). There may be vertebral scalloping, even without tumours (Riccardi, 1981).

Café-au-lait spots (Figure 7.1), axillary freckling and Lisch nodules (Figure 7.2) become more prominent during childhood. In a series of 41 children who had six or more café-au-lait macules at their first visit and were followed yearly, NF1 was eventually diagnosed in 26, by the development of skin crease freckling in 18, Lisch nodules in five, and neurofibromas in three (Korf, 1992). Short stature is

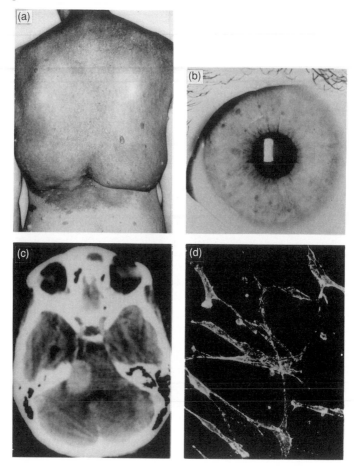

Figure 7.2 Phenotypic and other findings in NF1 and NF2. (a) A massive region of skin hyperpigmentation and multiple dermal and plexiform neurofibromas on the back of an adult with NF1. (b) Lisch nodules in the iris of a child with NF1. (c) Enhanced CT scan of a young adult with NF2, showing a large vestibular schwannoma. (d) A monolayer culture prepared from a dissociated dermal neurofibroma from an adult with NF1, immunostained with a monoclonal antibody against the low affinity nerve growth factor receptor, showing spindle-shaped and multipolar Schwann cells.

common, while about 10% of patients develop scoliosis (Akbarnia *et al.*, 1992). There is marked heterogeneity in clinical severity of NF1 even with a family.

Headaches, macrocephaly and learning disability are frequent. Brain imaging may show non-specific brain enlargement, enlarged ventricles or central nervous system (CNS) hamartomas and glial rests. Optic glioma may develop, and present with visual field defect (Riccardi, 1981; DiMario *et al.*, 1993).

The incidences of benign neural crest-derived tumours such as pheochromocytoma, carcinoid and somatostatinoma, and of malignancies arising from neural crest (neurofibrosarcoma) or other embryological origins (childhood leukaemia, rhabdomyosarcoma) are increased in NF1 patients (Bader and Miller, 1978; Perilongo *et al.*, 1993). The propensity for malignant tumours was studied in 212 patients with NF1 followed for 42 years in Denmark (Sorensen *et al.*, 1986). Eighty-four severely affected probands and 128 mildly affected relatives had a relative risk of new malignant tumours of 4.0 and 1.5 times, respectively. Second tumours occurred in 33% of the NF1 probands, compared with 4% of the general population.

PATHOLOGY OF NF1

Café-au-lait spots and axillary freckles in NF1 are caused by increased synthesis of melanin by skin melanocytes (Kaufmann *et al.*, 1991). Lisch nodules are hamartomas enriched in iris melanocytes. Dermal neurofibromas, which arise in continuity with small subcutaneous nerves, contain Schwann cells interspersed with unmyelinated axons, fibroblasts, small blood vessels, mast cells and collagen fibrils. Activation of neurofibroma mast cells may be responsible for the pruritus sometimes associated with these lesions. Neurofibroma Schwann cells resemble Schwann cells in traumatic neuromas; they are bi- to multipolar, and stain immunohistologically with antibodies against the low affinity nerve growth factor receptor (Sobue *et al.*, 1985; see Figure 7.2), 2',3'-cyclic nucleotide-3'-phosphohydrolase, S-100 protein, or cell adhesion molecules expressing HNK-1 carbohydrate epitopes.

Plexiform neurofibromas arise in deeper nerves, and resemble dermal neurofibromas in cellular composition, but may also contain regions in which Schwann cells have formed onion bulb-like arrays around en passant axons. Sarcomatous transformation of plexiform neurofibroma may occur; this should be suspected when there is a rapid increase in size, and can be confirmed histologically by the demonstration of aggregates of pleomorphic Schwann cells with frequent mitotic figures.

Patients with NF1 are at increased risk of developing spinal root and peripheral nerve schwannomas. Fibroblasts are far less common in schwannomas than in neurofibromas, and axons are rare or absent. The Schwann cells in schwannomas are arranged in two patterns: bundles of bipolar, spindle-shaped cells, sometimes in palisades (Antoni type A tissue); and loosely packed whorls (Antoni type B tissue) (Rubinstein and Korf, 1990).

Pilocytic astrocytomas of the optic nerves and third ventricular region are common in NF1. Even more frequent are dysplastic lesions of the CNS, including subependymal glial nodules, regions of proliferative gliosis, and neuronal heterotopias (Russell and Rubinstein, 1989; Rubinstein and Korf, 1990).

Meningioangiomatosis (Drut *et al.*, 1993) is a benign lesion of the meninges made up of neural crest-derived meningeal cells with blood vessels, psammoma bodies (spherical, laminated concretions with osteoid deposition) and macrophages. It is rare but associated with NF1 in more than half the 30 reported cases. Resection is curative.

MOLECULAR GENETICS OF NF1

With its high incidence and rate of mutation, it could be speculated that the NF1 gene would be unusually large or might have one or more so-called 'hotspots' for mutation. It appears that the former case is more likely true. The initial gene assignment by linkage analysis for NF1 was made to the region of chromosome 17q11.2 through the use of linked anonymous DNA markers (Barker *et al.*, 1987). The attempt to identify the NF1 gene through positional cloning strategies was greatly expedited by the recognition of two NF1 patients with associated cytogenetically detectable lesions involving chromosome 17q11.2. One patient had a t(1;17) (Schmidt *et al.*, 1987), and the other a t(17;22) (Ledbetter *et al.*, 1989). In both situations, the translocation breakpoint fell within band 17q11.2, the region of the NF1 locus as defined by studies with tightly linked flanking markers. Subsequently, it was shown that the translocation breakpoints actually could be localized to the same 600-kb (kilobase) *Nru*I DNA fragment. Further cloning and mapping of the translocation breakpoint region showed that the two breakpoints in the NF1 patients fell within a 60-kb interval (O'Connell *et al.*, 1989a,b) and detected small deletions in this region in other patients (Viskochil *et al.*, 1990), leading to the identification of the NF1 gene. Sequence analysis using transcripts from the break-point region detected single-base change mutations, predicted to inactivate the NF1 gene in patients (Cawthon *et al.*, 1990a), and provided additional evidence that the NF1 gene was in hand. Independently, two cDNA clones (Wallace *et al.*, 1990) were isolated from the translocation breakpoint region and demonstrated sequence identity to that reported associated with point mutations in NF1 patients (Cawthon *et al.*, 1990a).

Interestingly, during the process of investigating the translocation breakpoint region for NF1 candidate genes, three additional genes (EVI2A, EVI2B and OMgp) mapping to the translocation breakpoint region were detected (Cawthon *et al.*, 1990b, 1991; Viskochil *et al.*, 1991). These three genes are entirely contained within the NF1 gene and are transcribed in the opposite direction from which transcription occurs in the NF1 gene. The relationships of the NF1 gene to these other genes contained within it are illustrated in Figure 7.2. EVI2A and EVI2B are human homologues of mouse protooncogenes and are thought to possibly play a role in the genesis of murine leukemias (Buchberg *et al.*, 1988). OMgp (oligodendrocyte–myelin glycoprotein) was briefly an exciting candidate for NF1 as it is an abundantly expressed myelin protein (Mikol *et al.*, 1990). However, no OMgp-specific mutations were found to be associated with NF1 (Viskochil *et al.*, 1991). The significance, if any, of the location and orientation of these three genes within the NF1 gene remains unknown.

The NF1 gene is unusually large, spanning approximately 350 kb and encoding a 13-kb messenger RNA. The predicted NF1 protein is composed of 2818 amino acids and has a molecular mass of 327 kDa (Marchuk *et al.*, 1991). It is composed of 49 exons, with two alternately spliced forms (Gutmann and Collins, 1993). The NF1 gene is ubiquitously expressed (Wallace *et al.*, 1990) and its protein product is known as neurofibromin. Neurofibromin carries sequence homology with the GTPase-activating protein (GAP) superfamily of genes (Ballester *et al.*, 1990; Martin *et al.*, 1990; Xu *et al.*, 1990a,b), including mammalian GAP, yeast IRA1, IRA2, and sar1 and *Drosophila* Gap1.

Because of the large size of the NF1 gene and the apparent degree of heterogeneity in type of mutations, abnormalities have not been detected in the overwhelming majority (>90%) of patients. Furthermore, the high spontaneous mutation rate for NF1 may increase the difficulties of molecular genetic diagnosis in many cases. Locus genetic heterogeneity for NF1 has not been found, and a study of 34 families in Italy confirmed linkage to chromosome 17q11.2 markers for all pedigrees (Clementi *et al.*, 1991). For the majority of presumed *de novo* mutations in NF1,

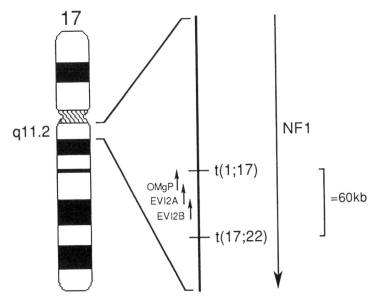

Figure 7.3 Idiogram of chromosome 17 with expanded view depicting the region of the NF1 locus in band 17q11.2. Relative positions of two known translocations in NF1 patients are shown. Orientation and direction of transcription for the EVI2A, EVI2B and OMgp genes are given.

most are of paternal origin, implicating problems during male germ cell meiosis (Jadeyel *et al.*, 1990).

Aside from the two previously mentioned chromosomal translocations involving band 17q11.2, various deletions in the NF1 gene have been found (Upadhyaya *et al.*, 1990; Viskochil *et al.*, 1990). A 320-bp Alu repetitive element insertion resulting in a splice site disruption and frameshift mutation has been described (Wallace *et al.*, 1991). Point mutations have included Lys to Glu or Lys to Gln substitutions at position 1423 (Li *et al.*, 1992) and an Arg to stop codon at positions 1610 (Cawthon *et al.*, 1990a) or 365 (Estivill *et al.*, 1991).

With direct analysis for specific NF1 mutations available for only a small portion of patients, DNA-based diagnosis relying upon polymorphic intragenic and closely linked markers becomes a mainstay for families seeking either presymptomatic or prenatal diagnosis of NF1. However, the currently available DNA markers for diagnosis are only informative in approximately 75% of pedigrees (Vivarelli *et al.*, 1991; Upadhyaya *et al.*, 1992; Rodenhiser *et al.*, 1993), and linkage dysequilibrium which serves to limit the usefulness of a clustered set of markers has been found for the NF1 region (Messiaen *et al.*, 1993).

The often extreme variability in expression of NF1 within a family contributes to the difficulty of genetic counselling in this disorder. Environmental factors may contribute to this variability. However, analysis of the correlation between numbers of café-au-lait spots or neurofibromas and the degree of relatedness within a family suggests that as yet unidentified genes influence penetrance of NF1 mutations (Ponder, 1992).

A mutation in the NF1 gene has been demonstrated recently in a family with features of Watson and Noonan syndromes, consisting of a tandem duplication of 42 base pairs in an exon (Allanson *et al.*, 1985; Tassabenji *et al.*, 1993). Patients with Watson syndrome have many of the clinical features of NF1, including café-au-lait spots and short stature in 80%, Lisch nodules in 58%, retardation or learning difficulties in 68%, neurofibromas in 30% and axillary freckling (Allanson *et al.*, 1991; Stern *et al.*, 1992).

CELL BIOLOGY OF NF1

NF1 is characterized by multifocal Schwann cell hyperplasia. Neurofibromas are frequent, and are often excised for cosmetic reasons. Despite this abundance of tissue for study, and the advances in molecular genetics of NF1 summarized above, we as yet poorly understand the cell biology of NF1.

Because of the admixture of cell types within neurofibromas, it is unclear whether the Schwann cells in these benign tumours are monoclonal or polyclonal. In either case, a local change in Schwann cells or their environment must be present to explain the occurrence of foci or Schwann cell hyperplasia in some regions of the PNS, and not others. The nature of this local factor is not known, although it has been established that neurofibrosarcoma arising from a plexiform neurofibroma or schwannoma is monoclonal, and that the tumour cells lack a normal copy of the NF1 gene because of a 'second hit' (Skuse *et al.*, 1989, 1991; Ponder, 1992).

While there are obviously too many Schwann cells in neurofibromas and schwannomas of patients with NF1, and these Schwann cells have a mutation affecting one copy of the NF1 gene, tissue culture studies have failed to demonstrate any abnormal behaviours of NF1 Schwann cells. These is one report that Schwann cells isolated from NF1 neurofibromas and transplanted to a chick egg chorioallantoic membrane are better able to induce angiogenesis and to penetrate basement membranes than are normal Schwann cells (Sheela *et al.*, 1990), but this observation has not yet been confirmed. While it might seem self-evident that an abnormality in NF1 Schwann cells causes neurofibromas and schwannomas to develop, it is too early to discard an alternative scenario, in which there is a failure by NF1 neurons to drive Schwann cells to their terminally differentiated states.

Neurofibromin catalyses the conversion of GTP bound to the signal transduction protein, p-21 *ras*, to GDP. This causes inhibition of the interaction between *ras* and the next protein in this signalling cascade, *raf*, and prevents *ras* from influencing cell proliferation and differentiation (Warne *et al.*, 1993). It is of interest that the gene mutated in another phakomatosis, tuberous sclerosis, may also have GTPase activity (Nellist *et al.*, 1993).

Neurofibrosarcomas, which have markedly depressed levels of neurofibromin, demonstrate increased ratios of activated to inactivated p21–*ras*. Neurofibromin deficiency and increased levels of activated p22–*ras* have also been observed in some human neuroblastoma and melanoma cell lines (Menon *et al.*, 1990; Andersen *et al.*, 1993; The *et al.*, 1993). Proliferation of these cultured tumour cells is inhibited, and their differentiation enhanced, by transfection with complementary DNA encoding normal neurofibromin (DeClue *et al.*, 1992). These observations support the concept that the NF1 gene is a tumour suppressor gene. Further support for this comes from the finding that the normal NF1 allele was lost from marrow cell DNA in five children with malignant myeloid syndromes and NF1 (Shannon *et al.*, 1994).

Most embryonic tissues express neurofibromin, but later in development, expression becomes progressively restricted to neurons and glia of the CNS and PNS, and to adrenal medulla (Daston and Ratner, 1992; Daston *et al.*, 1992; Nordlund *et al.*, 1993). The mechanism of this tissue-specific regulation of neurofibromin protein expression is not known. Neurofibromin GAP enzyme activity in the various tissues is also regulated at the level of RNA processing. Two forms of neurofibromin RNA are formed by alternative splicing. Neurofibromin type 1, which predominates during the first 20 weeks of human gestation, is a more potent inactivator of p21-*ras* than is neurofibromin type 2, which is the preferred transcript later in development (Gutmann and Collins, 1993). The level of expression of neurofibromin type 2 by Schwann cells is subject to modulation by the environment; agents which markedly raise intracellular $3',5'$-cyclic adenosine-$3'$-phosphohydrolase (cAMP) levels, and induce the synthesis of myelin lipids and proteins (Sobue *et al.*, 1986; Shuman *et al.*, 1988), also induce expression of neurofibromin type 2 (Gutmann *et al.*, 1993). An additional way in which neurofibromin GAP activity is modulated is by association with microtubules. Tubulin partially inhibits neurofibromin GAP. Targeting to microtubules is conferred by regions of the neurofibromin molecule in or adjacent to the GAP domain (Bollag *et al.*, 1993; Gregory *et al.*, 1993).

The GAP domain accounts for only about 10% of the neurofibromin sequence. Most of the mutations of the NF1 gene thus far recognized do not directly affect this region of the protein (Ponder, 1992). It is reasonable to speculate, therefore, that some of the tissue abnormalities in NF1 result from defects in non-GAP-related functions of neurofibromin. This speculation is supported by two recent observations: (1) that over-expression of neurofibromin in 3T3 fibroblasts inhibits growth of the cells without altering the level of activity of *ras* in the cells; and (2) that transformation of cells with v-*ras*, an oncogenic member of the *ras* family resistant to inactivation by neurofibromin GAP, is suppressed by transfection with neurofibromin (Johnson *et al.*, 1994).

NF2

NF2 is a dominantly inherited disorder with an incidence of 1 in 35 000 births and at least a 50% new mutation rate. Criteria for diagnosis of NF2 (Stumpf *et al.*, 1988) include:

(1) Bilateral vestibular schwannomas or
(2) Family history of NF2 plus
    (a) unilateral vestibular schwannoma or
    (b) any two of: meingioma, glioma, neurofibroma, schwannoma, posterior subcapsular lenticular opacities
    (c) cerebral calcification

Symptoms and signs of vestibular schwannoma (tinnitus, deafness, headache) usually appear in early adulthood, between 18 and 26 years on average. Bilateral vestibular schwannomas eventually appear in 95% of patients. Posterior lenticular opacities may be noted as early as birth in NF2, eventually affecting 80% of patients

Table 7.1 Comparison of major findings in NF1 and NF2

	NF1	*NF2*
Inheritance	AD	AD
Incidence	1 in 3000	1 in 35 000
Chromosome location	17 q11.2	22 q12
	translocations, point mutations, insertions, deletions	
New mutation frequency	50% of probands; > 90% paternal chromosome origin	50–75% of probands
Prenatal diagnosis	Genetic linkage Ultrasound	–
Age recognized	At birth in 50% cases	Mean = 22 years 10% at < 10 years 11% at > 40 years
Gene product	Neurofibromin, tumour suppressor – a GAP for p21 *ras* oncogene	Merlin tumour suppressor
Expressivity	Highly variable	Low variability
Clinical/Pathological		
Skin	CAL (> 5) in 95–100%; intertriginous freckling in 66%; subcutaneous NF (often > 10); plexiform NF	CAL (< 5, atypical) in 43% Subcutaneous NF (> 10 in 10%)
CNS pathology	Gliomas in 15% (90% optic tract); rare unilateral VS	Bilateral VS in > 90%; meningioma, ependymoma, spinal cord astrocytoma in 53%
Eye	Lisch nodules (> 2) in > 90% adults; enlarged orbit; glaucoma	Posterior subcapsular cataracts in 80%, occasionally at birth
Learning disability	In > 40%	None associated
Skeletal	Absent sphenoid wing; pseudoarthrosis in 0.5–1%; kyphoscoliosis in 2%; short stature: mean 34%tile, median 25%tile	–
Cancer potential	Neurofibrosarcoma in 5%, malignant schwannoma, Wilm's, leukaemia, etc.	–
Variant forms	Watson, Noonan, segmental, etc.	–

*Data from Riccardi (1981), Rubinstein and Korf (1990) and Evans *et al.* (1992).
AD, autosomal dominant; CAL, café-au-lait macules; GAP, GTPase activating protein; NF, neurofibroma; VS, vestibular schwannoma.

(Rubinstein and Korf, 1990). General features of NF2 are contrasted with those of NF1 in Table 7.1.

Among 100 patients in a registry spanning from 1989 to 1992, the prevalence of multiple skin tumours was 68%, averaging six per patient with a maximum of 27. These were papillary intradermal or fusiform neurofibromas located on peripheral nerves, but no plexiform or areolar neurofibromas were found. Café-au-lait spots occurred in 43% of patients, but were fewer than six in number. Intelligence was normal. The prevalence of cataracts was 38%, but might be considerably higher if routine slit-lamp examination were done (Evans *et al.*, 1992). There is a tendency toward increased severity with successive generations and with inheritance of the mutation from the mother (Evans *et al.*, 1992).

The critical differential for the patient with a unilateral vestibular schwannoma is between an NF2-associated lesion yet to become bilateral and the more common unilateral tumour occurring in the general population. Both originate in the superior vestibular branch of the eighth nerve but NF2 tumours are multilobar and enmesh other cranial nerves (Rubinstein and Korf, 1990). All cranial nerves except the olfactory have been affected in this manner in NF2 patients (Evans *et al.*, 1992). Magnetic resonance imaging is superior to computed tomography (CT) imaging for visualization of small schwannomas developing in the cerebellopontine angles.

Management of the tumours is critical to the outcome. Dramatically different growth rates for the tumours must be weighed against the exacting nature of the surgery with marked risks for alteration of seventh nerve as well as cochlear nerve function. Early screening of at risk family members should be undertaken, including an eye examination for cataracts, auditory evaluation with evoked potentials and an MRI scan. Death occurs in more than 40% by 50 years of age, on average at about 15 years after diagnosis is made (Evans *et al.*, 1992).

In some instances, the first tumour to be recognized is a spinal root schwannoma, meningioma, or glioma. The individual tumours do not have histological features that permit them to be distinguished from sporadic tumours of the same type. Peripheral neuropathy is rare. Rarely distal sensorimotor neuropathy occurs in NF2, and perhaps in NF1, too (Thomas *et al.*, 1990).

MOLECULAR GENETICS OF NF2

Linkage studies permitted assignment of the NF2 gene to chromosome 22, and subsequently to refine the localization to band 22q12. Somatic mutations affecting this region of chromosome 22 have also been documented in sporadic acoustic neuromas and ependymomas (Irving *et al.*, 1993; Rubio *et al.*, 1994). Identification of the NF2 gene was facilitated by study of NF2 families with non-overlapping germ-line deletions in this chromosomal segment.

CELL BIOLOGY OF NF2

The NF2 gene encodes a widely expressed protein, 'merlin', with a sequence homologous to that of moesin, ezrin, radixin, talin and protein 4.1. Members of this family of proteins are believed to link cytoskeletal elements with the plasma membrane in erythrocytes and other cell types (Rouleau *et al.*, 1993; Trofatter *et al.*, 1993; Hara *et al.*, 1994). Protein 4.1, for example, links the erythrocyte actin–spectrin network with the plasma membrane anion channel and glycophorin, and a protein 4.1 mutation is one of the causes of hereditary elliptocytosis.

Meningiomas from patients with NF2 demonstrate loss of heterozygosity on chromosome 22 (Trofatter *et al.*, 1993). This observation suggests that these tumours arise when both copies of the NF2 gene are mutated or lost, and that the NF2 gene, like the NF1 gene, encodes a protein with tumour suppressor activity (Knudsen, 1971).

REFERENCES

Akbarnia, B. A., Gabriel, K. R., Beckman, E. and Chalk, D. (1992). Prevalence of scoliosis in neurofibromatosis. *Spine*, **17**, S244–248

Allanson, J. E., Hall, J. G. and Van Allen, M. I. (1985). Noonan phenotype associated with neurofibromatosis. *Am. J. Med. Genet.*, **21**, 457–462

Allanson, J. E., Upadhyaya, M., Watson, G. H. *et al.* (1991). Watson syndrome: is it a subtype of type I neurofibromatosis? *J. Med. Genet.*, **28**, 752–756

Andersen, L. B., Fountain, J. W., Gutmann, D. H. *et al.* (1993). Mutations in the neurofibromatosis 1 gene in sporadic malignant melanoma cell ines. *Nature Genet.*, **3**, 118–121

Bader, J. L. and Miller, R. W. (1978). Neurofibromatosis and childhood leukemia. *J. Pediatr.*, **92**, 925–929

Ballester, R., Marchuk, D., Boguski, M. *et al.* (1990). The NF1 locus encodes a protein functionally related to mammalian GAP and yeast IRA proteins. *Cell*, **63**, 851–859

Barker, D. F., Wright, E., Nguyen, K. *et al.* (1987). Gene for NF1 von Recklinghausen neurofibromatosis is in the pericentromeric region of chromosome 17. *Science*, **236**, 1100–1102

Bollag, G., McCormack, F. and Clark, R. (1993). Characterization of full-length neurofibromin: tubulin inhibits Ras GAP activity. *EMBO J.*, **12**, 1923–1927

Buchberg, A., Bedigan, G.,Taylor, B. *et al.* (1988). Localization of EVI-2 to chromosome 11: linkage to other protooncogene and growth factor loci using interspecific backcross mice. *Oncogene Res.*, **2**, 149–165

Cawthon, R. M., Weiss, R., Xu, G. *et al.* (1990a). A major neurofibromatosis type 1 gene: cDNA sequence, genomic structure and point mutations. *Cell*, **62**, 193–201

Cawthon, R., O'Connell, P., Buchberg, A. *et al.* (1990b). Identification and characterization of transcripts from the neurofibromatosis region: the sequence and genomic structure of EVi-2 and mapping of other transcripts. *Genomics*, **7**, 555–565

Cawthon, R., Anderson, L., Buchberg, A. *et al.* (1991). cDNA sequence and genomic structure of EVI-2B, a gene lying within an intron of the neurofibromatosis type 1 gene. *Genomics*, **9**, 446–460

Clementi, M., Murgia, A., Anglani, F. *et al.* (1991). Linkage analysis of neurofibromatosis type 1. *Hum. Genet.*, **87**, 91–94

Craig, J. B. and Govender, S. (1992). Neurofibromatosis of the cervical spine. A report of eight cases. *J. Bone Joint Surg. [Br]*, **74**, 575–578

Daston, M. M., Scrable, H., Nordlund, M. *et al.* (1992). The protein product of the neurofibromatosis type 1 gene is expressed in highest abundance in neurons, Schwann cells, and oligodendrocytes. *Neuron*, **8**, 415–428

Daston, M. M. and Ratner, N. (1992). Neurofibromin, a predominantly neuronal GTPase activating protein in the adult, is ubiquitously expressed during development. *Developmental Dynamics*, **195**, 216–226

DeClue, J. E., Papageorge, A. G., Fletcher, J. A. *et al.* (1992). Abnormal regulation of mammalian p21ras contributes to malignant tumor growth in von Recklinghausen (type 1) neurofibromatosis. *Cell*, **69**, 265–273

DiMario, F. J., Ramsby, G., Greenstein, R. *et al.* (1993). Neurofibromatosis Type 1: magnetic resonance imaging findings. *J. Child. Neurol.*, **8**, 32–39

Drut, M. M., Miles, J. M. and Gilbert-Barness, E. (1993). Pathological cases of the month. Meningioangiomatosis. *Am. J. Dis. Child.*, **147**, 1009–1010

Estivill, X., Lazaro, C., Casals, T. *et al.* (1991). Recurrence of a nonsense mutation in the NF1 gene causing classical neurofibromatosis type 1. *Hum. Genet.*, **88**, 185–188

Evans, D. G. R., Huson, S. M., Donnai, D. *et al.* (1992). A clinical study of type 2 neurofibromatosis. *Q. J. Med.*, **84**, 603–618

Gregory, P. E., Gutmann, D. H., Mitchell, A. *et al.* (1993). Neurofibromatosis type 1 gene product (neurofibromin) associates with microtubules. *Somatic Cell Mol. Genet.*, **19**, 265–274

Gutmann, D. H. and Collins, F. S. (1993). The neurofibromatosis type 1 gene and its protein product, neurofibromin. *Neuron*, **10**, 335–343

Gutmann, D. H., Tennekoon, G. I., Cole, J. L. *et al.* (1993). Modulation of the neurofibromatosis type 1 gene product, neurofibromin, during Schwann cell differentiation. *J. Neurosci. Res.*, **36**, 216–223

Hara, T., Bianchi, A. B., Seizinger, B. R. and Kley, N. (1994). Molecular cloning and characterization of alternatively spliced transcripts of the mouse neurofibromatosis 2 gene. *Cancer Res.*, **54**, 330–335

Irving, R. M., Moffat, D. A., Hardy, D. G. *et al.* (1993). Molecular genetic analysis of the mechanism of tumorigenesis in acoustic neuroma. *Arch. Otolaryngol. Head Neck Surg.*, **119**, 1222–1228

Jadayel, D, Fain, P., Upadhyaya, M. *et al.* (1990). Paternal origin of new mutations in Von Recklinghausen neurofibromatosis. *Nature*, **343**, 558–559

Johnson, M. R., DeClue, J. E., Felzmann, S. *et al.* (1994). Neurofibromin can inhibit Ras-dependent growth by a mechanism independent of its GTPase-accelerating function. *Mol. Cell. Biol.*, **14**, 641–645

Kaufmann, D., Wiandt, S., Veser, J. and Krone, W. (1991). Increased melanogenesis in cultured epidermal melanocytes from patients with neurofibromatosis 1 (NF1). *Hum. Genet.*, **87**, 144–150

Knudsen, A. G. (1971). Mutation and cancer: statistical study of retinoblastoma. *Proc. Natl Acad. Sci. USA*, **68**, 820–823

Korf, B. R. (1992). Diagnostic outcome in children with multiple café-au-lait spots. *Pediatrics*, **90**, 924–927

Li, Y., Bollag, G., Clark, R. *et al.* (1992). Somatic mutations in the neurofibromatosis 1 gene in human tumors. *Cell*, **69**, 275–281

Ledbetter, D. H., Rich, D. C., O'Connell, P. *et al.* (1989). Precise localization of NF1 to 17q11.2 by balanced translocation. *Am. J. Hum. Genet.*, **44**, 20–24

Marchuk, D., Saulino, A., Tavakkol, R. *et al.* (1991). cDNA cloning of the type 1A neurofibromatosis gene: complete sequence of the NF1 gene product. *Genomics*, **11**, 931–940

Martin, G., Viskochil, D., Bollag, G. *et al.* (1990). The GAP-related domain of the neurofibromatosis type 1 gene product interacts with ras p21. *Cell*, **63**, 843–849

Menon, A. G., Anderson, K. M., Riccardi, V. M. *et al.* (1990). Chromosome 17p deletion and p53 gene mutations associated with the formation of malignant neurofibrosarcomas in von Recklinghausen neurofibromatosis. *Proc. Natl Acad. Sci. USA*, **87**, 5435–5439

Messiaen, L., De Bie, S., Moens, T. *et al.* (1993). Lack of independence between five DNA polymorphisms in the NF1 gene. *Hum. Mol. Genet.*, **2**, 485

Mikol, D., Gulcher, J. and Stefansson, K. (1990). The oligodendrocyte–myelin glycoprotein belongs to a distinct family of proteins and contains the HNK-1 carbohydrate. *J. Cell Biol.*, **110**, 471–480

Nellist, M. and other members of the European Chromosome 16 Tuberous Sclerosis Consortium (1993). Identification and characterization of the tuberous sclerosis gene on chromosome 16. *Cell*, **75**, 1305–1315

Nordlund, M., Gu, X., Shipley, M. T. and Ratner, N. (1993). Neurofibromin is enriched in the endoplasmic reticulum of CNS neurons. *J. Neurosci.*, **13**, 1588–1600

O'Connell, P., Leach, R. J. Cawthon, R. M. *et al.* (1989a). Two NF1 translocations map within a 600-kilobase segment of 17q11.2. *Science*, 244, 1087–1088

O'Connell, P., Leach, R. J., Ledbetter, D. H. *et al.* (1989b). Fine structure DNA mapping studies of the chromosomal region harboring the genetic defect in neurofibromatosis type 1. *Am. J. Hum. Genet.*, **44**, 51–57

Perilongo, G., Felix, C. A., Meadows, A. T. *et al.* (1993). Sequential development of Wilms tumor, T-cell acute lymphoblastic leukemia, medulloblastoma and myeloid leukemia in a child with type 1 neurofibromatosis: a clinical and cytogenetic case report. *Leukemia*, **7**, 912–915

Pleasure, J. R. and Geller, S. A. (1967). Neurofibromatosis in infancy presenting with congential stridor. *Am. J. Dis. Child.*, **113**, 390–393

Ponder, B. A. J. (1992). Neurofibromatosis: from gene to phenotype. *Cancer Biology*, **3**, 115–120

Riccardi, V. M. (1981). Von Recklinghausen neurofibromatosis. *N. Engl. J. Med.*, **305**, 1617–1627

Rodenhiser, D. I., Ainsworth, P. J., Coulter-Mackie, M. B. *et al.* (1993). A genetic study of neurofibromatosis type 1 (NF1) in south-western Ontario. II A PCR based approach to molecular and prenatal diagnosis using linkage. *J. Med. Genet.*, **30**, 363–368

Rouleau, G. A., Merel, P., Lutchman, M. *et al.* (1993). Alteration in a new gene encoding a putative membrane-organizing protein causes neurofibromatosis type 2. *Nature*, **363**, 515–521

Rubinstein, A. E. and Korf, B. R. (1990). Neurologic aspects of neurofibromatosis. In *Neurofibromatosis: a Handbook for Patients, Families and Health-Care Professionals* (A. E. Rubinstein and B. R. Korf, eds), pp. 40–54, New York: Thieme Medical Publishers, Inc

Rubio, M. P., Correa, K. M., Ramesh, V. *et al.* (1994). Analysis of the neurofibromatosis 2 gene in human ependymomas and astrocytomas. *Cancer Res.*, **54**, 45–47

Russell, D. S. and Rubinstein, L. J. (1989). *Pathology of Tumours of the Nervous System*, 5th edn. Williams and Wilkins

Schmidt, M. A., Michels, V. V. and Dewald, G. W. (1987). Cases of neurofibromatosis with rearrangements of chromosome 17 involving band 17q11.2. *Am. J. Med. Genet.*, **28**, 771–777

Shannon, K. M., O'Connell, P., Martin, G. A. *et al.* (1994). Loss of the normal NF 1 allele from the bone marrow of children with type 1 neurofibromatosis and malignant myeloid disorders. *N. Engl. J. Med.*, **330**, 597–601

Sheela, S., Riccardi, V. M. and Ratner, N. (1990). Angiogenic and invasive properties of neurofibroma Schwann cells. *J. Cell. Biol.*, **111**, 645–653

Shuman, S., Hardy, M., Sobue, G. and Pleasure, D. (1988). A cyclic adenosine 3′,5′-monophosphate (cAMP) analogue induces synthesis of a myelin-specific glycoprotein by cultered Schwann cells. *J. Neurochem.*, **50**, 190–194

Skuse, G. R., Kosciolek, B. A. and Rowley, P. T. (1989). Molecular genetic analysis of tumors in von Recklinghausen neurofibromatosis: loss of heterozygosity for chromosome 17. *Genes Chromosom. Cancer*, **1**, 36–41

Skuse, G. R., Kosciolek, B. A. and Rowley, P. T. (1991). The neurofibroma in von Recklinghausen neurofibromatosis has a unicellular origin. *Am. J. Hum. Genet.*, **49**, 507–510

Sobue, G., Sonnenfeld, K., Rubenstein, A. and Pleasure, D. (1985). Tissue culture studies of neurofibromatosis: effects of axolemmal fragments and cyclic adenosine 3′,5′-monophosphate analogues on proliferation of Schwann-like and fibroblast-like neurofibroma cells. *Ann. Neurol.*, **18**, 68–73

Sobue, G., Shuman, S. and Pleasure, D. (1986). Schwann cell responses to cyclic AMP: proliferation, change in shape, and appearance of surface galactocerebroside. *Brain Res.*, **362**, 23–32

Sorensen, S. A., Mulvihill, J. J. and Nielsen, A. (1986). Long term follow-up of von Recklinghausen's neurofibromatosis. *N. Engl. J. Med.*, **314**, 1010–1015

Stern, H. J., Saal, H. M., Lee, J. S. *et al.* (1992). Clinical variability of type I neurofibromatosis: is there a neurofibromatosis–Noonan syndrome? *J. Med. Genet.*, **29**, 184–187

Stumpf, D. A., Alksne, J. F. and Annegers, J. F. (1988). Neurofibromatosis. *Arch. Neurol.*, **45**, 575–579

Tassabenji, M., Strachan, T., Sharland, M. *et al.* (1993). Tandem duplication within a neurofibromatosis type 1 (NF1) gene exon in a family with features of Watson syndrome and Noonan syndrome. *Am. J. Hum. Genet.*, **53**, 90–95

The, I., Murthy, A. E., Harrigan, G. E., Jacoby, L. B., Menon, A. G., Gusella, J. F. and Bernards, A. (1993). Neurofibromatosis type 1 gene mutations in neuroblastoma. *Nat, Genet.*, **3**, 62-66.

Thomas, P. K., King, R. H. M., Chiang, T. R. *et al.* (1990). Neurofibromatous neuropathy. *Muscle Nerve*, **13**, 93–101

Trofatter, J. A., MacCollin, M. M., Rutter, J. L. *et al.* (1993). A novel moesin-, ezrin-, radixin-like gene is a candidate for the neurofibromatosis 2 tumor suppressor. *Cell*, **72**, 791–800

Upadhyaya, M., Cheryson, A., Broadhead, W. *et al.* (1990). A 90 kilobase deletion associated with neurofibromatosis type 1. *J. Med. Genet.*, **27**, 738–741

Upadhyaya, M., Fryer, A., MacMillan, J. *et al.* (1992). Prenatal diagnosis and presymptomatic detection on neurofibromatosis type 1. *J. Med. Genet.*, **29**, 180–183

Viskochil, D., Buchberg, A. M., Xu, G. *et al.* (1990). Deletions and a translocation interrupt a cloned gene at the neurofibromatosis type locus. *Cell*, **62**, 187–192

Viskochil, D., Cawthon, R., O'Connell, P. *et al.* (1991). The gene encoding the oligodendrocyte–myelin glycoprotein is embedded within the neurofibromatosis type 1 gene. *Mol. Cell. Biol.*, **11**, 909–912

Vivarelli, R., Bartalini, G., Calistri, L. *et al.* (1991). Molecular study in von Recklinghausen neurofibromatosis (NF1). *Childs Nerv. Syst.*, **7**, 98–99

Wallace, M. R., Marchuk, D. A., Anderson, L. B. *et al.* (1990). Type 1 neurofibromatosis gene: identification of a large transcript disrupted in three NF1 patients. *Science*, **249**, 181–186

Wallace, M. R., Anderson, L. B., Saulino, A. M. *et al.* (1991). A de novo Alu insertion results in neurofibromatosis 1. *Nature*, **353**, 864–866

Warne, P. H., Viciana, P. R. and Downward, J. (1993). Direct interaction of Ras and the amino-terminal region of Raf-1 in vitro. *Nature*, **364**, 352–355

Xu, G., O'Connell, P., Viskochil, D. *et al.* (1990a). The neurofibromatosis type 1 gene encodes a protein related to GAP. *Cell*, **62**, 599–608

Xu, G., Lim, K., Tanaka, D. *et al.* (1990b). The catalytic domain of the neurofibromatosis gene product stimulates ras GTPase and complements IRA mutants of S cerevisiae. *Cell*, **63**, 835–841

8
Neuropathies associated with anti-glycoconjugate antibodies and IgM monoclonal gammopathies

N. Latov and A. J. Steck

INTRODUCTION

Increased titres of IgM antibodies that react with oligosaccharide determinants of glycolipids and glycoproteins (glycoconjugates) in peripheral nerve are associated with chronic progressive neuropathies. These antibodies may be polyclonal or occur as IgM monoclonal gammopathies. For some of the autoantibodies, there is an association between the antigenic specificities of the antibodies and the associated clinical syndromes. In the neuropathy associated with anti-myelin-associated glycoprotein (MAG) antibodies, there is good evidence that the autoantibodies cause the disease. In some of the other syndromes, it is not yet known whether the antibodies are pathogenic or whether they are only associated with the diseases.

Increased titres of IgG or IgA antibodies that react with glycoconjugate antigens are usually associated with acute neuropathies or the Guillain–Barré syndrome and its variants. As in the chronic neuropathies associated with IgM autoantibodies, there is frequently a correlation between the antibody specificities and the clinical syndrome. IgG or IgA anti-GM1 antibodies, for example, are associated with acute motor axonal neuropathy, and anti-GQ1b antibodies are associated with the Miller–Fisher variant of the syndrome. It is not yet known whether these antibodies have a role in the causation of the neuropathy.

IgM anti-glycoconjugate antibodies may occur as monoclonal gammopathies, whereas the IgG or IgA anti-glycoconjugate antibodies are typically polyclonal. A majority of the IgM monoclonal gammopathies from patients with neuropathy exhibit anti-glycoconjugate activity. The monoclonal gammopathies are thought to result from transformation of single clones of B cells which then proliferate and secrete the autoantibodies in excess. These antibodies are also called M-proteins or paraproteins, and are detectable by serum protein immunoelectrophoresis or immunofixation electrophoresis. Most IgM monoclonal gammopathies are non-malignant, but in some cases they are associated with Waldenström's macroglobulinaemia or chronic lymphocytic leukaemia. The non-malignant monoclonal gammopathies have also been called monoclonal gammopathies of undetermined significance (MGUS) because they sometimes progress to malignancy (Kyle, 1978). However, these antibodies are frequently significant in patients with neuropathy, so that the term MGUS is incorrect.

The neuropathies that are associated with IgM monoclonal gammopathies are generally distinct from those associated with IgG or IgA monoclonal gammopathies (Gosselin *et al.*, 1991; Yeung *et al.*, 1991; Suarez and Kelly, 1993; Latov, 1994). IgG or IgA monoclonal gammopathies in patients with neuropathy have not been shown to react with glycoconjugates, and they may be associated with such distinct syndromes as the POEMS syndrome (Polyneuropathy, Organomegally, Endocrinopathy, Myeloma and Skin changes) which is not usually associated with IgM monoclonal gammopathies. Monoclonal gammopathy of any isotype may also be found in normal individuals, especially with increasing age or with chronic inflammation or infection, so that in some patients they may be coincidental and unrelated to the neuropathy.

This chapter reviews the clinical syndromes that are associated with anti-glycoconjugate antibodies and IgM monoclonal gammopathies, and discusses the evaluation, pathophysiology and therapy of patients with these disorders.

DETECTION AND MEASUREMENT OF MONOCLONAL GAMMOPATHIES AND ANTI-GLYCOCONJUGATE ANTIBODIES

Monoclonal gammopathies are routinely detected and characterized into heavy and light chain types by serum protein immunoelectrophoresis or immunofixation electrophoresis. Other abnormal laboratory tests such as an increase in the concentration of a particular immunoglobulin isotype, a decrease in background immunoglobulins, or the presence of cryoglobulins or urinary Bence-Jones protein may alert the physician to the possible presence of an occult monoclonal gammopathy. If a monoclonal protein is detected, haematological studies, including bone marrow aspiration, skeletal survey and bone scan, and appropriate tissue biopsies may be done to help determine whether the monoclonal gammopathy is associated with multiple myeloma, Waldenström's macroglobulinaemia, chronic lymphocytic leukaemia, or lymphoma, or whether it is non-malignant.

Antibody binding to normal peripheral nerve can be determined by immunofluorescence microscopy or immunocytochemistry. Several assay systems are available for detecting and quantitating anti-glycoconjugate antibodies. The Western blot system allows detection of antibody binding to glycoprotein antigens, and was initially used to identify myelin associated glycoprotein (MAG) as a target antigen in demyelinating neuropathies. The thin layer chromatography (TLC) overlay system allows identification of glycolipid antigens, and was initially used to identify GM1 as a target antigen in motor neuropathies. In the Western blot system, glycoproteins are separated by size using polyacrylamide gel electrophoresis, transferred to nitrocellulose sheets, and immunostained by the antibodies. In the TLC overlay system, glycolipids are separated according to charge, and stained directly on the TLC plates by the antibodies. Both these systems are useful for identifying target antigens in tissue extracts containing multiple glycolipids or glycoproteins, but are inconvenient for measuring antibody titres to specific antigens.

The Enzyme-Linked Immunosorbent Assay (ELISA) system is most commonly used for quantitation of antibody titres. Microwells in the titre plate are coated with the glycolipid or glycoprotein antigen, the patient serum added to the antigen-coated microwells, and the serum antibodies that bind to the immobilized antigen are then measured by the addition of enzyme-conjugated anti-human immunoglobulins in a colorimetric reaction using added substrate. Sera are tested at multiple dilutions in triplicate, and for each serum dilution, readings in control microwells without antigen, are subtracted from readings in the corresponding antigen-coated wells. Titres are usually expressed as the highest serum dilution at which binding is detected, or in comparison with standard curves. Because low levels of circulating anti-glycoconjugate antibodies are present in many normal individuals, elevated titres are defined in comparison with titres in normal subjects and in patients with other neurological and immunological diseases (van den Berg *et al.*, 1993a).

False positives in the ELISA system can result from non-specific binding of low-affinity antibodies if sera are tested at too low dilutions, or if readings in control, non-antigen-coated wells, are not subtracted from values in the antigen-coated wells. False negative readings can occur if detergent is used or if determinations are made at non-optimal temperatures (McGinnis *et al.*, 1988; Marcus *et al.*, 1989; van den Berg *et al.*, 1993; Willison *et al.*, 1994a). Also, some antibodies are better detected by Western blot or TLC than by ELISA (van den Berg *et al.*, 1992b), and the ELISA system favours detection of multivalent IgM antibodies and is less favourable for the detection of IgG or IgA anti-glycoconjugate antibodies of the same affinities (Spatz *et al.*, 1992a; Ogino *et al.*, 1994).

Results of antibody assays are used to help evaluate patients with neuropathy, but do not by themself make a diagnosis. Any serological assays only approximate the *in vivo* conditions, and do not measure such variables as the state of the blood–nerve barrier, the concentration of antibodies in the endoneurial compartment, the activity of the autoantibodies at physiological temperatures, and the ability of the antibodies to activate complement or recruit effector cells. These could all influence the effect of the antibodies *in vivo*. The antibody assays should always be interpreted in the light of the clinical presentation and results of other laboratory investigations.

CLINICAL SYNDROMES ASSOCIATED WITH ANTI-GLYCOCONJUGATE ANTIBODIES

Demyelinating neuropathy and anti-MAG antibodies

In approximately 50% of patients with neuropathy and IgM monoclonal gammopathy, the M-proteins bind to myelin and to an oligosaccharide determinant that is shared by the myelin-associated glycoprotein and the glycolipids sulphoglucuronyl paragloboside (SGPG) and sulphoglucuronyl lactosaminyl paragloboside (SGLPG) (Latov *et al.*, 1988a; Nobile-Orazio *et al.*, 1989; van den Berg *et al.*, 1992b). The incidence of this type of neuropathy is estimated to be between 1 to 5 per 10 000 adult population, with symptoms usually beginning in later life, but with age of onset as early as the fourth decade. Males appear to be affected more frequently than females. Patients typically present with a slowly progressive distal and symmetrical sensory or sensorimotor neuropathy, usually affecting the arms and then the legs. An intention tremor may be present, sometimes early in the disease. Cranial nerves and autonomic functions are preserved. Many patients have a predominantly sensory neuropathy, sometimes with pain. A few patients may present with a predominantly motor neuropathy (van den Berg *et al.*, 1992b), and rapid progression with profound weakness and fatal outcome has been described (Antoine *et al.*, 1993). The cerebrospinal fluid (CSF) is acellular and protein concentration is frequently increased. Visual evoked responses may reveal subclinical involvement of the optic nerves, particularly if the antibodies are present in the CSF (Barbieri *et al.*, 1987).

Electrophysiological studies typically show demyelinating features with slowed nerve conduction velocities, dispersed action potential amplitudes, and prolonged distal latencies (Kelly, 1990). In some patients, there is disproportionate prolongation of the distal latencies in comparison with proximal motor conduction velocities, an electrophysiological abnormality which may be peculiar to this disease (Kaku and Sumner, 1992).

Pathological studies of biopsied nerves usually display loss of myelinated fibres (Figure 8.1), thinned myelin sheaths, segmental demyelination, and onion bulbs (Figure 8.2). Two pathological alterations are characteristic of the neuropathy associated with anti-MAG antibodies. These are: (1) the presence of deposits of the monoclonal IgM and complement on myelin sheaths (Takatsu *et al.*, 1985; Hays *et al.*, 1988; Monaco *et al.*, 1990); and (2) widening of the myelin lamellae at the minor dense line, with IgM deposits in the areas of widened myelin loops (Figures 8.3a,b) (Mendell *et al.*, 1985; Mata *et al.*, 1988; Vital *et al.*, 1989; Jacobs and Scadding, 1990; Lach *et al.*, 1993).

The anti-MAG M-proteins from patients with neuropathy and IgM monoclonal gammopathy were first demonstrated to bind to peripheral nerve myelin using a complement fixation assay and by immunocytochemistry (Figure 8.4). The antibodies were then shown to bind to the MAG by the Western blot system, and to two sulphated glucuronic acid-containing glycolipids, SGPG and SGLPG, by immunostaining on thin layer chromatographs. The epitope which is recognized by the human antibodies is also recognized by several mouse monoclonal antibodies, including HNK-1 and L2, and is shared also by the peripheral myelin proteins P_0 and PMP-22 (Bollensen *et al.*, 1988; Snipes *et al.*, 1993). The HNK-1 bearing glycoproteins function as adhesion molecules, and the disruption of these functions may contribute to the neuropathy in affected patients.

Anti-MAG antibodies in patients with neuropathy almost always occur as IgM monoclonal gammopathies. These are usually non-malignant, and serum IgM may remain constant for years or decades, but in some cases the gammopathy is associated with Waldenström's macroglobulinaemia or chronic lymphocytic leukaemia.

The M-proteins are thought to cause the neuropathy because pathological studies show demyelination, corresponding to the antigenic specificity of the autoantibodies, and because deposits of the anti-MAG M-proteins and complement are found on the affected myelin sheaths. Passive transfer of patient's serum intraneurally into cat

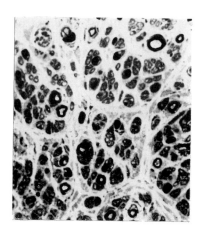

Figure 8.1 Sural nerve biopsy from a patient with a demyelinating neuropathy and monoclonal IgM anti-MAG antibodies. A methylene blue-stained semithin cross-section shows a severe loss of myelinated fibres. (Reproduced with permission from Steck *et al.*, 1983.)

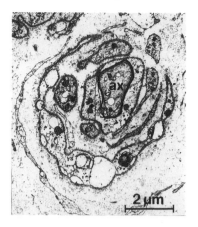

Figure 8.2 Sural nerve biopsy from a patient with a demyelinating neuropathy and monocolonal IgM anti-MAG antibodies. Electronmicrograph showing a thinly myelinated axon surrounded by an onion bulb formation of Schwann cell processes. (Reproduced with permission from Steck *et al.*, 1983.)

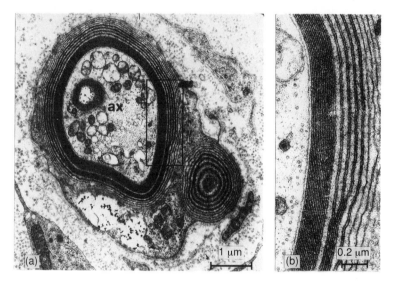

Figure 8.3 Sural nerve biopsy from a patient with a demyelinating neuropathy and monocolonal IgM anti-MAG antibodies. (a) Electronmicrograph showing widening of the external myelin lamellae. (b) At higher magnification, the splitting occurs in some of the middle layers of the myelin and affects the minor dense line. ax, axon. (Reproduced with permission from Steck *et al.*, 1983.)

nerve induces demyelination (Hays *et al.*, 1987; Willison *et al.*, 1988; Trojaborg *et al.*, 1989), and systemic administration of anti-MAG antibodies in the chicken causes neuropathy and demyelination with separation of the myelin lamellae at the minor dense line, similar to that seen in the human disease (Tatum, 1993).

The neuropathy associated with anti-MAG antibodies usually improves with therapy directed at lowering the autoantibody concentrations. Clinical improvement has been reported to follow therapy with plasmapheresis or chemotherapy using chlorambucil, cyclophosphamide or fludarabine (Haas and Tatum, 1988; Latov *et al.*, 1988a; Nobile-Orazio *et al.*, 1988; Leger *et al.*, 1993; Sherman *et al.*, 1994). IVIg has also been reported to be beneficial in some patients (Cook *et al.*, 1990).

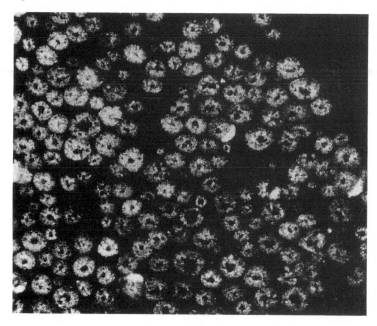

Figure 8.4 Binding of human IgM anti-MAG antibodies to myelin in normal human peripheral nerve by indirect immunofluorescence microscopy. (Reproduced with permission from Nobile-Orazio *et al.*, 1984.)

IgM anti-GM1 antibodies and motor neuropathy

Increased titres of anti-GM1 antibodies were first reported in a patient with IgM monoclonal gammopathy and lower motor neuron disease (Freddo *et al.*, 1986a), and in patients with motor neuropathy and multifocal conduction block (Pestronk *et al.*, 1988). Other patients with increased titres of monoclonal or polyclonal IgM anti-GM1 antibodies and motor neuropathy or motor neuron disease syndromes were later described (reviewed in Pestronk *et al.*, 1990, 1991; Pestronk, 1991; Adams *et al.*, 1991; Apostolski and Latov, 1993; Kinsella *et al.*, 1994). Patients with highly elevated anti-GM1 antibody titres typically have progressive weakness with muscle atrophy and fasciculations, absent or active deep tendon reflexes but without definite upper motor neuron signs, and with electromyographic evidence of denervation. The weakness is frequently asymmetric, involves the arms more than the legs, and bulbar muscles may occasionally be affected. Conduction studies frequently show one or more areas of conduction block in motor nerves, although in some patients motor conduction is normal or diffusely slowed. Sensory conduction is typically normal, including through the regions of motor conduction block. Some of the patients have mild paraesthaesias and sensory loss distally in the hands or feet, or less commonly, frank sensorimotor neuropathy. CSF protein is frequently normal but may be elevated. In most cases the IgM anti-GM1 antibodies are polyclonal, but in some, they occur as monoclonal gammopathies, or they may be oligoclonal (Willison *et al.*, 1994a). Serum IgM concentration may be elevated or normal. The clinical presentation frequently resembles that of motor neuron disease, but patients can be recognized by the presence of conduction abnormalities or increased titres of anti-GM1 antibodies. Estimates of the frequency of increased anti-GM1 antibody titres in patients with motor neuropathy and multifocal motor conduction block range from 18% to 84% (Kinsella *et al.*, 1994).

In most patients, the anti-GM1 antibodies recognize the Gal(β1-3)GalNAc determinant which is shared by asialo GM1 (GA1) and the ganglioside GD1b (Table 8.1). The same determinant is also present on some glycoproteins and is recognized by the lectin peanut agglutinin (PNA). Some of the antibodies, however, are highly specific for GM1 or recognize internal determinants shared by GM1 and GM2 (Ilyas *et al.*, 1988a; Baba *et al.*, 1989; Kusunoki *et al.*, 1989; Sadiq *et al.*, 1990; Willison *et al.*, 1994a).

Although GM1 and other Gal(β1-3)GalNAc-bearing glycoconjugates are highly concentrated and widely distributed in the central and peripheral nervous systems, they are mostly cryptic and unavailable to the antibodies except where they are exposed on the surface of cells. Studies using anti-GM1 antibodies from patients with neuropathy show that the antibodies bind to spinal cord grey matter, and to GM1 on the surface of isolated bovine spinal motor neurons (Figure 8.5), but not to dorsal root ganglion neurons (Corbo *et al.*, 1992). In peripheral nerve, GM1 and Gal(β1-3)GalNAc-bearing glycoproteins are expressed at the nodes of Ranvier as determined by the binding of human anti-GM1 antibodies (Gregson *et al.*, 1989) or cholera toxin and PNA (Figure 8.6) (Corbo *et al.*, 1993), and to the presynaptic region of motor fibres at the motor endplates (Thomas *et al.*, 1991). Two Gal(β1-3)GalNAc-bearing glycoproteins have been identified as potential targets for anti-GM1 antibodies at the nodes of Ranvier. One is the oligodendroglial–myelin glycoprotein (OMgp) which is localized at the paranodal region, and the second is a versican-like glycoprotein which is at the nodal gap (Apostolski *et al.*, 1994). GM1 itself is present on myelin sheaths at the paranodal region, but it is not yet known whether it is also present on motor axons.

Pathological studies at post mortem in a patient who died with motor neuropathy and elevated titres of anti-GM1 antibodies revealed degeneration of the anterior roots, immunoglobulin deposits on myelin sheaths, and chromatolytic changes in spinal motor neurons (Adams *et al.*, 1993). The anterior roots were more affected than the more distal nerves. Preferential involvement of the anterior roots might explain the lack of correlation between the extent and distribution of the weakness and the presence of conduction block in most patients. The motor neuron involvement is likely to be secondary to the degeneration of the anterior roots, as suggested by the presence of chromatolysis.

It is not known whether the anti-GM1 antibodies cause or contribute to the disease, or whether they are only an associated abnormality. The binding to motor, but not sensory, neurons correlates with the clinical syndrome, and GM1 is highly enriched and has a different fatty acid composition in myelin sheaths of motor nerves in comparison with sensory nerves (Ogawa-Goto *et al.*, 1990, 1992), which might make the anterior roots more susceptible to the effects of autoantibodies. Anti-GM1 antibodies have also been shown to damage cultured motor neurons (Heiman-Patterson *et al.*, 1993) and to interfere with neuromuscular transmission (Willison *et al.*, 1994b), and immunization of rabbits with GM1 or Gal(β1-3)GalNAc–BSA resulted in a reduction in the amplitudes of the motor compound action potentials with immunoglobulin deposits at the nodes of Ranvier (Thomas *et al.*, 1991). In another study, serum from a patient with increased titres of anti-GM1 antibodies and IgM deposits at the nodes of Ranvier induced demyelination and conduction block when injected into rat sciatic nerve (Santoro *et al.*, 1992). It might

Table 8.1 Structure of common ganglioside antigens*

Compound	Carbohydrate sequence	
GD1b	Gal(β1-3) GalNAc (β1-4)	Gal (β1-4) Glc (β1-1) Ceramide (α2–3) NeuNAc (α2–8) NeuNAc
GT1b	Gal(β1–3) GalNAc (β1–4) (α2–3) NeuNAc	Gal (β1–4) Glc (β1–1) Ceramide (α2–3) NeuNAc (α2–8) NeuNAc
GQ1b	Gal(β1–3) GalNAc (β1–4) (α2–3) NeuNAc (α2–8) NeuNAc	Gal (β1–4) Glc (β1–1) Ceramide (α2–3) NeuNAc (α2–8) NeuNAc
GD3		Gal (β1–4) Glc (β1–1) Ceramide (α2–3) NeuNAc (α2–8) NeuNAc
GD1a	Gal(β1–3) GalNAc (β1–4) (α2–3) NeuNAc	Gal (β1–4) Glc (β1–1) Ceramide (α2–3) NeuNAc
GM3		Gal (β1–4) Glc (β1–1) Ceramide (α2–3) NeuNAc
LM1 (= SPG)	Gal(β1–4) GlcNAc (β1–4) (α2–3) NeuNAc	Gal (β1–4) Glc (β1–1) Ceramide
GM1	Gal(β1–3) GalNAc (β1–4)	Gal (β1–4) Glc (β1–1) Ceramide (α2–3) NeuNAc
GM2	GalNAc (β1–4)	Gal (β1–4) Glc (β1–1) Ceramide (α2–3) NeuNAc
Asialo-GM1	Gal(β1–3) GalNAc (β1–4)	Gal (β1–4) Glc (β1–1) Ceramide

*Reproduced with permission from Willison *et al.* (1993a).

be that anti-GM1 antibodies have multiple sites of action along the peripheral nerves, explaining the clinical presentations.

Therapy with chemotherapeutic agents such as chlorambucil, cyclophosphamide or fludarabine (Latov *et al.*, 1988b; Pestronk *et al.*, 1988; Shy *et al.*, 1990; Feldman *et al.*, 1991; Kinsella *et al.*, 1994), or with infusion of human gammaglobulins (IVIg) (Kaji *et al.*, 1992; Chaudhry *et al.*, 1993; Nobile-Orazio *et al.*, 1993; Yuki *et al.*,

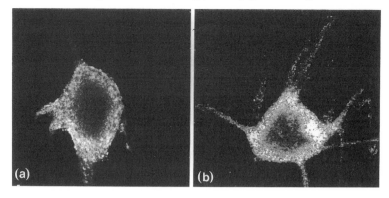

Figure 8.5 Confocal fluorescence imaging of motor neuron stained by (a) human IgM anti-GM1 antibodies, or (b) cholera toxin which binds specifically to GM1. The staining is restricted to the cell membrane and its processes. (Reproduced with permission from Corbo *et al.*, 1992.)

1993b; Azulay *et al.*, 1994) has been reported to result in clinical improvement. The most rational therapeutic approach would be to use IVIg to attain a quick therapeutic response, and then to add a chemotherapeutic agent to help sustain the response, decrease the dependence on IVIg, and eventually be able to discontinue all medications.

IgM anti-GD1b or disialosyl ganglioside antibodies and predominantly sensory demyelinating neuropathy

Ilyas *et al.* (1985) first described a patient with a predominantly sensory demyelinating neuropathy with circulating monoclonal IgM antibodies that recognized gangliosides containing disialosyl groups. The monoclonal IgM reacted best with GD3 and GT1b but showed strong cross-reactivity with GD1b and GD2 (Table 8.1). Six other patients with predominantly sensory neuropathy and monoclonal IgM antibodies to one or more gangliosides of the same series have since been reported (Arai *et al.*, 1992; Daune *et al.*, 1992; Obi *et al.*, 1992; Younes-Chennoufi *et al.*, 1992; Yuki *et al.*, 1992a; Willison *et al.*, 1993b). All seven monoclonals reacted strongly with GD1b, and in addition, five showed strong cross-reactivity with GT1b, three with GD3, two with GD1a, and two with GQ1b. Four of the patients showed strong cross-reactivity with four of the disialosyl-containing gangliosides, one with three, and one with two; one patient reacted strongly with GD1b only. Two of the antibodies exhibited anti-Pr2 activity and functioned as cold agglutinins (Arai *et al.*, 1992; Willison *et al.*, 1993a). All had large-fibre sensory loss with areflexia, and most had gait ataxia and elevated CSF proteins. The neuropathy was demyelinating in six and mixed axonal and demyelinating in one. IgM deposits were not detected in biopsied nerves using direct immunofluorescence. In one of the studies, the human monoclonal IgM bound to myelin in cross-sections of normal peripheral nerve (Younes-Chennoufi *et al.*, 1992), and in another study a mouse monoclonal antibody to GD1b was shown to bind to dorsal root ganglia neurons, possibly explaining the

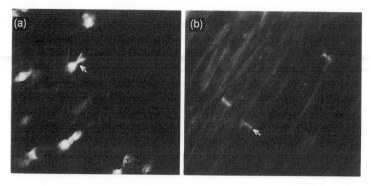

Figure 8.6 Localization of (b) peanut agglutinin (PNA) which binds to Gal(B1-3)GalNAc-bearing glycoproteins, and (a) cholera toxin (CT) which binds specifically to GM1, by fluorescence microscopy following intraneural injection into rat sciatic nerve. PNA binds at the nodal gap and CT binds to the paranodal myelin at the nodes of Ranvier in peripheral nerves (arrow). (Reproduced with permission from Corbo *et al.*, 1993.)

predominant sensory involvement (Kusunoki *et al.*, 1993). One of the patients developed an acute neuropathy as in the Guillain–Barré syndrome, but following initial improvement, the disease progressed in a stepwise fashion (Yuki *et al.*, 1992a). Response to therapy was generally poor, although some improvement was reported with plasmapheresis and prednisone (Arai *et al.*, 1992; Obi *et al.*, 1992).

Anti-sulfatide antibodies and sensory neuropathy

Increased titres of monoclonal or polyclonal IgM anti-sulfatide antibodies have been reported in association with predominantly sensory neuropathy (Pestronk *et al.*, 1991; Quattrini *et al.*, 1992; Nemni *et al.*, 1993; van den Berg *et al.*, 1993). Several of the patients appeared to have a small-fibre sensory neuropathy or a syndrome resembling ganglioneuritis, with electrophysiological or nerve biopsy studies showing no abnormalities or evidence of axonal degeneration. Immunocytochemical studies in these patients revealed that the antibodies bound to the surface of rat dorsal root ganglia neurons (Figure 8.7) (Quattrini *et al.*, 1992; Nemni *et al.*, 1993). Other patients with IgM anti-sulfatide antibodies had sensorimotor neuropathies with demyelination, widened myelin lamellae, and deposits of IgM on myelin sheaths (van den Berg *et al.*, 1993; Nobile-Orazio *et al.*, 1994). In some patients with demyelinating neuropathy the anti-sulfatide antibodies cross-reacted with MAG (Ilyas *et al.*, 1992a; Nobile-Orazio *et al.*, 1994), whereas in others with axonal neuropathy, the antibodies cross-reacted with chondroitin sulphate C (Nemni *et al.*, 1993). Sulfatide is highly concentrated in peripheral nerve myelin, but is also present on dorsal root ganglia neurons, and the anti-sulfatide antibodies might bind to either myelin or sensory neurons, depending on the orientation of sulfatide in the cell membrane and the fine specificity of the anti-sulfatide antibodies. It is not yet known whether the anti-sulfatide antibodies have a role in the pathogenesis of the neuropathy.

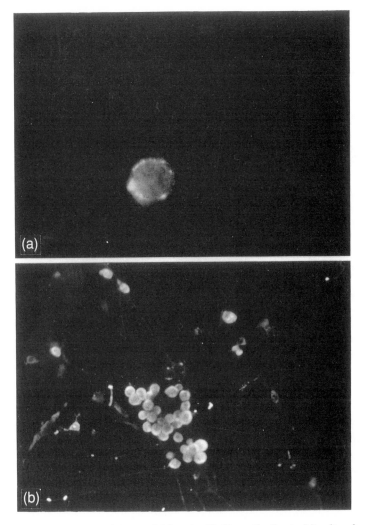

Figure 8.7 Binding of human IgM anti-sulfatide antibodies to (a) cultured human neuroblastoma cells and (b) isolated rat dorsal root ganglia neurons, by immunofluororescence microscopy. (Reproduced with permission from Quattrini *et al.*, 1992.)

Anti-chondroitin sulphate antibodies and neuropathy

Several patients with monoclonal or polyclonal IgM anti-chondroitin sulphate antibodies and axonal neuropathy have been described (Sherman *et al.*, 1983; Kabat *et al.*, 1984; Freddo *et al.*, 1985, 1986c; Yee *et al.*, 1989; Quattrini *et al.*, 1991; Nemni *et al.*, 1993; Nobile-Orazio *et al.*, 1994). The neuropathies varied ranging from predominantly sensory to sensorimotor, or predominantly motor. In some, there were deposits of IgM in the endoneurium. Some of the chondroitin C antibodies cross-reacted with sulfatide (Nemni *et al.*, 1993).

Other autoantigens in neuropathy with IgM monoclonal antibodies

Isolated cases of neuropathy associated with monoclonal IgM antibodies to other glycolipids have been reported. One patient had a monoclonal IgM that bound to sialosyllactosaminyl paragloboside (Baba *et al.*, 1985; Miyatani *et al.*, 1987). Two patients had IgM M-proteins specific for GM2, GM1b–GalNAc, and GD1a–GalNAc (Ilyas *et al.*, 1988b). One patient had a motor neuropathy with IgM antibodies to GD1a (Bollensen *et al.*, 1989). Another monoclonal IgM from a patient with chronic lymphocytic leukaemia and neuropathy bound to myelin and cross-reacted with denatured DNA and with a conformational epitope of phosphatidic acid and gangliosides (Freddo *et al.*, 1986b; Spatz *et al.*, 1990). Several patients with neuropathy and IgM antibodies to intermediate filaments have also been described (Dellagi *et al.*, 1982).

IgM monoclonal gammopathies without autoreactivity in neuropathy

In many patients with neuropathy and IgM monoclonal gammopathy, the IgM antibodies could not be demonstrated to react with self antigens. Many of these patients responded to immunosuppressive therapy, similar to patients with autoreactive antibodies, indicating that the neuropathies in these cases may also be immune-mediated (Kelly *et al.*, 1988). In some patients, the monoclonal IgMs could function as cryoglobulins and be associated with vasculitic neuropathy (Thomas *et al.*, 1992). In others, the monoclonal B cells may directly infiltrate the peripheral nerves (Ince *et al.*, 1987), or they may be associated with amyloid infiltration of nerve (Kelly *et al.*, 1979). In other cases the IgM may be reactive with an as yet unidentified antigen, or it may be coincidental and unrelated to the neuropathy.

IgG and IgA antibodies to glycoconjugates in the Guillain–Barré syndrome

Increased titres of antibodies to several glycolipids have been reported in association with the Guillain–Barré syndrome and its variants. Antibodies to the gangliosides LM1, GD1b, GD1a or GT1b (Ilyas *et al.*, 1988c, 1991, 1992c; Fredman *et al.*, 1991), to a Forssman-like glycolipid (Koski *et al.*, 1989) or to sulfatide (Svennerholm and Fredman, 1990; Fredman *et al.*, 1991) were described in some patients with typical Guillain–Barré syndrome.

Several studies reported increased titres of IgG or IgA anti-GM1 antibodies in Guillain–Barré syndrome (Gregson *et al.*, 1991, 1993; Garcia-Guijo *et al.*, 1992; Ilyas *et al.*, 1992b), particularly in patients with the motor axonal variant of the syndrome, and following infection with *Campylobacter jejuni* (Yuki *et al.*, 1990; Walsh *et al.*, 1991; van den Berg *et al.*, 1992; McKhann *et al.*, 1993; Kornberg *et al.*, 1994). The Penner 0:19 strain of *Campylobacter jejuni*, whose lipopolysaccharides bear GM1-like oligosaccharides (Aspinall *et al.*, 1992; Yuki *et al.*, 1992b), is most frequently associated with Guillain–Barré syndrome in Japan (Fujimoto *et al.*, 1992; Kuroki *et al.*, 1993). It is likely that the anti-GM1 antibodies in these patients are induced by the bacterial lipopolysaccharides (Wirguin *et al.*, 1994). The acute disease has features in common with the chronic disease associated with IgM anti-GM1 antibodies in that both are predominantly motor and associated with axonal degeneration and denervation, and both exhibit pathological changes of anterior root degeneration and chromatolysis of spinal motor neurons.

The motor axonal variant of Guillain–Barré syndrome with increased titres of anti-GM1 antibodies was also reported to occur following parenteral administration of a mixture of gangliosides or of GM1 ganglioside alone (Latov *et al.*, 1991; Figeuras *et al.*, 1992; Nobile-Orazio *et al.*, 1992; Schonhoffer, 1992; Landi *et al.*, 1993). Induction of IgG anti-GM1 antibodies without clinical weakness has also been reported following ganglioside injection (Ala *et al.*, 1994), suggesting that the anti-ganglioside antibodies may be coincidental. Alternatively, some anti-GM1 antibodies may not be pathogenic (Willison *et al.*, 1994b), or other factors such as presence of a cellular response or perturbation of the blood–nerve barrier could be important for the development of neurological disease. One patient developed GBS with anti-GM2 antibodies following administration of gangliosides (Yuki *et al.*, 1991).

Several patients, who developed an acute motor axonal neuropathy following gastrointestinal infection, were found to have increased titres of anti-N-acetylgalactosaminyl GD1a antibodies. It was not known whether these patients had a preceding infection with *Campylobacter jejuni* (Kusunoki *et al.*, 1994).

Anti-GQ1b antibodies were reported to be elevated in most patients with the Miller Fisher variant of Guillain–Barré syndrome with ophthalmoplegia (Chiba *et al.*, 1992, 1993; Willison *et al.*, 1993b; Yuki *et al.*, 1993a). Titres decreased following the acute phase of the illness. The anti-GQ1b antibodies selectively immunostained the paranodal regions of the extramedullary portion of human oculomotor, trochlear and abducens nerves, which biochemically had a higher content of GQ1b than spinal nerves. In electrophysiological studies, serum from patients with anti-GQ1b antibodies inhibited the release of acetyl choline from motor nerve terminals, suggesting that the antibodies have a role in the disease (Roberts *et al.*, 1994).

The anti-glycolipid antibodies in Guillain–Barré syndrome are typically of the IgG or IgA isotypes, compared with the IgM isotype found in patients with the slowly progressive neuropathies. The IgG antibodies appear to be restricted to the IgG1 and IgG3 subclasses (Ogino *et al.*, 1995; Willison and Veitch, 1994). This suggests that T cells participate in the anti-glycolipid immune response in patients with the acute neuropathies.

DEVELOPMENT OF ANTI-GLYCOCONJUGATE ANTIBODIES

Antibodies to glycoconjugates such as MAG or GM1 are present at low titres in most normal individuals, and B cells that express these antibodies are common constituents of the human immune repertoire (Mizutamari *et al.*, 1994). These B cells are thought to express the CD5+ phenotype (Lee *et al.*, 1991; Graves and Ravindranath, 1992), and are normally suppressed or rendered anergic, but might be activated by cross-reactive antigens or infectious agents, by T cell-dependent or independent mechanisms, to secrete antibodies at high titres. Activating antigens might include bacterial lipopolysaccharides such as the *Campylobacter jejuni* lipopolysaccharide which contains GM1-like oligosaccharides, parenteral preparations which may contain gangliosides or other oligosaccharide-bearing molecules (Offner *et al.*, 1985; Knorr-Held *et al.*, 1986), exposure to insects which bear HNK-1 reactive glycoconjugates (Dennis *et al.*, 1988), or viral particles which can incorporate host cell glycolipids or glycoprotein oligosaccharides into their membranes (Pathak *et al.*, 1990).

Monoclonal gammopathies are likely to result from transformation of activated B cells, occurring spontaneously or through viral or chemical mechanisms (Gelman and Dennis, 1981; Hanto *et al.*, 1983; Mann *et al.*, 1987; Jack *et al.*, 1992; Konrad *et al.*, 1993). Monoclonal gammopathies with anti-MAG activity have also been reported to develop following the onset of neuropathy, and in a patient with Charcot–Marie–Tooth disease, possibly due to chronic antigenic stimulation and coincidental inflammation (Julien *et al.*, 1987; Gregory *et al.*, 1993; Valldeoriola *et al.*, 1993). Genetic factors and alterations in immunoregulation are also important determinants in the development of monoclonal gammopathies (Radl *et al.*, 1986; Jensen *et al.*, 1988; Stall *et al.*, 1988). Regardless of their aetiology, once the auto-antibodies are present, they could damage the nerves and contribute to the neuropathy.

Although oligosaccharides are thought to be recognized by the immune system as a T cell-independent antigens, and anti-MAG antibodies have been found to exhibit low intrinsic affinities similarly to naturally occurring antibodies derived by a T-independent mechanisms (Brouet *et al.*, 1992; Ogino *et al.*, 1994), there is evidence to suggest that T cells are involved in the development of both IgM and IgG anti-glycoconjugate antibodies in patients with neuropathy. Both anti-MAG and anti-GM1 antibody-secreting B cells respond to stimulation by activated T cells (Latov *et al.*, 1985; Heidenreich *et al.*, 1994), and investigations of the anti-MAG and anti-GM1 monoclonal gammopathies indicate that they are encoded by immunoglobulin variable region genes which contain significant mutations as is seen in an antigen-driven, T cell-dependent immune response (Mihaesco *et al.*, 1989; Ayadi *et al.*, 1992; Spatz *et al.*, 1992b; Weng *et al.*, 1992; Lee *et al.*, 1994). Also, an association between the presence of anti-MAG monoclonal gammopathy and the presence of a tryptophan amino acid residue at position 9 of the DRβ chain, has been reported, suggesting that antigen presentation by HLA–DR is a factor in the anti-MAG antibody response (Vrethem *et al.*, 1993). It is not known whether effector T cells that recognize the same oligosaccharide determinants in peripheral nerve are also present in patients with neuropathy (Henningsson *et al.*, 1987), and if so, whether these could have a role in the disease.

THERAPEUTIC CONSIDERATIONS

The chronic neuropathies which are associated with IgM anti-glycoconjugate antibodies or with IgM monoclonal gammopathies are thought to be caused by auto-immune mechanisms, as has been shown for patients with anti-MAG antibodies. Therapy has therefore been directed at lowering the antibody concentrations or interfering with their effector mechanisms.

In patients with anti-MAG antibodies, therapy with chemotherapeutic agents including chlorambucil, cyclophosphamide or fludarabine has been reported to lower the IgM concentrations and result in clinical improvement (Latov *et al.*, 1988a; Nobile-Orazio *et al.*, 1988; Leger *et al.*, 1993; Sherman *et al.*, 1994).

Plasmapheresis has been reported to be helpful in some patients, but frequent exchanges are required to sustain a significant reduction in IgM concentration, so that it is usually used as an adjunct to chemotherapy rather than as sole therapy (Haas and Tatum, 1988; Leger *et al.*, 1993). Intravenous infusion of human gammaglobulins (IVIg) has also been reported to be beneficial (Cook *et al.*, 1990), and may exert its effects by inhibiting effector mechanisms, such as the activation of complement or macrophages, rather than by lowering the antibody concentration (Thornton and Griggs, 1994). Occasionally, symptoms may improve with chemotherapy before a fall in IgM concentrations, possibly due to a decrease in inflammation, stabilization and reduced permeability of the blood–nerve barrier, or inhibition of effector mechanisms in the peripheral nerves (Ernerudh *et al.*, 1992). In some cases the response to therapy has been poor (Gosselin *et al.*, 1991; Yeung *et al.*, 1991).

IVIg has been reported to be particularly effective in patients with motor neuropathies which are associated with IgM anti-GM1 antibodies (Chaudhry *et al.*, 1993; Nobile-Orazio *et al.*, 1993). These patients also respond to therapy with chemotherapeutic agents including cyclophosphamide, chlorambucil or fludarabine (Latov *et al.*, 1988b; Feldman *et al.*, 1991; Sherman *et al.*, 1994). A combination of IVIg and a chemotherapeutic agent may also be used.

There is less experience with therapy in the other types of neuropathy associated with IgM anti-glycoconjugate antibodies or IgM monoclonal gammopathies. The neuropathies in patients with IgM gammopathies without known specificities also improve with chemotherapy, similarly to patients with anti-MAG or GM1 antibodies (Kelly *et al.*, 1988). Painful symptoms which may be associated with anti-sulphatide antibodies or amyloidosis can be particularly resistant to therapy. Plasmapheresis and corticosteroids may be beneficial in patients with cryoglobulinaemia (Berkman and Orlin, 1980).

Patients with the motor axonal variant of the Guillain–Barré syndrome, which is associated with IgG or IgA anti-GM1 antibodies, are said to have a worse prognosis than patients with typical Guillain–Barré syndrome, and it is not known whether the disease in these patients is responsive to plasmapheresis or IVIg as in patients with typical Guillain–Barré syndrome (Thornton and Griggs, 1994). These therapies have also not been tested in patients with the Miller Fisher variant of the syndrome which is associated with IgG or IgA anti-GQ1b antibodies.

The available therapies often result in clinical improvement or halt the progression of the disease, but are rarely curative. Patients are frequently left with significant residual motor or sensory deficits and require further help in the form of physical therapy, supportive devices, or pain relief.

REFERENCES

Adams, D., Kuntzer, T., Burger, D. *et al.* (1991). Predictive value of anti-GM1 ganglioside antibodies in neuromuscular diseases; a study of 181 sera. *J. Neuroimmunol.*, **32**, 223–230

Adams, D., Kuntzer, T., Steck, A. *et al.* (1993). Motor conduction block and high titers of anti-GM1 ganglioside antibodies: pathological findings in a case of multifocal motor neuropathy in a patient with lower motor neuron syndrome. *J. Neurol. Neurosurg. Psychiatry*, **56**, 982–987

Ala, T. A., Perfetti, P. A. and Frey, II, W. H. (1994). Two cases of acute anti-GM1 antibody elevations in response to exogenous GM1 without neurological symptoms. *J. Neuroimmunol.*, **53**, 109–113

Antoine, J. C., Steck, A. and Michel, D. (1993). Neuropathie périphérique mortelle avec predominance motrice associée à une IgM monoclonale anti-MAG. *Rev. Neurol. (Paris)*, **149**, 496–499

Apostolski, S. and Latov, N. (1993). Clinical syndromes associated with anti-GM1 antibodies. *Semin. Neurol.*, **13**, 364–368

Apostolski, S., Sadiq, S. A., Hays, A. *et al.* (1994). Identification of Gal(β1-3)GalNAc bearing glycoproteins at the nodes of Ranvier in peripheral nerve. *J. Neurosci. Res.*, **38**, 134–141

Arai, M., Yoshino, H., Kusano, Y. *et al.* (1992). Ataxic polyneuropathy and anti-Pr2 IgMk M-proteinaemia. *J. Neurol.*, **239**, 147–151

Aspinall, G. O., McDonald, A. G., Raju, T. S. *et al.* (1992). Serological diversity and chemical structure of *Campylobacter jejuni* low-molecular weight lipopolysaccharides. *J. Bacteriol.*, **174**, 1324–1332

Ayadi, H., Mihaesco, E., Congy, N. *et al.* (1992). H chain V region sequences of three human monocloncal IgMs with anti-myelin associated glycoprotein activity. *J. Immunol.*, **148**, 2812–2816

Azulay, J. P., Blin, O., Pouget, J. *et al.* (1994). Intravenous immunoglobulin treatment in patients with motor neuron syndromes associated with anti-GM1 antibodies. *Neurology*, **44**, 429–432

Baba, H., Miyatani, N., Sato, S. *et al.* (1985). Antibody to glycolipid in a patient with IgM paraproteinemia and polyradiculoneuropathy. *Acta Neurol. Scand.*, **72**, 218–221

Baba, H, Daune, G. C., Ilyas, A. A. *et al.* (1989). Anti-GM1 ganglioside antibodies with differing specificities in patients with multifocal motor neuropathy. *J. Neuroimmunol.*, **25**, 143–150

Barbieri, S., Nobile-Orazio, E., Baldini, L. *et al.* (1987). Visual evoked potentials in patients with neuropathy and macroglobulinemia. *Ann. Neurol.*, **12**, 663–666

Berkman, E. M. and Orlin, J. B. (1980). Use of plasmapheresis and partial plasma exchange in the management of patients with cryoglobulinemia. *Transfusion*, **20**, 171–178

Bollensen, E., Steck, A. J. and Schachner, M. (1988). Reactivity with the peripheral myelin glycoprotein Po in serum from patients with monoclonal IgM gammopathy and polyneuropathy. *Neurology*, **38**, 1266–1270

Bollensen, E., Schipper, H. I. and Steck, A. J. (1989). Motor neuropathy with activity of monoclonal IgM antibody to GD1a ganglioside. *J. Neurol.*, **236**, 353–355

Brouet, J. C., Mariette, X., Chevalier, A. and Hauttecoeur, B. (1992). Determination of the affinity of monoclonal IgM for myelin association glycoprotein and sulfated glucuronic paragloboside. *J. Neuroimmunol.*, **36**, 209–215

Chaudhry, V., Corse, A. M., Cornblath, D. R. *et al.* (1993). Multifocal motor neuropathy: response to human immune globulin. *Ann. Neurol.*, **33**, 237–242

Chiba, A., Kusunoki, S., Shimizu, T. and Kanzawa, I. (1992). Serum IgG antibody to ganglioside GQ1b is a possible marker of Miller–Fisher syndrome. *Ann. Neurol.*, **31**, 677–679

Chiba, A., Kusunoki, S., Obata, H. *et al.* (1993). Serum anti-GQ1b antibodies is associated with ophthalmoplegia in Miller–Fisher syndrome and Guillain–Barré syndrome. *Neurology*, **43**, 1911–1917

Cook, D., Dalakas, M., Galdi, A. *et al.* (1990). High-dose intravenous immunoglobulin in the treatment of demyelinating neuropathy associated with monoclonal gammopathy. *Neurology*, **40**, 212–214

Corbo, M., Quattrini, A., Lugaresi, A. *et al.* (1992). Patterns of reactivity of human anti-GM1 antibodies with spinal cord and motor neurons. *Ann. Neurol.*, **32**, 487–493

Corbo, M., Quattrini, A., Latov, N. and Hays, A. P. (1993). Localization of GM1 and Gal(β1-3)GalNAc antigenic determinants at the nodes of Ranvier in peripheral nerve. *Neurology*, **43**, 809–816

Daune, G. C., Farrer, R. G., Dalakas, M. C. and Quarles, R. H. (1992). Sensory neuropathy associated with immunoglobulin M to GD1b ganglioside. *Ann. Neurol.*, **31**, 683–685

Dellagi, K., Brouet, J. C., Perreau, J. and Paulin, D. (1982). Human monoclonal IgM with autoantibody activity against intermediate filaments. *Proc. Natl Acad. Sci. USA*, **79**, 446–450

Dennis, R. D., Antonicek, H., Wiegandt, H. and Schachner, M. (1988). Detection of the L2/HNK-1 carbohydrate epitope on glycoproeteins and acidic glycolipids of the insect *Calliphora vicina*. *J. Neurochem.*, **51**, 1490–1496

Ernerudh, J. H., Vrethem, M., Andersen, O. *et al.* (1992). Immunochemical and clinical effects of immunosuppressive treatment in monoclonal IgM neuropathy. *J. Neurol. Neurosurg. Psychiatry*, **55**, 930–934

Feldman, E. L., Bromberg, M. B., Albers, J. W. and Pestronk, A. (1991). Immunosuppressive treatment of multifocal motor neuropathy. *Ann. Neurol.*, **30**, 397–401

Figeuras, A., Morales-Olivas, F. J., Capella, D. *et al.* (1992). Bovine gangliosides and acute motor polyneuropathy. *Br. Med. J.*, **305**, 1330–1331

Freddo, L., Hays, A. P., Sherman, W. H. and Latov, N. (1985). Axonal neuropathy in a patient with IgM M-protein reactive with nerve endoneurium. *Neurology*, **35**, 1321–1325

Freddo, L, Yu, R. K., Latov, N. *et al.* (1986a). Gangliosides GM1 and GD1b are antigens for IgM M-proteins in a patient with motor neuron disease. *Neurology*, **36**, 454–458

Freddo, L., Hays, A. P., Nickerson, K. G. *et al.* (1986b). Monoclonal anti-DNA IgMk in neuropathy binds to myelin and to a conformational epitope formed by phosphatidic acid and gangliosides. *J. Immunol.*, **137**, 3821–3825

Freddo, L., Sherman, W. H. and Latov, N. (1986c). Glycosaminoglycan antigens in peripheral nerve; studies with antibodies from a patient with neuropathy and monoclonal gammopathy. *J. Neuroimmunol.*, **12**, 57–64

Fredman, P., Vedeler, C. A., Nyland, H. *et al.* (1991). Antibodies in sera from patients with inflammatory demyelinating polyradiculoneuropathy react with ganglioside LM1 and sulfatide of peripheral nerve myelin. *J. Neurol.*, **238**, 75–79

Fujimoto, S., Yuki, N., Itoh, T. and Amako, K. (1992). Specific serotypes of *Campylobacter jejuni* associated with Guillain–Barré syndrome. *J. Infect. Dis.*, **165**, 183

Garcia-Guijo, C., Garcia-Merino, A., Rubio, G. *et al.* (1992). IgG anti-ganglioside antibodies and their subclass distribution in two patients with acute and chronic motor neuropathy. *J. Neuroimmunol.*, **37**, 141–148

Gelman, E. P. and Dennis, L. H. (1981). Plasma cell dyscrasia after alkylating agent therapy for Hodgkins disease (letter). *N. Engl. J. Med.*, **35**, 135

Gosselin, S., Kyle, R. A. and Dyck, P. J. (1991). Neuropathy associated with monoclonal gammopathies of undetermined significance. *Ann. Neurol.*, **30**, 54–61

Graves, M. C. and Ravindranath, R. M. H. (1992). Do CD5+ B cells secrete anti-GM1 and asialo-GM1 antibodies in lower motor neuron disease (abstract). *Ann. N. Y. Acad. Sci.*, **651**, 570–571

Gregory, R., Thomas, P. K., King, R. H. M. *et al.* (1993). Coexistence of hereditary motor and sensory neuropathy type Ia and IgM paraproteinemic neuropathy. *Ann. Neurol.*, **33**, 649–652

Gregson, N. A., Jones, D., Thomas, P. K. and Willison, H. J. (1991). Acute motor neuropathy with antibodies to GM1 ganglioside. *J. Neurol.*, **238**, 447–451

Gregson, N. A., Koblar, S. and Hughes, R. A. C. (1993). Antibodies to gangliosides in Guillain–Barré syndrome: specificity and relationship to clinical features. *Q. J. Med.*, **86**, 111–117

Hanto, D., Frizzera, G., Gajl-Peczalska, K. J. *et al.* (1983). Epstein–Barr virus induced B-cell lymphoma after renal transplantation. Acyclovir therapy and transition from polyclonal to monoclonal B-cell proliferation. *N. Engl. J. Med.*, **306**, 913–918

Haas, D. C. and Tatum, A. H. (1988). Plasmapheresis alleviates neuropathy accompanying IgM anti-myelin associated glycoprotein paraproteinemia. *Ann. Neurol.*, **23**, 394–396

Hays, A. P., Latov, N., Takatsu, M. and Sherman, W. H. (1987). Experimental demyelination of nerve induced by serum of patients with neuropathy and anti-MAG proteins. *Neurology*, **37**, 242–256

Hays, A. P., Lee, S. L. and Latov, N. (1988). Immunoreactive C3d on the surface of myelin sheaths in neurology. *J. Neuroimmunol.*, **18**, 231–244

Heidenreich, F., Leifeld, L. and Jovin, T. (1994). T-cell dependent activity of ganglioside GM1 specific B-cells in Guillain-Barré syndrome and multifocal motor neuropathy *in vitro*. *J. Neuroimmunol.*, **49**, 97–108

Heiman-Patterson, T., Krupa, T., Thompson, P. *et al.* (1993). Anti-GM1/GD1b M-proteins damage human spinal cord neurons co-cultured with muscle. *J. Neurol. Sci.*, **20**, 38–45

Henningsson, C. M., Selvaraj, S., MacLean, G. D. *et al.* (1987). T-cell recognition of a tumor-associated glycoprotein and its synthetic carbohydrate epitopes: stimulation of anticancer T-cell immunity *in vivo*. *J. Immunol. Immunother.*, **25**, 231–241

Ilyas, A. A., Quarles, R. H., Dalakas, M. C. *et al.* (1985). Monoclonal IgM in a patient with parapro-teinemic polyneuropathy binds to gangliosides containing disialosyl groups. *Ann. Neurol.*, **18**, 655–659

Ilyas, A. A., Willison, H. J., Dalakas, M. *et al.* (1988a). Identification and characterization of gangliosides reacting with IgM paraproteins in three patients with neuropathy and biclonal gammopathy. *J. Neurochem.*, **51**, 851–858

Ilyas, A. A., Li, S.-C., Chou, D. K. H. *et al.* (1988b). Gangliosides GM2, IVGalNAcGm1b, and IVGalNAcGd1a as antigens for monoclonal immunoglobulin M in neuropathy associated with gammapathy. *J. Biol. Chem.*, **263**, 4369–4373

Ilyas, A. A., Willison, H. J., Quarles, R. H. *et al.* (1988c). Serum antibodies to gangliosides in Guillain–Barré syndrome. *Ann. Neurol.*, **23**, 440–447

Ilyas, A. A., Mithen, F. A., Chen, Z. W. and Cook, S. D. (1991). Search for antibodies to neutral glycolipids in sera of patients with Guillain–Barré syndrome. *J. Neurol. Sci.*, **102**, 67–75

Ilyas, A. A., Cook, S. D., Dalakas, M. C. and Mithen, F. A. (1992a). Anti-MAG IgM paraproteins from some patients with polyneuropathy associated with IgM paraproteinemia also react with sulfatide. *J. Neuroimmunol.*, **37**, 85–92

Ilyas, A. A., Mithen, F. A., Chen, Z. W. and Cook, S. D. (1992b). Anti-GM1 antibodies in Guillain–Barré syndrome. *J. Neuroimmunol.*, **36**, 69–76

Ilyas, A. A., Mithen, F. A., Dalakas, M. C. *et al.* (1992c). Antibodies to acidic glycolipids in Guillain–Barré syndrome and chronic inflammatory demyelinating neuropathy. *J. Neurol. Sci.*, **107**, 111–121

Ince, P. G., Shaw, P. J., Fawcett, P. R. and Bates, D. (1987). Demyelinating neuropathy due to primary IgM kappa B-cell lymphoma of peripheral nerve. *Neurology*, **37**, 1231–1235

Jack, H.-M., Beck-Engeser, G., Lee, G. *et al.* (1992). Tumorigenesis mediated by an antigen receptor. *Proc. Natl Acad. Sci. USA*, **89**, 8482–8486

Jacobs, J. M. and Scadding, J. W. (1990). Morphological changes in IgM paraproteinemic neuropathy. *Acta Neuropathol. (Berl)*, **80**, 77–84

Jensen, T. S., Schroder, H. D., Ionsson, V. *et al.* (1988). IgM monoclonal gammapathy and neuropathy in two siblings. *J. Neurol. Neurosurg. Psychiatry*, **51**, 1308–1315

Julien, J., Vital, C., Vallat, J. M. *et al.* (1984). Chronic demyelinating neuropathy with IgM producing lymphocytes in peripheral nerve and delayed appearance of "benign" monoclonal gammapathy. *Neurology*, **34**, 1387–1389

Kabat, K. A., Liao, J., Sherman, W. H. and Osserman, E. F. (1984). Immunological characterization of the specificities of two human monoclonal IgMs reacting with chondroitin sulfates. *Carbohydrate Res.*, **130**, 289–298

Kaji, R., Shibasaki, H. and Kimura, J. (1992). Multifocal demyelinating motor neuropathy: cranial nerve involvement and immunoglobulin therapy. *Neurology*, **42**, 506–509

Kaku, D. A. and Sumner, A. J. (1992). Characteristic electrophysiological findings in anti-MAG polyneuropathy. *Neurology*, **42**(suppl. 3), 408

Kelly, J. J., Jr. (1990). The electrodiagnostic findings in polyneuropathies associated with IgM monoclonal gammapathies. *Muscle Nerve*, **13**, 1113–1117

Kelly, J. J., Jr., Kyle, R. A., O'Brien, P. C. and Dyck, P. J. (1979). The natural history of peripheral neuropathy in primary systemic amyloidosis. *Ann. Neurol.*, **6**, 1–7

Kelly, J. J., Jr., Adelman, L. S., Berkman, E. and Bhan, I. (1988). Polyneuropathies associated with IgM monoclonal gammapathies. *Arch. Neurol.*, **45**, 1355–1359

Kinsella, L. J., Lange, D. J., Trojaborg, W. *et al.* (1994). The clinical and electrophysiological correlates of elevated anti-GM1 antibody titers. *Neurology*, **44**, 1278–1282

Knorr-Held, S., Brendel, W., Kiefer, H. *et al.* (1986). Sensitization against brain gangliosides after therapeutic swine brain implantation in a multiple sclerosis patient. *J. Neurol.*, **233**, 54–56

Konrad, R. J., Kricka, L. J., Goodman, D. B. P. *et al.* (1993). Myeloma associated paraprotein directed against the HIV-1 p24 antigen in an HIV-1 seropositive patient. *N. Engl. J. Med.*, **328**, 1817–1819

Kornberg, A., Pestronk, A., Bieser, K. *et al.* (1994). The clinical correlates of high-titer IgG anti-GM1 antibodies. *Ann. Neurol.*, **35**, 234–237

Koski, C. L., Chou, D. K. H. and Jungalwala, F. B. (1989). Anti-peripheral nerve myelin antibodies in Guillain–Barré syndrome bind a neutral glycolipid of peripheral myelin and cross reacts with Forssman antigen. *J. Clin. Invest.*, **84**, 280–287

Kuroki, S., Saida, T., Nukina, M. *et al.* (1993). *Campylobacter jejuni* strains from patients with Guillain–Barré syndrome belong mostly to Penner serogroup 19 and contain N-acetylglucosamine residues. *Ann. Neurol.*, **33**, 243–247

Kusunoki, S., Shimizu, T., Matsumura, K. *et al.* (1989). Motor dominant neuropathy and IgM paraproteinemia: the IgM M-protein binds to specific gangliosides. *J. Neuroimmunol.*, **21**, 177–181

Kusunoki, S., Chiba, A., Tai, T. and Kanazawa, I. (1993). Localization of GM1 and GD1b antigens in the human peripheral nervous system. *Muscle Nerve*, **16**, 752–756

Kusunoki, S., Chiba, A., Kon, K. *et al.* (1994). N-Acetylgalactosaminyl GD1a is a target molecule for serum antibody in Guillain–Barré syndrome. *Ann. Neurol.*, **35**, 570–576

Kyle, R. A. (1978). Monoclonal gammapathy of undetermined significance. Natural history in 241 cases. *Am. J. Med.*, **64**, 814–826

Lach, B., Rippstein, P., Atack, D. *et al.* (1993). Immunoelectron microscopic localization of monoclonal IgM antibodies in gammopathy associated with peripheral demyelinating neuropathy. *Acta Neuropathol. (Berl)*, **85**, 298–307

Landi, G., D'Alessandro, R., Dossi, B. C. *et al.* (1993). Guillain–Barré syndrome after exogenous gangliosides in Italy. *Br. Med. J.*, **307**, 1463–1464

Latov, N. (1994). Evaluation and treatment of patients with neuropathy and monoclonal gammopathy. *Semin. Neurol.*, **14**, 118–122

Latov, N., Godfrey, M., Thomas, Y. *et al.* (1985). Neuropathy and anti-MAG M-proteins; T-cell regulation of M-protein secretion *in vitro*. *Ann. Neurol.*, **18**, 182–188

Latov, N., Hays, A. P. and Sherman, W. H. (1988a). Peripheral neuropathy and anti-MAG antibodies. *CRC Crit. Rev. Neurobiol.*, **3**, 301–332

Latov, N., Hays, A. P., Donofrio, P. D. *et al.* (1988b). Monoclonal IgM with unique reactivity to gangliosides GM1 and GD1b and to lacto-N-tetraose in two patients with motor neuron disease. *Neurology*, **38**, 763–768

Latov, N., Koski, C. L. and Walicke, P. A. (1991). Guillain–Barré syndrome and parenteral gangliosides (letter). *Lancet*, **338**, 757

Lee, G., Ware, R. R. and Latov, N. (1994). Somatically mutated member of human V-lambda VII gene family encodes anti-myelin associated glycoprotein (MAG) activity. *J. Neuroimmunol.*, **51**, 45–52

Lee, K. W., Inghirami, G., Spatz, L. *et al.* (1991). The B cells that express anti-MAG antibodies in neuropathy and non-malignant IgM monoclonal gammopathy belong to the CD5 population. *J. Neuroimmunol.*, **31**, 83–88

Leger, J. M., Oksenhendler, E., Bussel, A. *et al.* (1993). Treatment by chlorambucil with/without plasma exchanges of polyneuropathy associated with monoclonal IgM: a prospective randomized control study in 44 patients. *Neurology*, **43**, A215

Mata, M., Kahn, S. N. and Fink, D. J. (1988). A direct electron microscopic immuno-cytochemical study of IgM paraproteinemic neuropathy. *Arch. Neurol.*, **45**, 693–697

Mann, J. L., DeSantis, P., Mark, G. *et al.* (1987). HTLV-I-associated B-cell CLL: indirect role for retrovirus in leukemogenesis. *Science*, **236**, 1103–1106

Marcus, D. M., Latov, N., Hsi, B. P. and Gillard, B. K. (1989). Report of a conference on measurement and significance of antibodies against GM1 ganglioside, *J. Neuroimmunol.*, **25**, 255–259

McGinnis, S., Kohriyama, T., Yu, R. K. *et al.* (1988). Antibodies to sulfated glucuronic acid containing glycosphingolipids in neuropathy associated with anti-MAG antibodies and in normal subjects. *J. Neuroimmunol.*, **17**, 119–126

McKhann, G. M., Cornblath, D. R., Griffin, J. W. *et al.* (1993). Acute motor axonal neuropathy: a frequent cause of acute flaccid paralysis in China. *Ann. Neurol.*, **33**, 333–342

Mendell, J. R., Zahenk, Z., Whitaker, J. N. *et al.* (1985). Polyneuropathy and IgM monoclonal gammopathy: studies on the pathogenetic role of anti-myelin associated glycoprotein antibody. *Ann. Neurol.*, **17**, 243–254

Mihaesco, E., Ayadi, H., Congy, N. *et al.* (1989). Multiple mutations in the variable region of the k light chains of three monoclonal human IgM with anti-myelin associated glycoprotein activity. *J. Biol. Chem.*, **264**, 21481–21485

Miyatani, N., Baba, H., Sato, S. *et al.* (1987). Antibody to sialosyllactosaminylparagloboside in patient with IgM paraproteinemia and polyradiculoneuroapthy. *J. Neuroimmunol.*, **14**, 189–196

Mizutamari, R. K., Wiegant, H. and Nores, G. A. (1994). Characterization of anti-ganglioside antibodies present in normal human plasma. *J. Neuroimmunol.*, **50**, 215–220

Monaco, S., Bonetti, B., Ferrari, S. *et al.* (1990). Complement dependent demyelination in patients with IgM monoclonal gammopathy and polyneuropathy. *N. Engl. J. Med.*, **322**, 649–652

Nemni, R., Fazio, R., Quattrini, A. *et al.* (1993). Antibodies to sulfatide and to chondroitin sulfate C in patients with chronic sensory neuropathy. *J. Neuroimmunol.*, **43**, 79–86

Nobile-Orazio, E., Hays, A. P., Latov, N. *et al.* (1984). Reactivity of mouse and human anti-MAG antibodies; antigenic specificity and immunofluorescence studies. *Neurology*, **34**, 1336–1342

Nobile-Orazio, E., Baldini, L., Barbieri, S. *et al.* (1988). Treatment of patients with neuropathy and anti-MAG IgM M-proteins. *Ann. Neurol.*, **24**, 93–97

Nobile-Orazio, E., Francomano, E., Daverio, E. *et al.* (1989). Anti-myelin associated glycoprotein IgM antibody titers in neuropathy associated with macroglobulinemia. *Ann. Neurol.*, **26**, 543–550

Nobile-Orazio, E., Carpo, M., Meucci, N. *et al.* (1992). Guillain–Barré syndrome associated with high titers of anti-GM1 antibodies. *J. Neurol. Sci.*, **109**, 200–206

Nobile-Orazio, E., Meucci, N., Barbieri, S. *et al.* (1993). High dose intravenous immunoglobulin therapy in multifocal motor neuropathy. *Neurology*, **4**, 537–543

Nobile-Orazio, E., Manfredini, E., Carpo, M. *et al.* (1994). Frequency and clinical correlates of anti-neural IgM antibodies in neuropathy associated with IgM monoclonal gammopathy. *Ann. Neurol.*, **36**, 416–424

Obi, T., Kusunoki, S., Takatsu, M. *et al.* (1992). IgM M-protein in a patient with sensory-dominant neuropathy binds preferentially to polysialogangliosides. *Acta Neurol. Scand.*, **86**, 215–218

Offner, H., Standage, B. A., Burger, D. R. and Vandenbark, A. A. (1985). Delayed type hypersensitivity to gangliosides in the Lewis rat. *J. Neuroimmunol.*, **9**, 145–157

Ogawa-Goto, K., Funamoto, N., Abe, T. and Nagashima, K. (1990). Different ceramide compositions of gangliosides between human motor and sensory nerves. *J. Neurochem.*, **55**, 1486–1492

Ogawa-Goto, K., Funamoto, N., Ohta, Y. *et al.* (1992). Myelin gangliosides of human peripheral nervous system: an enrichment of GM1 in the motor nerve myelin associated from cauda equina. *J. Neurochem.*, **59**, 1844–1848

Ogino, M., Tatum, A. H. and Latov, N. (1994). Affinity of human anti-MAG antibodies in neuropathy. *J. Neuroimmunol.*, **52**, 41–46

Ogino, M., Nobile-Orazio, E., Latov, N. (1995). IgG anti-GM1 antibodies from patients with acute motor neuropathy are restricted and predominantly IgG1 and IgG3 (abstract). *J. Neuroimmundol.* (in press)

Pathak, S., Illavia, S. J., Kahlili-Shirazi, A. and Webb, H. E. (1990). Immunoelectron microscopic labeling of a glycolipid in the envelopes of brain cell-derived budding viruses, Semliki Forest, influenza, and measles, using a monoclonal antibody directed chiefly against galactocerebroside resulting from Semliki Forest virus infection. *J. Neurol. Sci.*, **96**, 293–302

Pestronk, A. (1991). Motor neuropathies, motor neuron disorders, and antiglycolipid antibodies. *Muscle Nerve*, **14**, 927–935

Pestronk, A., Cornblath, D. R., Ilyas, A. A. *et al.* (1988). A treatable multifocal motor neuropathy with antibodies to GM1 ganglioside. *Ann. Neurol.*, **24**, 73–78

Pestronk, A., Chaudhry, V., Feldman, E. L. *et al.* (1990). Lower motor neuron syndromes defined by patterns of weakness, nerve conduction abnormalities and high titers of antiglycolipid antibodies. *Ann. Neurol.*, **27**, 316–326

Pestronk, A., Li, F., Griffin, J. *et al.* (1991). Polyneuropathy syndromes associated with serum antibodies to sulfatide and myelin associated glycoprotein. *Neurology*, **41**, 357–362

Quattrini, A., Nemni, R., Fazio, R. *et al.* (1991). Axonal neuropathy in a patient with monoclonal IgM kappa reactive with Schmidt–Lanterman incisures. *J. Neuroimminol.*, **33**, 73–79

Quattrini, A., Corbo, M., Dhaliwal, S. K. *et al.* (1992). Anti-sulfatide antibodies in neurological disease; binding to rat dorsal root ganglia neurons. *J. Neurol. Sci.*, **112**, 152–159

Radl, J., DeGlopper, E., van den Berg, P. and Wanzwieten, M. J. (1986). Idiopathic paraproteinemia III. Increased frequency of paraproteinemia in thymectomized, aging C57GL/Kahukig and CBA/Brarij mice. *J. Immunol.*, **125**, 31–35

Roberts, M., Willison, H., Vincent, A. and Newsom-Davis, J. (1994). Serum factor in Miller-Fisher variant of Guillain–Barré syndrome and neurotransmitter release. *Lancet*, **343**, 454–455

Sadiq, S. A., Thomas, F. P., Kilidireas, K. *et al.* (1990). The spectrum of neurological disease associated with anti-GM1 antibodies. *Neurology*, **40**, 1067–1072

Santoro, M., Uncini, A., Corbo, M. *et al.* (1992). Experimental conduction block induced by serum from a patient with anti-GM1 antibodies. *Ann. Neurol.*, **31**, 385–390

Schonhoffer, P. S. (1992). GM1 ganglioside for spinal cord injury (letter). *N. Engl. J. Med.*, **326**, 493

Sherman, W. H., Latov, N., Hays, A. P. *et al.* (1983). Monoclonal IgMk antibody precipitating with chondroitin sulfate C from patients with axonal polyneuropathy and epidermolysis. *Neurology*, **33**, 192–201

Sherman, W. H., Latov, N., Lange, D. E. *et al.* (1994). Fludarabine for IgM antibody mediated neuropathies (abstract). *Ann. Neurol.*, **36**, 326

Shy, M. E., Heiman-Patterson, T., Parry, G. J. *et al.* (1990). Lower motor neuron disease in a patient with antibodies against Gal(β1-2)GalNAc in gangliosides Gm1 and GD1b: improvement following immunotherapy. *Neurology*, **40**, 842–844

Snipes, G. J., Suter, U. and Shooter, E. M. (1993). Human peripheral myelin protein-22 carries the L2/HNK-1 carbohydrate adhesion epitope. *J. Neurochem.*, **61**, 1961–1964

Spatz, L. A., Wong, K. K., Williams, M. *et al.* (1990). Cloning and sequence analysis of the variable heavy and light chain regions of an anti-myelin/DNA antibody from a patient with peripheral neuropathy and chronic lymphocytic leukemia. *J. Immunol.*, **144**, 2821–2828

Spatz, L. A., Williams, M., Brender, B. *et al.* (1992a). DNA sequence analysis and comparison of the variable heavy and light chain regions of the two IgM monoclonal anti-MAG antibodies. *J. Neuroimmunol.*, **36**, 29–39

Spatz, L.A., Daugherty, B. L., DeMartino, J. A. *et al.* (1992b). Expression of recombinant human anti-MAG antibodies in non-lymphoid mammalian cells. *Hum. Antibod. Hybrid.*, **3**, 107–111

Stall, A. M., Farinas, C., Tarlington, D. M. *et al.* (1988). Ly-1 B-cell clones similar to human chronic lymphocytic leukemia routinely develop in older normal mice and young autoimmune (New Zealand Black-related) animals. *Proc. Natl Acad. Sci. USA*, **85**, 7312–7316

Steck, A. J., Murray, N., Meier, C. *et al.* (1983). Demyelinating neuropathy and monoclonal IgM antibody to myelin associated glycoprotein. *Neurology*, **33**, 19–23

Suarez, G. A. and Kelly, J. J., Jr. (1993). Polyneuropathy associated with monoclonal gammopathy of undetermined significance: further evidence that IgM-MGUS neuropathies are different than IgG-MGUS. *Neurology*, **43**, 1304–1308

Svennerholm, L. and Fredman, P. (1990). Antibody detection in the Guillain–Barré syndrome. *Ann. Neurol.*, **27**(suppl), 36–40

Takatsu, M., Hays, A. P., Latov, N. *et al.* (1985). Immunofluorescence study of patients with neuropathy and IgM M-proteins. *Ann. Neurol.*, **18**, 173–181

Tatum, A. H. (1993). Experimental paraprotein neuropathy, demyelination by passive transfer of human IgM anti-myelin associated glycoprotein. *Ann. Neurol.*, **33**, 502–506

Thomas, F. P., Adapon, P. H., Goldberg, G. P. *et al.* (1989). Localization of neural epitopes that bind to IgM monoclonal autoantibodies (M-proteins) from two patients with motor neuron disease. *J. Neuroimmunol.*, **21**, 31–39

Thomas, F. P., Trojaborg, W., Nagy, C. *et al.* (1991). Experimental autoimmune neuropathy with anti-GM1 antibodies and immunoglobulin deposits at the nodes of Ranvier. *Acta Neuropathol.*, **82**, 378–383

Thomas, F. P., Lovelace, R. E., Ding, X. S. *et al.* (1992). Vasculitis, axonal degeneration, and demyelinating neuropathy with cryoglobulinemia and anti-MAG monoclonal gammopathy. *Muscle Nerve*, **15**, 891–898

Thornton, C. and Griggs, R. C. (1994). Plasma exchange and intravenous immunoglobulin treatment of neuromuscular disease. *Ann. Neurol.*, **35**, 260–268

Trojaborg, W., Galassi, G., Hays, A. P. *et al.* (1989). Electrophysiologic study of experimental demyelination induced by serum of patients with IgM M-proteins and neuropathy. *Neurology*, **39**, 1581–1586

Valldeoriola, E., Graus, F., Steck, A. J. *et al.* (1993). Delayed appearance of anti-myelin associated glycoprotein antibodies in a patient with chronic demyelinating polyneuropathy. *Ann. Neurol.*, **34**, 394–396

van den Berg, L. H., Marrink, J., de Jager, A. E. J. *et al.* (1992a). Anti-GM1 antibodies in patients with Guillain–Barré syndrome. *J. Neurol. Neurosurg. Pyschiatry*, **55**, 6–11

van den Berg, L. H., Lankamp, C. L. A. M., de Jager, A. E. J. *et al.* (1993). Anti-sulfatide antibodies in peripheral neuropathy. *J. Neurol. Neurosurg. Psychiatry*, **56**, 1164–1168

van den Berg, L. H., Kinsella, L. J., Corbo, M. *et al.* (1992b). Antibodies to MAG and SGPG in neuropathy. *Ann. Neurol.*, **32**, 251

Vrethem, M. Ernerudh, J., Cruz, M. *et al.* (1993). Susceptibility to demyelinating polyneuropathy in plasma cell dyscrasia may be influenced by amino acid position 9 of the HLA-DR β chain. *J. Neuroimmunol.*, **43**, 139–144

Vital, A., Vital, C., Julien, J. *et al.* (1989). Polyneuropathy associated with IgM monoclonal gammopathy; immunological and pathological study in 31 patients. *Acta Neuropathol.*, **79**, 160–167

Walsh, F. S., Cronin, M., Koblar, S. *et al.* (1991). Association between glycoconjugate antibodies and *Campylobacter* infection in patients with Guillain–Barré syndrome. *J. Neuroimmunol.*, **34**, 43–51

Weng, N., Yu-Lee, L., Sanz, I. *et al.* (1992). Structure and specificities of anti-ganglioside autoantibodies associated with motor neuropathies. *J. Immunol.*, **149**, 2518–2529

Willison, H. J. and Veitch, J. (1994). Immunoglobulin subclass distribution and binding characteristics of anti-GQ1b antibodies in Miller–Fisher syndrome. *J. Neurochem.*, **50**, 159–165

Willison, H. J., Trapp, B. D., Bacher, J. D. *et al.* (1988). Demyelination induced by intraneural injection of human anti-myelin associated glycoprotein antibodies. *Muscle Nerve*, **11**, 1169–1176

Willison, H. J., Paterson, G., Veitch, J. *et al.* (1993a). Peripheral neuropathy associated with monoclonal IgM anti-Pr2 cold agglutinin. *J. Neurol. Neurosurg. Psychiatry*, **56**, 1178–1181

Willison, H. J., Veitch, J., Patterson, G. and Kennedy, P. G. E. (1993b). Miller–Fisher syndrome is associated with serum antibodies to GQ1b ganglioside. *J. Neurol. Neurosurg. Psychiatry*, **56**, 204–206

Willison, H. J., Paterson, G., Kennedy, P. G. E. and Veitch, J. (1994a). Cloning of human anti-GM1 antibodies from motor neuropathy patients. *Ann. Neurol.*, **35**, 471–478

Willison, H. J., Roberts, M., O'Hanlon, G. *et al.* (1994b). Human monoclonal anti-GM1 ganglioside antibodies interfere with neuromuscular transmission (abstract). *Ann. Neurol.*, **36**, 289

Wirguin, I., Suturkova-Milosevic, L. J., Della-Latta, P. *et al.* (1994). Monoclonal IgM antibodies to GM1 and asialo-GM1 in chronic neuropathies cross-react with *Campylobacter jejuni* lipopolysaccharides. *Ann. Neurol.*, **35**, 698–703

Yee, W. C., Hahn, A. F., Hearn, S. A. and Rupar, A. R. (1989). Neuropathy in IgM paraproteinemia; immunoreactivity to neural proteins and chondroitin sulfate. *Acta Neuropathol.*, **78**, 57–64

Yeung, K. B., Thomas, P. K., King, R. H. *et al.* (1991). The clinical spectrum of peripheral neuropathies associated with benign monoclonal IgM, IgG and IgA paraproteinemia. Comparative clinical, immunological and nerve biopsy findings. *J. Neurol.*, **238**, 383–391

Younes-Chennoufi, A. B., Leger, J. M., Hauw, J. J. *et al.* (1992). Ganglioside GD1b is the target antigen for a biclonal IgM in a case of sensory–motor axonal neuropathy. *Ann. Neurol.*, **32**, 18–23

Yuki, N., Yoshino, H., Sato, S. and Miyatake, T. (1990). Acute axonal polyneuropathy associated with anti-GM1 antibodies following *Campylobacter* enteritis. *Neurology*, **40**, 1900–1902

Yuki, N., Sato, S., Miyatake, T. *et al.* (1991). Motor neuron disease-like disorder after ganglioside therapy. *Lancet*, **337**, 1109–1110

Yuki, N., Miyatani, N., Sato, S. *et al.* (1992a). Acute relapsing sensory neuropathy associated with IgM antibody against B-series gangliosides. *Neurology*, **42**, 686–689

Yuki, N., Handa, S., Taki, T. *et al.* (1992b). Cross-reactive antigen between nervous tissue and a bacterium elicits Guillain–Barré syndrome: molecular mimickry between ganglioside GM1 and lipopolysaccharide from Penner's serotype 19 of *Campylobacter jejuni*. *Biomed. Res.*, **13**, 451–453

Yuki, N., Sato, S., Tsuji, S. *et al.* (1993a). Frequent presence of anti-GQ1b antibody in Fisher's syndrome. *Neurology*, **43**, 414–417

Yuki, N., Yamazaki, M., Kondo, H. *et al.* (1993b). Treatment of multifocal motor neuropathy with a high dosage of intravenous immunoglobulin (letter). *Muscle Nerve*, **16**, 220–221

9
Guillain–Barré syndrome and chronic inflammatory demyelinating polyradiculoneuropathy

R. A. C. Hughes

INTRODUCTION

Guillain–Barré syndrome (GBS) is a clinically defined syndrome of acute weakness of the limbs attributable to disorder of the peripheral nerves not due to systemic disease. The syndrome was described by Guillain, Barré and Strohl (1916) who emphasized the accompanying rise in CSF albumin concentration while the cell count remained normal. Its diagnostic boundaries have been re-described in modern terms by Asbury and Cornblath (1990) but continue to defy strict definition. The clinical syndrome is classically an acute monophasic sensory and motor polyradiculoneuropathy. Variants include pure motor or rarely pure sensory forms, chronic or relapsing disease and the Miller Fisher syndrome (MFS) of ophthalmoplegia, ataxia and areflexia (Table 9.1). The classical syndrome is usually due to an endoneurial inflammatory process whose distribution determines the clinical features. When the inflammation is particularly severe, axons as well as myelin sheaths are destroyed. In some cases axonal or neuronal disorder is the primary event (see Chapter 4). Immune responses against myelin glycolipids and proteins have been discovered which could explain the pathogenesis of some of these syndromes. In advance of a full understanding of the aetiology, empirical trials have shown that immunomodulatory treatment is helpful.

GBS reaches its nadir within 4 weeks (Asbury and Cornblath, 1990) and forms one end of a spectrum of disorders of which the most chronic is chronic inflammatory (or idiopathic) demyelinating polyradiculoneuropathy (CIDP). This too has been defined by an international committee and has a relapsing or progressive course which evolves over at least 2 months (Ad Hoc Subcommittee of the American Academy of Neurology AIDS Task Force, 1991). Patients with an intermediate monophasic course have been described as having subacute idiopathic demyelinating polyradiculoneuropathy (SIDP) (Hughes *et al.*, 1992a).

GUILLAIN–BARRÉ SYNDROME
Typical clinical picture

Typically GBS develops over the course of a few days. Tingling and slight impairment of sensation of the hands and feet appear at the same time as limb weakness.

Table 9.1 Classification of Guillain–Barré syndrome

- Acute inflammatory demyelinating polyradiculoneuropathy

- Acute motor axonal neuropathy

- Acute motor and sensory axonal neuropathy

- Acute pandysautonomia

- Miller–Fisher syndrome

- Subacute inflammatory demyelinating polyradiculoneuropathy

- Chronic inflammatory demyelinating polyradiculoneuropathy
    Relapsing
    Recurrent
    Progressive

- Chronic relapsing axonal neuropathy

The symptoms are usually approximately symmetrical and more marked at first in the lower limbs so that the paralysis appears to ascend. The tingling may be painful and pain may also occur in the limb and back muscles. In children the pain is sometimes so severe as to resemble meningism and cause diagnostic confusion. The advancing disease may involve the cranial nerves, especially the facial and bulbar nerves, and sometimes the nerves to the external ocular muscles. In about 25% of cases the innervation of the respiratory muscles is so severely affected as to require ventilatory support. Such patients appear superficially comfortable at rest but become tired and breathless on slight exertion. They use the accessory muscles of respiration (elevators of the nostrils, sternomastoids and pectorals). If the diaphragm is paralysed abdominal wall movement becomes paradoxical and if the intercostal muscles are affected chest expansion becomes impaired (Hughes and Bihari, 1993). Typically the progressive phase lasts from 3 days up to about 3 weeks. The distribution of the duration of the progressive phase is unimodal with the modal value being between 1 and 3 weeks and is skewed with a long tail (Gibbels and Giebisch, 1992). The separation of inflammatory neuropathy into acute, subacute and chronic subgroups is based on the arbitrary decisions of international committees and not on any sound epidemiological basis.

The cerebrospinal fluid (CSF) protein usually becomes increased during the second week of the illness and the CSF cell count usually remains normal or only slightly increased (Hughes, 1990). However when GBS is associated with HIV infection, the CSF cell count may be increased. A slight CSF pleocytosis is not uncommon in HIV-infected subjects without overt neurological disease (Cornblath *et al.*, 1987b).

Variants

The evolution of GBS is sometimes much more rapid than in the typical case, with weakness becoming so severe that walking becomes impossible within 2 days, sometimes even within a few hours. A very rapid onset is associated with a worse prognosis (Winer *et al.*, 1988a) and is probably due to very severe inflammation causing axonal damage as well as demyelination. However this 'hyperacute' variant of GBS probably includes patients with what has been called the 'axonal' form of GBS (Feasby *et al.*, 1986) but which would be better described as acute motor and sensory axonal neuropathy (AMSAN) or acute motor axonal neuropathy (AMAN) depending on the presence or absence of sensory involvement. Proving that the underlying pathological process is an axonal neuropathy and not inflammation and demyelination with secondary axonal degeneration is difficult. Until recently cases in which this had been rigorously done were few (Feasby *et al.*, 1993). AMAN has now been clearly described as the cause of an epidemic paralytic illness occurring in the summer months in children in China (McKhann *et al.*, 1991, 1993). Acute motor axonal neuropathy also occurs in sporadic form in both paediatric and adult patients but is rare (see Chapter 4).

A sensory form of GBS has been postulated and a few cases have been reported in which the neurophysiological findings suggest that the underlying pathological process is demyelination (Dawson *et al.*, 1988; Miralles *et al.*, 1992a). Such cases are difficult to distinguish from acute sensory neuronopathy (Sterman *et al.*, 1986) (see Chapter 3).

Miller Fisher syndrome has been regarded as a variant of GBS and consists of ophthalmoplegia, ataxia and tendon areflexia. This syndrome is usually due to an acute neuropathy affecting a subset of peripheral nerve fibres. Neurophysiological studies suggest that the underlying pathological process is an axonopathy (see below).

In most patients with GBS, the upper as well as the lower limbs are affected and the weakness usually starts and is maximal in the lower limbs. Ropper has drawn attention to variants with different distributions of weakness (Ropper *et al.*, 1991; Ropper, 1992). In the commonest variant the weakness descends from the cranial nerves to the shoulder girdle, a pattern which should give rise to consideration of botulism or diphtheria. Rarely the weakness remains confined to the lower limbs and resembles a compressive cauda equina lesion. In AIDS a syndrome of cytomegalovirus-induced cauda equina radiculoneuropathy is an important differential diagnosis. Finally a syndrome of acute pandysautonomia associated with absent tendon reflexes, sensory symptoms and raised CSF protein has been regarded as a variant of GBS (Young *et al.*, 1975; Ropper *et al.*, 1991).

Differential diagnosis

The neurologist has no reason to be scornful of the doctor who first sees a patient with GBS and fails to make the correct diagnosis. Apart from a banal infection a few days earlier, the patient is likely to have been otherwise well and the tendon reflexes may still be present. Hysteria is a common misdiagnosis at this stage. When the onset is very rapid the possibility of a stroke is sometimes entertained. Depressed tendon reflexes do occur with brainstem lesions, as in brainstem encephalitis, and also in spinal shock. In the purely motor forms of GBS, muscle disease, electrolyte disturbance (especially hypo- or hyperkalaemia), and neuromuscular conduction block (myasthenia, botulism) need to be considered (Hughes and Bihari, 1993). It is usually clear to the neurologist that the differential diagnosis is limited to that of an acute neuropathy (Table 9.2).

Table 9.2 Causes of acute motor or acute motor and sensory neuropathy*

Alcohol

Critical illness polyneuropathy (see Chapter 13)

Toxins
  Organophosphates
  Thallium
  Arsenic
  Lead
  Gold
  Lithium

Drugs
  Vincristine
  Nitrofurantoin

Neurotoxic fish poisoning

Lymphoma

Vasculitis
  Systemic lupus erythematosus
  Polyarteritis nodosa
  Churg–Strauss syndrome

Metabolic
  Acute intermittent porphyria
  Hereditary tyrosinaemia
  Leigh's disease

Diphtheria

Cytomegalovirus lumbosacral radiculopathy

Buckthorn neuropathy (Central America)

---

*After Hughes and Bihari (1993).

Neurophysiological features

The characteristic neurophysiological abnormalities develop during the first week and consist of multifocal conduction block and slowing of nerve conduction, especially in the spinal roots, proximal nerve segments, nerve trunks at sites of compression and terminal motor nerve branches (Cornblath, 1990). The changes are compatible with the typical pathological substrate of multifocal endoneurial inflammation (see next section). Criteria for the neurophysiological diagnosis of GBS have been published (Cornblath, 1990) but may need modification as the best diagnostic index for conduction block is refined (Oh *et al.*, 1994). The electrophysiological features of GBS have been particularly clearly reviewed and explained in a recent book (Parry, 1993). During the first day or two of the disease it may be difficult to identify any neurophysiological abnormalities which is unfortunate because this is the time when treatment decisions have to be made. The earliest changes are absent or impersistent F waves, because of spinal root involvement, and diminished compound muscle action potentials (CMAPs) because of the terminal motor nerve involvement. Next, where conduction can be tested across an affected nerve segment, the proximally evoked CMAP falls in amplitude relative to the distally evoked CMAP from which the presence of conduction block can be deduced. As the regions of inflammation and conduction block accumulate, conduction at each demyelinated segment is slowed and slow motor conduction velocities become detectable. The F wave latencies are prolonged and show marked dispersion due to variation in conduction velocity between normal or nearly normal fibres and less or more severely demyelinated fibres (Parry, 1993). Sensory nerves may be relatively spared. When sensory action potentials are affected, those from the sural nerve are relatively preserved although the upper limb sensory nerve action potentials become diminished, delayed or absent (Albers *et al.*, 1985; Albers and Kelly, 1989).

In many cases of severe GBS the motor nerves become inexcitable, and denervation changes are found on electromyography. In most patients these changes are preceded by evidence of conduction block or slowing of conduction, when it has been looked for, and the underlying pathological substrate is acute inflammatory demyelinating polyradiculoneuropathy (AIDP) (Hall *et al.*, 1992). However, in the small proportion of patients with AMAN or AMSAN, the nerves become inexcitable without a preliminary period of slowed conduction, electromyography shows profuse fibrillation, and the muscles become severely wasted (Feasby *et al.*, 1986).

Pathology

The pathological substrate of the typical case of GBS is an acute multifocal inflammatory process throughout the peripheral nervous system, especially affecting the anterior roots (Asbury *et al.*, 1969). During the first few days lymphocytes usually predominate in the inflammatory infiltrate, although in some cases lymphocytes are sparse (Honavar *et al.*, 1991). Ultrastructural studies have shown that the demyelination is mediated by macrophages which invade the basal lamina, penetrate and ingest the myelin lamellae and strip the axon bare (Figure 9.1) (Prineas, 1972, 1981). The macrophages have Fc receptors which attach to the Fc portion of antibodies bound to myelin or Schwann cell antigens (see below). This picture of the pathological changes in GBS has been largely built up from autopsy studies. Sural nerve biopsies often show very little change (Hughes *et al.*, 1992b). Biopsy of terminal motor nerves is not usually a reasonable diagnostic procedure but did show demyelination of almost all nerve fibres in one patient who had inexcitable motor nerves at the time of biopsy (Figure 9.2) (Hall *et al.*, 1992). In severe cases of GBS, biopsies and autopsy may show severe axonal degeneration, sometimes with little or no inflammation. This can usually be explained by inflammation and axonal damage at a more proximal site (Honavar *et al.*, 1991).

In some severe cases of GBS, usually with a very rapid onset, electrophysiological features, biopsy and autopsy all indicate primary axonal pathology (Feasby *et al.*, 1986, 1993; Honavar *et al.*, 1991; McKhann *et al.*, 1993). This condition may be entirely motor and is appropriately called AMAN (see Chapter 4) or may also affect sensory fibres (AMSAN).

Epidemiology

The incidence of GBS is uniformly within the range 1–2 per 100 000 in all countries where it has been studied. It is 1.5 to 2 times more common in males than females.

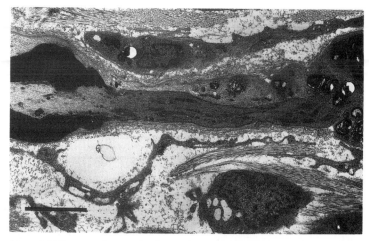

Figure 9.1 Electron micrograph of a partly demyelinated nerve fibre from a sural nerve biopsy of a patient with Guillain–Barré syndrome. The myelin of the right internode has been stripped and one macrophage containing myelin debris remains within the basal lamina while another lies nearby. Bar = 5 μm. (Reproduced from Hughes (1990), with permission.)

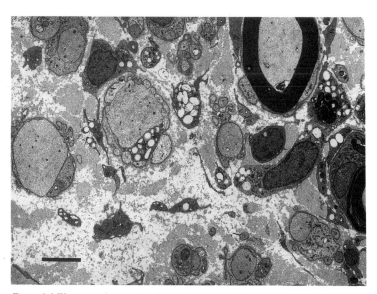

Figure 9.2 Electron micrograph of a terminal branch of the nerve to long head of biceps from a patient with Guillain–Barré syndrome and inexcitable motor nerves. The axons are preserved but most have lost their myelin sheaths. Bar = 5 μm. (Reproduced from Hall *et al.* (1992), with permission.)

The incidence gradually rises with age with a minor hump in the age distribution indicating a slightly increased incidence in young adults. Diagnosis in small children is difficult but it has been reported throughout the paediatric age range including neonates. The disease is very uncommon under the age of 2 years (Ropper *et al.*, 1991; Bradshaw and Jones, 1992).

Table 9.3 Infections and other events commonly reported as preceding Guillain–Barré syndrome

*Campylobacter jejuni**
Cytomegalovirus*
Epstein–Barr virus
Varicella zoster virus
Measles
Human immunodeficiency virus
Mycoplasma
Semple or mouse-brain-containing rabies vaccine
Swine-influenza vaccine
Surgical operation

*Only the associations with *Campylobacter jejuni* and cytomegalovirus have been proved with case-control studies: the other associations are based on the much weaker evidence of published case reports and uncontrolled case series. (See Hughes, 1990; Arnason and Soliven, 1993.)

The characteristic epidemiological feature of GBS is the occurrence of a previous event, usually an infection but sometimes an immunization or operation, during the previous few weeks. In a case control study Winer *et al.* (1988c) found that 55% of 100 patients compared with 15% of hospital controls had symptoms of an infection, and 6% of the patients and 5% of the controls had had an immunization during the previous 4 weeks. These percentages are compatible with uncontrolled reports in the literature. The infections were respiratory in 38% of patients and gastrointestinal in 17%. Serological tests showed evidence of recent cytomegalovirus infection in 11% of patients and *Campylobacter* in 14%. In subsequent series there has been evidence of *Campylobacter* infection from stool culture or serological tests in 14% to 42% of patients (Yuki *et al.*, 1992a; Mishu *et al.*, 1993; Vriesendorp *et al.*, 1993). A huge number of other bacterial, viral and parasitic infections have been reported as preceding GBS with the implication that they may actually precipitate it. Those for which there is evidence from case-controlled studies or from strikingly numerous reports are listed in Table 9.3.

Pathogenesis

Non-specific evidence of inflammation

Abundant evidence of an ongoing inflammatory response in AIDP has been obtained without resort to biopsy or post-mortem examination. Concentrations of the important cell adhesion molecule E-selectin are increased in the serum, indicating activation of the endothelium which will permit the adhesion and penetration by T cells (Hartung *et al.*, 1994). There is an increased number of circulating T cells bearing the activation markers IL-2 and transferrin receptors (Taylor and Hughes, 1989) and an increased serum concentration of soluble IL-2 receptors which are shed by activated T cells (Hartung *et al.*, 1990). Concentrations of the activated complement components C3a and C5a are increased in the CSF, indicating activation of complement (Hartung *et al.*, 1987). Activated T cells release many different cytokines including tumour necrosis factor alpha (TNFα) and the concentration of this is also increased in the serum in the acute stage of GBS (Sharief *et al.*, 1993). The concentration of TNFα in the serum is correlated with disease severity (Exley *et al.*, 1994). This cytokine is potentially important since it induces demyelination following injection into rat sciatic nerves (K. J. Smith, personal communication). Every arm of the immune response is involved in AIDP and the problem is to discover the target of all this activity.

Experimental allergic neuritis

Thinking about the pathogenesis of GBS was dominated until recently by the resemblance of the pathological changes of AIDP to experimental allergic neuritis induced in rabbits, rats or guinea-pigs by immunization with peripheral nerve tissue and Freund's adjuvant (Waksman and Adams, 1955, 1956). The inflammatory response in this experimental disease is induced by T cells directed against specific epitopes on either P_2 basic protein or P_0 glycoprotein (Kadlubowski and Hughes, 1979; Linington *et al.*, 1984, 1992) but the demyelination is enhanced by the presence of antibodies directed against the major myelin glycolipid galactocerebroside (Hahn *et al.*, 1993). The final common pathway of demyelination in experimental allergic neuritis, as in AIDP, is macrophage invasion of the basal lamina and stripping of myelin (Lampert, 1969).

T cell-mediated immunity

An explanation of how AIDP could be triggered in an immunogenetically susceptible individual can readily be constructed from experimental allergic neuritis. T cells activated by an antecedent infection or other event will cross the blood–nerve barrier more readily than non-activated T cells because of the up-regulation of the cell adhesion molecules on their surface. If the activated T cells recognize an endoneurial antigen, they will be stimulated, release cytokines, attract macrophages and initiate an endoneurial inflammatory response. T cell responses to P_2 and P_0 proteins have been identified in only a small proportion of patients with GBS (Khalili-Shirazi *et al.*, 1992; Giegerich *et al.*, 1994) but the bulk culture techniques so far used to detect these responses may be too insensitive or the target proteins may be different in humans compared with rats. It is possible that the T cell-mediated endoneurial inflammatory response *per se* releases cytokines and can induce demyelination in the absence of antibody but this has not been proved (Hughes, 1990). However it is more likely that both arms of the immune response are involved in AIDP and that an initial T cell response breaks down the blood–nerve barrier and initiates the inflammation while a subsequent antibody response contributes to the myelin and axon damage.

The role of antibody

The most obvious and direct way in which antibody might damage Schwann cells and myelin is by fixing complement and initiating the inflammatory cascade. The main glycolipid in myelin which stimulates the formation of complement fixing antibodies is galactocerebroside. Injection of galactocerebroside with Freund's adjuvant into rabbits induces a peripheral neuropathy with macrophage-associated demyelination without a marked inflammatory response (Saida *et al.*, 1981). However, significant titres of complement-fixing antibody to galactocerebroside have not been found in GBS. The only condition in which high titres of complement-fixing antibody to myelin antigens have been found by conventional techniques is IgM paraproteinaemic demyelinating neuropathy, in which the antigenic epitopes are the carbohydrate residues shared by myelin-associated glycoprotein (MAG), P_0 glycoprotein, sulphated glucuronyl paragloboside (SGPG) and sulphated glucuronyl lactosyl paragloboside (SGLPG) (Gregson and Leibowitz, 1985: McGinnis *et al.*, 1988). Low titres of complement-fixing antibody to myelin are found with a conventional complement-fixation test in only 10% of patients with GBS (Winer *et al.*, 1988b). However, with a more sensitive complement C1 fixation and transfer test Koski has found antibodies to human myelin in almost all patients with GBS. The antibodies are predominantly IgM and directed at least partly against an incompletely identified neutral glycolipid resembling Forssman antigen. The antibodies are present in their highest concentration when the patient is admitted to hospital and rapidly disappear during the next 4 weeks, especially following plasma exchange, only to reappear if there is a relapse (Koski *et al.*, 1985, 1986, 1989; Vriesendorp *et al.*, 1991, 1993). Antibodies with these characteristics are likely to be major players in the pathogenesis of GBS. Unfortunately this version of the complement-fixation test is so complex that the test has not been widely adopted and is not readily available as a diagnostic test or for further research.

The major recent research interest has been in antibodies to gangliosides which can be relatively easily measured by ELISA. There has been some difficulty about standardizing results between laboratories. Strict criteria for scoring a test as 'positive' are necessary, and positive results should be checked by immuno-overlay. To perform an immuno-overlay, lipids are separated on a thin layer chromatogram, overlaid with the test serum and then developed with an antibody to the appropriate human immunoglobulin class. With this combination of techniques we have found antibodies to ganglioside GM1 in 29% of patients with GBS (Gregson *et al.*, 1993). We have found that IgG antibodies are more common in patients with disease with a poor outcome reflecting severe axonal degeneration (Walsh *et al.*, 1991; Gregson *et al.*, 1993) and in patients who have serological evidence of *Campylobacter* infection preceding their GBS. Yuki *et al.* (1990, 1992b) have identified the same association in Japanese patients but two other groups, although also finding anti-ganglioside GM1 antibodies in some patients, have failed to identify the same relationship with *Campylobacter* infection and axonal degeneration (Enders *et al.*, 1993; Vriesendorp *et al.*, 1993). In a case-control study of 103 patients we have confirmed the association between *Campylobacter* infection, IgG antibodies to ganglioside GM1, and severe axonal degeneration (J. H. Rees, personal communication, 1994).

The bacterial wall of some *Campylobacter* strains contains lipopolysaccharides having glycoconjugate epitopes which are shared by ganglioside GM1 and might induce an antibody response which causes the axonal damage (Oomes *et al.*, 1991; Jacobs *et al.*, 1993; Yuki *et al.*, 1993b). However, our latest information is that the story is not so simple in that affinity-purified anti-ganglioside GM1 antibodies from patients with GBS react with the purified *Campylobacter* lipopolysaccharide from some but not all *Campylobacter* strains isolated from patients with GBS (J. H. Rees, personal communication, 1994). There is a further difficulty that antibodies to ganglioside GM1 have not so far been shown experimentally to induce demyelination or axonal damage. There is one report that GBS serum containing antibodies to ganglioside GM1 induced conduction block following injection into rat nerves (Santoro *et al.*, 1992) whereas the clinical association described by us suggests that these antibodies would be more likely to cause axonal degeneration. There are individual case reports of an association between AMAN or AMSAN and antibodies to ganglioside GD1a (Yuki *et al.*, 1993c) and GD1b (Fujii *et al.*, 1993). Antibodies to a novel ganglioside *N*-acetylgalactosaminyl GD1a have recently been identified in the serum of six out of 50 GBS patients but not in any normal or disease controls (Kusunoki *et al.*, 1994). All these patients had had gastroenteritis and the electrophysiological features were consistent with an axonal neuropathy. These observations raise the possibility that bacterial infections stimulate a family of different antibodies to glycoconjugates which can cause either the axonal or the demyelinating component of GBS or both.

Prognostic features

The prognosis of GBS is extremely variable. In large surveys about 12% of patients have died of GBS or other causes not necessarily directly related to GBS (Raphael *et al.*, 1984; Winer *et al.*, 1988a). In recent multicentre trials the mortality has only been 2–3% (The Guillain–Barré Syndrome Study Group, 1985; French Cooperative Group on Plasma Exchange in Guillain–Barré Syndrome, 1987; Guillain–Barré Syndrome Steroid Trial Group, 1993). This difference could be due to failure to admit the most severe patients to the randomized trials or to improved care of patients in the context of a trial where patients were moved to tertiary referral centres with special expertise.

About 20% of patients are left disabled and 10% of these are still severely disabled after a year. Improvement continues during the second year and, in my experience, during subsequent years as well, but at a much slower rate. Accurate predictions of prognosis are difficult but algorithms have been devised which offer helpful guidelines. Table 9.4 shows the simple algorithm computed from a study of 100 patients (Winer *et al.*, 1988a). The factors associated with a poor outcome in that study were old age, absent or small distally evoked CMAPs and need for ventilation. Analysis of 75 recent personal patients showed that six of the nine with very severe disability (still needing walking aids after a year) had a previous diarrhoeal illness and a very rapid onset of their neuropathy becoming unable to walk within 24 hours. Adverse prognostic factors in other series have included antibodies to *Campylobacter*,

Table 9.4 Prognosis of Guillain–Barré syndrome: the percentage probability of not being able to return to work or unrestricted activities 1 year later according to speed of onset, age, need for ventilation and median nerve distal CMAP amplitude. (Reproduced from Winer *et al.*, 1988a, with permission.)

	Bedbound 0–4 days		Bedbound >4 days	
	Age < 40 years	*Age ≥ 40 years*	*Age < 40 years*	*Age ≥ 40 years*
CMAP APB ≤ 1 mV				
Not ventilated	36	71	15	44
Ventilated	59	86	31	67
CMAP APB > 1 mv				
Not ventilated	12	39	4	17
Ventilated	27	62	11	34

antibodies to ganglioside GM1 (see previous paragraph and F. van der Meché, personal communication, 1994), and non-treatment with plasma exchange (Cornblath *et al.*, 1987a; McKhann *et al.*, 1988).

Treatment

The first essential in the management of GBS is to recognize and avoid the risks of respiratory failure, autonomic disturbance and venous thromboembolism which have caused death in 12% of patients in large surveys. Every patient should be monitored carefully after diagnosis until it is clear that the plateau has been reached, improvement has started and the patient has been extubated. The vast majority require admission to hospital and about one-third need admission to an intensive care unit. Intensive care units which specialize in the management of GBS will have more experience of dealing with the special problems posed by prolonged artificial ventilation of conscious, paralysed patients with autonomic disturbances (Hughes and Bihari, 1993; Hund *et al.*, 1993). Whether transfer of patients to such units results in better outcomes has not been demonstrated but the mortality from GBS has only been 2–3% in multicentre trials and in recent series from the specialist centres (The Guillain–Barré Syndrome Study Group, 1985; French Cooperative Group on Plasma Exchange in Guillain–Barré Syndrome, 1987; Smith and Hughes, 1992).

The recognition of respiratory failure by monitoring vital capacity and assessment of bulbar function and fatigue are particularly important. It is a common misconception that monitoring arterial or digital oxygen saturation or peak expiratory flow are adequate substitutes. With neuromuscular causes of respiratory failure, by the time arterial oxygen desaturation has occurred the patient is in imminent danger of a cardiorespiratory arrest. Peak expiratory flow measures the speed of respiration, which is useful in asthma but not in GBS. As a rule of thumb intubation and ventilatory support will be needed if the vital capacity falls to 15 ml/kg. Bulbar palsy or fatigue may make this necessary at an earlier stage. The management of neuromuscular respiratory failure was discussed in the first volume of this book (Ropper and Shahani, 1984) and has recently been reviewed (Hughes and Bihari, 1993; Hund *et al.*, 1993). The essential points are summarized in Table 9.5.

Neither a small randomized open trial of oral prednisolone (Hughes *et al.*, 1978) nor a large double-blind trial of intravenous methylprednisolone (500 mg daily for 5 days in 124 treated patients) showed any beneficial effect (Guillain–Barré Syndrome Steroid Trial Group, 1993). The possibility of a beneficial interaction between intravenous immunoglobulin (IVIg) and steroids has been raised by the apparent beneficial effect of intravenous methylprednisolone added to IVIg in a group of 25 patients compared with historical controls (The Dutch Guillain–Barré Study Group, 1994). At present the balance of evidence is against the use of steroids in GBS. This result is surprising because steroids are effective in experimental allergic neuritis and also in CIDP (see below). The anti-inflammatory effect of steroids may be too minor to have a clinical effect or be outweighed by adverse effects such as inhibiting axonal regrowth, macrophage removal of myelin debris, Schwann cell proliferation and remyelination.

Plasma exchange became the standard treatment for GBS soon after two large controlled trials (The Guillain–Barré Syndrome Study Group, 1985; French Cooperative Group on Plasma Exchange in Guillain–Barré Syndrome, 1987, 1992) demonstrated its efficacy. Its use was associated with a shortening of time on a

Table 9.5 Important aspects of intensive care management of Guillain–Barré syndrome

---

- Monitor vital capacity, swallowing, fatigue
  Intubate and ventilate prophylactically
  Ventilation usually necessary if vital capacity < 15 ml/kg

- Monitor ECG continuously
  Watch for bradycardia/asystole during tracheal suction

- Except in children give subcutaneous heparin 5000 units twice daily

- Chest physiotherapy

- Passive limb movements through a full range

- Skin pressure areas: turning/special mattresses

- Analgesia (beware unstable autonomic system)

- Gastrointestinal stasis

- Nutrition

- Constipation

- Reassurance

- Plasma exchange or intravenous immunoglobulin

---

ventilator by about 2 weeks and of time to walk unaided by about a month in the North American trial in which 242 patients were randomized. Plasma exchange should be given within the first 2 weeks since there is no evidence of benefit after that time. It is logical to regard establishing the diagnosis of GBS as an emergency so that treatment can start as early as possible. We use a series of 50 ml/kg exchanges (approximately one plasma volume) on alternate days for a total of five exchanges. Albumin should be used as the exchange fluid since fresh-frozen plasma may cause allergic reactions and is no more efficacious (French Cooperative Group on Plasma Exchange in Guillain–Barré Syndrome, 1987). A continuous-flow machine is more efficacious than an intermittent-flow machine (McKhann *et al.*, 1988). There is no evidence whether centrifugation machines are better than filtration machines or whether immunoadsorption columns are as effective. The main problem with plasma exchange is venous access. We prefer to use a peripheral vein rather than central catheters which can cause life-threatening complications (Grishaber *et al.*, 1992).

In a randomized trial 75 patients treated with IVIg recovered the ability to walk unaided as fast or slightly faster than 75 patients treated with plasma exchange (Van der Meché, Schmitz and Dutch Guillain–Barré Study Group, 1992). Other reports of the use of IVIg have been variable. One group reported prompt and sustained improvement in all of seven patients (Jackson *et al.*, 1993). In another series five of seven deteriorated after initial improvement and required treatment with plasma exchange (Irani *et al.*, 1993). In a third series, seven of 15 consecutively treated patients deteriorated within 5 days after treatment (Castro and Ropper, 1993). None of these series provided evidence as powerful as the controlled trial but, before abandoning plasma exchange as the standard treatment of GBS, it seems prudent to confirm the conclusion from the first trial. The Plasma Exchange Sandoglobulin Trial Group are comparing the effects of IVIg, plasma exchange and plasma exchange followed by IVIg in a trial with 130 patients in each group.

Possible mechanisms of any beneficial effect of IVIg include blockade of T cell receptors, blockade of Fc receptors on macrophages, and an anti-idiotype action (Ronda *et al.*, 1993). Anti-idiotypic antibodies directed against anti-neuroblastoma cell-line antibodies were found in the serum of all 12 patients convalescent from GBS (Lundkvist *et al.*, 1993). Although the relevance of these autoantibodies to the pathogenesis of the disease is unknown, the presence of anti-idiotypic antibodies against relevant antineural antibodies in normal pooled immunoglobulin would explain any beneficial effect of IVIg.

We clearly need new ideas to improve the outcome for the most severely affected patients. It may be possible to exploit antibodies to ICAM-1 which have proved effective in experimental allergic neuritis (Archelos *et al.*, 1993). Alternatively it may be possible to use neurotrophic factors at an early stage to reverse the degenerative process of axons undergoing what would otherwise have been an irreversible change. The neurotrophic analogue of ACTH (4–9), Org 2766, has been shown to protect against experimental allergic neuritis (Duckers *et al.*, 1993) and against *cis*-platinum induced neuropathy (van der Hoop *et al.*, 1990). This or similar agents will be worth testing in GBS.

Excellent nursing, physiotherapy and occupational therapy are important throughout the course of GBS. Although plasma exchange in the acute stage reduces the severity of persistent motor deficit (French Cooperative Group on Plasma Exchange in Guillain–Barré Syndrome, 1992), at least 10% of patients are left severely disabled after a year and most of these are probably left with permanent disability (de Jager and Minderhoud, 1991). The reasons for persistent disability are often complex (Lennon *et al.*, 1993) and may be related to avoidable physical consequences, such as contractures, and treatable emotional consequences of the illness, such as anxiety. One concern is whether the illness will recur, as documented in 6.3% of a recent series of 238 patients (Combes and Goulon, 1992). Another concern is the safety of immunizations following GBS since immunizations are sometimes a triggering factor and immunization, especially with tetanus toxoid, has apparently triggered relapses of CIDP. It would be prudent to avoid immunizations during the first year after GBS and to be particularly cautious about tetanus toxoid thereafter.

MILLER FISHER SYNDROME

The term Miller Fisher syndrome (MFS) is properly reserved for an illness characterized by ophthalmoplegia, limb ataxia and tendon areflexia in the absence of weakness, long tract signs or alteration of consciousness (Fisher, 1956). The CSF protein is usually increased and post-mortem examination of one case showed an inflammatory radiculoneuropathy (Phillips *et al.*, 1984). The term is sometimes misused to describe patients with ophthalmoplegia superimposed on typical sensory and motor GBS. The condition can be mimicked by brainstem encephalitis but in such cases drowsiness and extensor plantar responses are usually present (Al-Din *et al.*, 1982). Published electrophysiological studies suggest that the pathological substrate of MFS is an axonal rather than a demyelinating neuropathy (Guiloff, 1977; Fross and Daube, 1987).

Several recent studies have shown a close association between antibodies to ganglioside GQ1b and MFS, strongly suggesting that the antibodies are related to the pathogenesis of the condition (Chiba *et al.*, 1993; Willison *et al.*, 1993; Yuki *et al.*, 1993a). Application of MFS serum containing antibodies to ganglioside GQ1b first increases and then blocks the firing of miniature endplate potentials in the mouse phrenic nerve diaphragm preparation consistent with an action upon receptors at or near the motor nerve terminal (Roberts *et al.*, 1994). The concentration of this ganglioside is greater in the nerves of the external ocular muscles than in other peripheral nerves or central nervous system (CNS) tissue (Chiba *et al.*, 1993). Serum containing antibodies to ganglioside GQ1b also has an adverse effect on rat dorsal root ganglion cultures (Yuki *et al.*, 1993e). These observations suggest that the antibodies to ganglioside GQ1b recognize an epitope on a glycolipid or glycoprotein which is shared by motor nerve terminals of the nerves to the external ocular muscles and by a subset of sensory neurons, probably primary cerebellar afferent nerve fibres.

Miller Fisher syndrome generally has a benign prognosis so that it is difficult to judge the efficacy of plasma exchange and other immune interventions which have been claimed to help (Gerard, 1981; Zifko *et al.*, 1994).

SUBACUTE DEMYELINATING POLYRADICULONEUROPATHY

It is arguable whether patients with SIDP have a long drawn-out form of AIDP or a mild form of CIDP. Their existence serves to confirm the continuity of the spectrum from AIDP to CIDP. During the period 1985–1990 we encountered seven patients fulfilling the criteria for SIDP at Guy's Hospital, 81 patients with GBS and 50 patients with CIDP, including patients with recurrent GBS. The patients with SIDP were all young adults and the progressive phase of their illnesses lasted between 32 and 56 days. Three had had recent upper respiratory tract infections. The clinical illnesses were relatively mild and although four patients were so weak that they were unable to walk even with assistance, none required ventilatory support. The clinical features consisted of a predominantly motor polyradiculoneuropathy affecting proximal and distal muscle groups in the upper and lower limbs in all, the facial nerves in two cases, and ophthalmoparesis in one. Neurophysiological investigations implicated demyelination in all seven cases. Sural nerve biopsies showed macrophage-associated demyelination. The CSF protein concentration was usually increased but the CSF cell count was normal. All patients made substantial or complete recoveries with or without steroid treatment (Hughes *et al.*, 1992a). These cases have had a benign course with no evidence of relapse during an average follow-up of 6 years. If such patients were to relapse subsequently they would have to be re-classified as having CIDP. The subdivision of acquired demyelinating neuropathy into subtypes is a semantic problem. These cases with an intermediate time course draw attention to the difficulties with present international criteria and the similarity between AIDP and CIDP.

CHRONIC INFLAMMATORY DEMYELINATING POLYRADICULONEUROPATHY

History

Austin (1958) described two patients with chronic relapsing steroid responsive neuropathy and reviewed the literature. Thomas *et al.* (1969) described five patients with recurrent and chronic relapsing polyneuritis and drew the analogy both with

Guillain–Barré syndrome and with chronic relapsing experimental allergic neuritis. Dyck *et al.* (1975) described 53 patients with what they called chronic inflammatory polyradiculoneuropathy and Prineas and McLeod (1976) 23 patients with chronic relapsing polyneuritis. These and later large series described the general concept of CIDP (McCombe *et al.*, 1987b; Barohn *et al.*, 1989) but had slightly different diagnostic criteria. The Ad Hoc Subcommittee of the American Academy of Neurology AIDS Task Force (1991) laid down stringent diagnostic clinical, neurophysiological, CSF and pathological criteria for definite, probable and possible CIDP (Table 9.6). Idiopathic cases are best segregated from those with associated diseases such as systemic lupus erythematosus (SLE), HIV infection, monoclonal gammopathy, diabetes mellitus and CNS demyelinating disease. The separation of patients with paraproteinaemia is a particular issue because about 10% of patients with undiagnosed neuropathy do have a paraprotein: this percentage is increased if a more sensitive test such as immunofixation or isoelectric focusing is used to seek the paraprotein instead of conventional electrophoresis (Vrethem *et al.*, 1993). In addition the clinical course of patients with paraproteinaemia and demyelinating neuropathy may be very similar to CIDP, especially if the paraprotein is IgG (Bleasel *et al.*, 1993). Neuropathy associated with paraproteinaemia is dealt with in the preceding chapter.

Typical course

Under the rubric of CIDP fall a number of entities which can sometimes be clearly distinguished but at other times merge into each other (Table 9.1). The course is usually relapsing – 65% of 92 patients in the largest published series (McCombe *et al.*, 1987a), but may be progressive, or monophasic and followed by remission (35% in the same series). The disease may start at any age from childhood onwards. The youngest age in this large series was 2 years. The relapsing cases tend to start at younger ages, especially between 10 and 30 years. The onset of relapses is usually more gradual than in GBS but there are some patients who have recurrent acute attacks, each of which resembles GBS, with complete or almost complete recovery between each (Grand'Maison *et al.*, 1992). The progressive or monophasic cases are more likely to begin in older age, especially 50 to 70 years. Males are affected almost twice as often as females, the same sex distribution as in GBS, but the opposite of that in multiple sclerosis and most organ-specific autoimmune disorders.

The typical case of CIDP is a patient with a motor and sensory polyradiculoneuropathy progressing gradually over several weeks, reaching a plateau and then improving with or without treatment, only to relapse again either spontaneously or as treatment is withdrawn. Weakness is present in almost all cases and usually predominates over sensory deficit. The lower limbs are usually more affected than the upper limbs and weakness is both proximal and distal, reflecting the combination of root and peripheral nerve involvement. Distal paraesthesias commonly accompany the weakness at presentation and the sensory symptoms are often more prominent than objective sensory loss. In some patients the sensory loss is severe, affecting both cutaneous and joint position sensation which may cause disabling incoordination. In other patients paraesthesias are painful. The facial nerves and sometimes other cranial nerves may be involved but much less often than in GBS. Respiratory failure and autonomic nerve involvement are both rare.

The presentation and clinical features of the primary progressive form of CIDP are similar to those of the relapsing–remitting form just described. In our own series

Table 9.6 Diagnostic criteria for chronic inflammatory demyelinating polyradiculoneuropathy*

I   Clinical
   A Mandatory
      1 Progressive or relapsing motor and sensory, rarely only motor or sensory, dysfunction of
         more than one limb of a peripheral nerve nature, developing over at least 2 months
      2 Hypo- or areflexia, usually involving all four limbs
   B Supportive
      1 Large predominating over small-fibre sensory loss
   C Exclusion
      1 Genetic, toxic or metabolic cause
      2 Significant sensory level or sphincter disturbance indicating spinal cord involvement

II Physiologic studies
   A Mandatory
   Nerve conduction studies including studies of proximal nerve segments in which the predominant
   process is demyelination
   Must have three of four:
      1 Reduction in conduction velocity (CV) in two or more motor nerves:
         a   < 80% of lower limit of normal (LLN) if amplitude > 80% of LLN
         b   < 70% of LLN if amplitude < 80% of LLN
      2 Partial conduction block or abnormal temporal dispersion in one or more motor nerves at
         sites not prone to compression:
         a   < 15% change in duration between proximal and distal sites
         b   > 15% change in duration between proximal and distal sites and > 20% drop in p-area
             or p–p amplitude
      3 Prolonged distal latencies in two or more nerves:
         a   > 125% of upper limit of normal (ULN) if amplitude > 80% of LLN
         b   > 150% of ULN if amplitude < 80% of LLN
      4 Absent F waves or prolonged minimum F-wave latencies (10–15 trials) in two or more motor
         nerves:
         a   > 120% of ULN if amplitude > 80% of LLN
         b   > 150% of ULN if amplitude < 80% of LLN
   B Supportive
      1 Reduction in sensory CV < 80% of LLN
      2 Absent H reflexes

III Pathologic features
   A Mandatory
   Nerve biopsy showing unequivocal evidence of demyelination and remyelination
   B Supportive
      1 Subperineurial or endoneurial oedema
      2 Mononuclear cell infiltration
      3 'Onion-bulb' formation
      4 Prominent variation in the degree of demyelination between fascicles
   C Exclusion
      1 Evidence of other specific cause

IV CSF Studies
   A Mandatory
      1 Cell count < 10/mm if HIV-seronegative or < 50/mm if HIV-seropositive
   B Supportive
      1 Elevated protein

---

*These criteria are a shortened form of those proposed by the Ad Hoc Subcommittee of the American Academy of Neurology AIDS Task
Force (1991).
Diagnostic categories for research purposes:
DEFINITE: Clinical A and C, Physiology A, Pathology A and C, and CSF A.
PROBABLE: Clinical A and C, Physiology A, and CSF A.
POSSIBLE: Clinical A and C and Physiology A.

there is an even more marked preponderance of males in the primary progressive form.

The presentation and clinical course of CIDP are extremely variable. Sometimes the presentation is markedly asymmetric and the deficit may even be confined to one limb for several months or years (Verma *et al.*, 1990). On rare occasions cranial nerve involvement has been the presenting feature (Donaghy and Earl, 1985). Papilloedema has been reported on a few occasions. Postural tremor is a well-recognized feature and may be disabling. It only occurred in three of the 92 patients in the series of McCombe *et al.* (1987a). The peripheral nerves are not usually thickened but remarkable hypertrophy of the lumbosacral nerve roots was demonstrated by myelography in one patient (De Silva *et al.*, 1994).

Multifocal motor neuropathy with conduction block

Multifocal motor neuropathy with conduction block (Lewis *et al.*, 1982) is probably a variant of CIDP and accounts for some of the patients with CIDP who have entirely motor symptoms and deficit (Pestronk *et al.*, 1988; Krarup *et al.*, 1990; Case Records of the Massachusetts General Hospital, Gominak and Cros, 1993). It presents with asymmetric weakness, usually of the upper limbs, often with wasting and fasciculation, which sometimes leads to confusion with motor neuron disease. Sensory symptoms are minor and sensory deficit is absent. The hallmark of the condition is multifocal conduction block. A biopsy of the site of conduction block in one case revealed onion bulb formation and chronic inflammatory changes (Kaji *et al.*, 1993). There is a loose association with IgM antibodies to ganglioside GM1 and some patients have a paraprotein, usually an IgM paraprotein (Baba *et al.*, 1989; Pestronk *et al.*, 1990; Kornberg and Pestronk, 1994). These patients are relatively unresponsive to treatment with steroids but have been reported to respond to intravenous cyclophosphamide (Pestronk *et al.*, 1988) and especially to IVIG (Charles *et al.*, 1992; Kermode *et al.*, 1992; Chaudhry *et al.*, 1993; Nobile-Orazio *et al.*, 1993; Yuki *et al.*, 1993d). A fuller account of this variant of CIDP is given in Chapter 4.

Sensory CIDP

About 5–10% of patients with CIDP have entirely sensory symptoms and deficits although multifocal slowing of motor nerve conduction is present (Oh *et al.*, 1992). The disease course and response to steroids are similar to the conventional sensory and motor form of CIDP (see also Chapter 4).

CIDP with CNS involvement

Patients are encountered who have clinical, electrophysiological and MRI features of CNS involvement suggestive of multiple sclerosis as well as CIDP (Rubin *et al.*, 1987; Thomas *et al.*, 1987). In large series this association is rare and clinical features of CNS involvment occur in only 3% of patients with CIDP (Barohn *et al.*, 1989). However, subclinical evidence of CNS involvement is obtainable from evoked response, central motor conduction or MRI studies in up to one-third of patients (Mendell *et al.*, 1987; Feasby *et al.*, 1990; Hawke *et al.*, 1990; Ormerod *et al.*, 1990).

Neurophysiological features

Multifocal neurophysiological abnormalities consisting of slowing of nerve conduction, conduction block or dispersion of CMAPs are the hallmarks of CIDP and the most important diagnostic tests (Albers and Kelly, 1989; Parry, 1993). Very strict criteria have been set by the Ad Hoc Subcommittee of the American Academy of Neurology AIDS Task Force (1991) and are partly reproduced in Table 9.6. In early cases the abnormalities are similar to those in AIDP but in advanced cases axonal degeneration may be superimposed and make the diagnosis more difficult. In hereditary demyelinating neuropathies slowing of nerve conduction is much more uniform, affecting every segment of the same nerve and affecting every nerve to a similar extent. Multifocal abnormalities in CIDP help to make the distinction but require testing of several nerves. The variable affection of different nerve fibres is sensitively demonstrated by the increased variation of F wave latencies (Panayiotopoulos *et al.*, 1992). Sensory nerve action potentials may be relatively preserved in the early stages of CIDP (Hughes *et al.*, 1992a) but are commonly absent in advanced cases. Patients with purely motor involvement have been separated as having 'multifocal motor neuropathy' (see above and Chapter 4).

Differential diagnosis

The establishment of demyelination as the underlying basis of a peripheral neuropathy considerably reduces the range of possible causes (Table 9.7). A long-standing history, pes cavus, claw toes and thickened nerves will suggest a hereditary neuropathy. A painstaking family history and clinical and neurophysiological examination of relatives are often necessary to identify or exclude a hereditary neuropathy. Many sporadic cases of Charcot–Marie–Tooth disease type I can now be diagnosed by

Table 9.7 Differential diagnosis of chronic demyelinating neuropathy

Hereditary
    Charcot Marie Tooth disease types Ia, Ib, X recessive, X dominant, III
    Hereditary liability to pressure palsies
    Refsum's syndrome
    Metachromatic leucodystrophy
    Globoid cell leucodystrophy

Paraproteinaemia (see text)
    Monoclonal gammopathy of undermined significance
    Solitary myeloma
    Multiple myeloma
    Waldenström's macroglobulinaemia
    Castleman's disease
    POEMS (usually associated with osteosclerotic myeloma)

Toxic
    Amiodarone
    Perhexilene

examining DNA extracted from blood leucocytes for a duplication of the PMP-22 gene on chromosome 17 (Hallam *et al.*, 1992; Hoogendijk *et al.*, 1992) (see Chapter 6). Careful electrophoresis of the serum proteins has revealed a paraprotein in 10% of patients with unexplained neuropathy and many of these have a demyelinating neuropathy (Kelly *et al.*, 1981). Since 10% of patients with osteosclerotic myeloma and neuropathy do not have a detectable paraprotein (Miralles *et al.*, 1992b), a case could be made for undertaking a skeletal survey in every patient with unexplained acquired demyelinating neuropathy. The rarity reduces the justification for this investigation unless there is hyperpigmentation or other features of POEMS syndrome.

An asymmetric presentation of CIDP can be difficult to distinguish from a vasculitic multiple mononeuropathy. This distinction can be made even more difficult in occasional patients in whom vasculitic lesions are accompanied by conduction block (Jamieson *et al.*, 1991). The neuropathy associated with SLE may be due either to vasculitis or inflammatory demyelinating polyradiculoneuropathy (Hughes *et al.*, 1982; Rechthand *et al.*, 1984). Both vasculitic neuropathy and CIDP occur in association with HIV infection, usually at or soon after seroconversion rather than after the development of AIDS (Cornblath *et al.*, 1987b; Chaunu *et al.*, 1989; Gherardi *et al.*, 1989; Leger *et al.*, 1989; Stricker *et al.*, 1992).

Pathology

In early or active phases of CIDP sural nerve biopsies may reveal multifocal mononuclear cell infiltration of the endoneurium and macrophage-associated demyelination (Figure 9.3). Usually, however, the inflammation is sparse or absent, probably because the disease is multifocal and the most florid changes are not in distal sensory nerves but proximal nerve trunks or spinal roots. This proximal location is supported by the few post-mortem examinations which have been published (Dyck *et al.*, 1975; Torvik and Lundar, 1977; review in Hughes, 1990) and by the characteristically delayed or absent F waves (see above). Although theoretically the hallmark of CIDP is segmental demyelination, in practice sural nerve biopsies often show depletion of nerve fibres, and a mixture of fibres undergoing axonal degeneration and demyelinated or remyelinated fibres. In the largest published series 48% of 56 sural nerve biopsies showed predominant demyelination, 21% axonal degeneration, 12% mixed changes and 18% were normal (Barohn *et al.*, 1989). What distinguishes CIDP from more acute inflammatory neuropathies is the presence of 'onion bulbs' in some severe cases (Figure 9.3). The layers of the onion are formed by supernumerary Schwann cells which develop during repeated bouts of demyelination and remyelination. Post-mortem examination of the CNS has usually only shown secondary changes attributable to damage to the ventral and dorsal roots, namely anterior horn cell chromatolysis and degeneration of the dorsal columns. In a few cases there has also been mononuclear cell infiltration of the spinal cord and brainstem (Borit and Altrocchi, 1971; Dyck *et al.*, 1975).

Pathogenesis

Symptomatic infections immediately preceding the onset of CIDP are reported in a relatively small proportion of cases compared with GBS. There were preceding

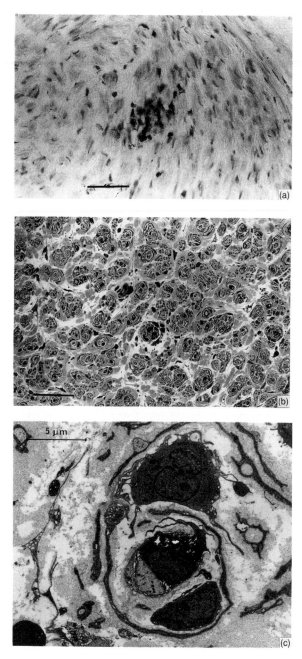

Figure 9.3 Sural nerve biopsy from a patient with chronic
inflammatory demyelinating polyradiculoneuropathy (CIDP).
(a) Light micrograph showing a small focal endoneurial infiltrate of T cells identified with a peroxidase-labelled pan T cell
monoclonal antibody; bar = 50 μm. (b) Light micrograph
showing 'onion bulbs' representing nerve fibres which have
undergone multiple cycles of demyelination and remyelination;
bar = 50 μm. (c) Electron micrograph showing two macrophages within an 'onion bulb', one containing myelin debris;
bar = 5 μm.

infections or immunizations within 6 weeks before onset in only 32% of 93 cases in the largest clinical series (McCombe *et al.*, 1987b). There is particular concern about tetanus toxoid immunization which immediately preceded onset in two cases and preceded relapse on two occasions in one case (Pollard and Selby, 1978). Relapses are more likely during a pregnancy year than a non-pregnancy year and the relapses occur especially in the last trimester or, as in multiple sclerosis, the puerperium (McCombe *et al.*, 1987a). The onset of CIDP soon after infections raises the possibility, as in AIDP, that an infective agent triggers or releases an immune response which in susceptible individuals cross-reacts with myelin antigens.

There have been relatively few attempts to identify immune responses to myelin antigens in CIDP compared with AIDP and those that have been made have not been very rewarding (Hughes, 1990). Antibodies to myelin antigens have not so far been consistently found in significant numbers of CIDP patients by complement-fixation, ELISA or other tests. A single report that demyelination can be induced in rat nerve following intraneural injection of CIDP serum has not been pursued (Dyck *et al.*, 1982a). Slowing of nerve conduction in the sciatic nerve of monkeys was reported following the systemic transfer of immunoglobulin from CIDP patients but was not accompanied by any morphological change (Heininger *et al.*, 1984). Antibodies to specific myelin antigens, such as P_0 glycoprotein, and ganglioside LM1 have been identified but only in a small percentage of patients with CIDP (Khalili-Shirazi *et al.*, 1993). Most recently antibodies to β-tubulin have been identified by ELISA in 57% of 70 CIDP patients, 29% of GBS and 3% of other neurlogical disease control subjects (Connolly *et al.*, 1993). The relevance of this finding to pathogenesis has yet to be explained since β-tubulin is a cytoskeletal element of many cells. Relevant autoantibodies would likely be directed against a component which is located predominantly or entirely in peripheral nerve myelin or Schwann cells. The response of CIDP to plasma exchange implicates autoantibodies in pathogenesis so that further efforts to identify specific antibodies would be worthwhile.

Surrogate markers of the presence of inflammation in CIDP can be identified in the blood. The percentage of circulating T cells bearing activation markers and the concentration of soluble IL-2 receptor are increased in active disease (Taylor and Hughes, 1989; Hartung *et al.*, 1990). Attempts to identify the antigens to which the activated T cells are responsive have been unsatisfactory although reponses to P_0 and P_2 myelin proteins or their peptides have been found in a small proportion of cases (Khalili-Shirazi *et al.*, 1992). The concentration of the soluble cell adhesion molecule ELAM-1 is also increased, indicating activation of the endothelium (Oka *et al.*, 1994), a necessary component of the complex reaction which permits T cells to cross the blood–nerve barrier and reach the endoneurium. The sequence of events which triggers the inflammatory process and the nature of the presumed autoimmune response still defies our understanding.

Treatment

In the absence of a clear understanding of pathogenesis treatment has been developed empirically. Since the classic paper of Austin (1958), clinical experience has confirmed the efficacy of steroids. The short-term benefit of oral prednisone was shown in a controlled trial (Dyck *et al.*, 1982b). In large series a worthwhile initial response has been reported in 65–95% of cases (McCombe *et al.*, 1987b; Barohn *et al.*, 1989). Unfortunately prolonged courses and high doses are often necessary and relapses following withdrawal are common. I start treatment with oral prednisolone 60 mg daily and continue with this dose until improvement occurs. If improvement does not occur within a month, I recommend either plasma exchange or IVIg (see below). After improvement begins the dose can be gradually reduced to an alternate-day regime by reducing to 60 mg alternating with 50 mg, 60/40, . . . 60/0 at weekly intervals with subsequent reductions to an alternate-day maintenance dose of 25 mg after 12 weeks. If complete recovery ensues it may be possible to wean the patient off steroids.

Plasma exchange has also found a place in the management of CIDP on the basis of favourable experience in published reports (Server *et al.*, 1979; Toyka *et al.*, 1980, 1982, 1992; Gross and Thomas, 1981; Donofrio *et al.*, 1985; Wrobel and Watson, 1992). This conclusion has been supported by a controlled trial of twice-weekly plasma exchange for 3 weeks versus a similar course of sham exchanges: the true plasma exchange was followed by significantly more improvement in several clinical and neurophysiological measures than was seen after sham exchange (Dyck *et al.*, 1986). It is possible to keep some patients with CIDP in remission for several years by repeating plasma exchange at intervals varying between 2 and 6 weeks. When venous access via antecubital veins is easy such repeated procedures may be reasonable despite the inconvenience and expense. When venous access requires the placement of an indwelling venous cannula the risks are unlikely to outweigh the potential benefits.

Intravenous immunoglobulin has become a popular alternative to plasma exchange on the basis of encouraging reports of at least temporary and sometimes long-lasting benefit following its use. The usual regime is 0.4g/kg daily for 5 consecutive days but no dose-ranging studies have been done. Some patients appear to need courses repeated every 2 to 6 weeks in which case it is more convenient to give 2.0 g/kg in a single dose over 24 hours. These regimes are based on published and personal experience and their efficacy has not been thoroughly established with controlled trials. In the only published trial involving patients who had not been treated with IVIg before, Vermeulen *et al.* (1993) found that 4/15 patients improved following IVIg compared with 3/13 patients improved following placebo. However, a more recent placebo-controlled cross-over trial in 30 patients showed that IVIg produced significantly more improvement in strength than placebo (A. F. Hahn, personal communication, 1994). IVIg was compared with plasma exchange in a cross-over trial and the effects of each were similar (P. J. Dyck, personal communication, 1994). In another controlled trial seven patients who were being treated with IVIg and appeared to respond were withdrawn from treatment and randomized to receive either IVIg or placebo. They were then crossed-over to receive the opposite treatment. All seven improved following IVIg, while none improved following placebo (van Doorn *et al.*, 1990). The evidence is that about two-thirds of patients with CIDP do respond to IVIg. However, spontaneous remissions do occur and the treatment is so expensive that patient and physician must beware of placebo responses. Future work must define more clearly which patients will respond and compare conventional steroid with IVIg regimes. The mechanism of action of IVIg in CIDP is obscure but the same mechanisms proposed in GBS may be operative.

Immunosuppressive drugs are commonly used in CIDP following an inadequate response to steroids, plasma exchange or IVIg. The most convenient and least toxic drug is azathioprine. A small controlled trial of azathioprine 2 mg/kg/day failed to show any benefit compared with prednisone alone (Dyck *et al.*, 1985). However, personal and published experience suggests benefit from 2.5–3.0 mg/kg/day. The disadvantages of azathioprine are the need for monthly monitoring of the blood count and liver function and the increased risk of developing a neoplasm, especially non-Hodgkin's lymphoma or skin cancer (about four cases per 100 per 10 years compared with a background risk of three cases; Kinlen, 1985). An alternative to azathioprine is cyclophosphamide but there is little published experience of its use in CIDP and it is more toxic (Rosen and Vastola, 1976). Remissions have been induced with cyclosporin A but in the rather high doses of 5–15 mg/kg which might be expected to produce renal damage (Kolkin *et al.*, 1987; Hodgkinson *et al.*, 1990). Lower doses are not, in my experience, effective.

Although a number of different treatments are effective in CIDP, scientific evidence for the superiority of one treatment over another and for the order in which they should be used is lacking. I prefer to start with prednisolone, add IVIg if necessary and use plasma exchange if that fails. If exchange or IVIg need to be repeated more than once I recommend adding azathioprine. This policy depends on the availability of plasma exchange and the ease of venous access in any individual.

Prognosis

The prognosis of CIDP is variable and difficult to discern from the literature because the available series of patients are all selected by referral to specialist centres and studied retrospectively. In the largest series 73% of 92 patients had made a good recovery at last follow-up, which was at a mean of 10 years after onset and had at most mild symptoms (McCombe *et al.*, 1987b). The mortality has ranged from 5–11% and the need for wheelchairs from 2–28% (Dyck *et al.*, 1975; McCombe *et al.*, 1987b; Barohn *et al.*, 1989).

ACKNOWLEDGEMENTS

I thank Action Research, the Wellcome Foundation, the Medical Research Council and the Guillain–Barré Syndrome Support Group for financial support, and Drs Norman Gregson, Susan Hall, Jeremy Rees and Kenneth Smith for their advice.

REFERENCES

Ad Hoc Subcommittee of the American Academy of Neurology AIDS Task Force. (1991). Research criteria for the diagnosis of chronic inflammatory demyelinating polyradiculoneuropathy (CIDP). *Neurology*, **41**, 617–618

Albers, J. W., Donofrio, P. D. and McGonagle, T. K. (1985). Sequential electrodiagnostic abnormalities in acute inflammatory demyelinating polyradiculoneuropathy. *Muscle Nerve*, **6**, 504–509

Albers, J. W.and Kelly, J. J. (1989). Acquired inflammatory demyelinating polyneuropathies: clinical and electrodiagnostic features. *Muscle Nerve*, **12**, 435–451

Al-Din, A. N., Anderson, M., Bickerstaff, E. R. and Harvey, I. (1982). Brainstem encephalitis and the syndrome of Miller–Fisher: a clinical study. *Brain*, **105**, 481

Archelos, J. J., Mäurer, M., Jung, S. *et al.* (1993). Suppression of experimental allergic neuritis by an antibody to the intercellular adhesion molecule ICAM-1. *Brain*, **116**, 1043–1058

Arnason, B. and Soliven, B. (1993). Acute inflammatory demyelinating polyradiculoneuropathy. In *Peripheral Neuropathy* (P. J. Dyck, P. K. Thomas, J. W. Griffin, P. A. Low, J. F. Poduslo, eds), pp. 1437–1497, Philadelphia: W. B. Saunders

Asbury, A. K. and Cornblath, D. R. (1990). Assessment of current diagnostic criteria for Guillain–Barré syndrome. *Ann. Neurol.*, **27** (suppl), S21–24

Asbury, A. K., Arnason, B. G. and Adams, R. D. (1969). The inflammatory lesion in idiopathic polyneuritis. Its role in pathogenesis. *Medicine*, **48**, 173–215

Austin, J. H. (1958). Recurrent polyneuropathies and their corticosteroid treatment. *Brain*, **81**, 157–192

Baba, H., Daune, G.C., Ilyas, A. A. *et al.* (1989). Anti GM1 ganglioside antibodies with differing fine specificities in patients with multifocal motor neuropathy. *J. Neuroimmunol.*, **25**, 143–150

Barohn, R. J., Kissel, J. T., Warmolts, J. R. and Mendell, J. R. (1989). Chronic inflammatory demyelinating polyradiculoneuropathy. Clinical characteristics, course, and recommendations for diagnostic criteria. *Arch. Neurol.*, **46**, 878–884

Bleasel, A.F., Hawke, S. H. B., Pollard, J. D. and McLeod, J. G. (1993). IgG monoclonal paraproteinaemia and peripheral neuropathy. *J. Neurol. Neurosurg. Psychiatry*, **56**, 52–57

Borit, A. and Altrocchi, P. H. (1971). Recurrent polyneuropathy and neurolymphomatosis. *Arch. Neurol.*, **24**, 40–47

Bradshaw, D. Y. and Jones, H. R. Jr. (1992). Guillain–Barré syndrome in children: clinical course, electrodiagnosis, and prognosis. *Muscle Nerve*, **15**, 500–506

Case Records of the Massachusetts General Hospital, Gominak S. C. and Cros, D. (1993). *N. Engl. J. Med.*, **329**, 1182–1190

Castro, L. H. M. and Ropper, A. H. (1993). Human immune globulin infusion in Guillain–Barré syndrome: worsening during and after treatment. *Neurology*, **43**, 1034–1036

Charles, N., Benoit, P., Vial, C. *et al.* (1992). Intravenous immunoglobulin treatment in multifocal motor neuropathy. *Lancet*, **340**, 182

Chaudhry, V., Corse, A. M., Cornblath, D. R. *et al.* (1993). Multifocal motor neuropathy: response to human immune globulin. *Ann. Neurol.*, **33**, 237–242

Chaunu, M.-P., Ratinahirana, H., Raphael, M. *et al.* (1989). The spectrum of changes on 20 nerve biopsies in patients with HIV infection. *Muscle Nerve*, **12**, 452–459

Chiba, A., Kusunoki, S., Obata, H. *et al.* (1993). Serum anti-GQ$_{1b}$ IgG antibody is associated with ophthalmoplegia in Miller Fisher syndrome and Guillain–Barré syndrome: clinical and immunohistochemical studies. . *Neurology*, **43**, 1911–1917

Combes, A. and Goulon, M. (1992). Recurrence of Guillain–Barré syndrome. *Ann. Med. Interne (Paris)*, **143**, 515–518

Connolly, A.M., Pestronk, A., Trotter, J. L. *et al.* (1993). High-titer selective serum anti-β-tubulin antibodies in chronic inflammatory demyelinating polyneuropathy. *Neurology*, **43**, 557–562

Cornblath, D. R. (1990). Electrophysiology in Guillain–Barré syndrome. *Ann. Neurol.*, **27** (suppl),, S17–20

Cornblath, D. R., Griffin, J. W., Fisher, R.S. *et al.* (1987a). Plasmapheresis and Guillain–Barré syndrome: II Analysis of electrodiagnostic data. *Neurology*, **37**, 252

Cornblath, D. R., McArthur, J. C., Kennedy, P. G. E. *et al.* (1987b). Inflammatory demyelinating peripheral neuropathies associated with human T-cell lymphotropic virus type III infection. *Ann. Neurol.*, **21**, 32–40

Dawson, D. M., Samuels, M. A. and Morris, J. (1988). Sensory form of acute polyneuritis. *Neurology*, **38**, 1728–1730

De Jager, A. E. J. and Minderhoud, J. M. (1991). Residual signs in severe Guillain–Barré syndrome: Analysis of 57 patients. *J. Neurol Sci.*, **104**, 151–156

De Silva, R. N., Willison, H. J., Doyle, D. *et al.* (1994). Nerve root hypertrophy in chronic inflammatory demyelinating polyneuropathy. *Muscle Nerve*, **17**, 168–170

Donaghy, M. and Earl, C. J. (1985). Ocular palsy preceding chronic relapsing polyneuropathy by several weeks. *Ann. Neurol.*, **17**, 49–50

Donofrio, P. D., Tandan, R. U. P. and Albers, J. W. (1985). Plasma exchange in chronic inflammatory demyelinating polyradiculoneuropathy. *Muscle Nerve*, **8**, 321–327

Duckers, H. J., Verhaagen, J. and Gispen, W. H. (1993). The neurotrophic analogue of ACTH (4-9), Org 2766, protects against experimental allergic neuritis. *Brain*, **116**, 1059–1075

Dyck, P. J., Lais, A. C., Ohta, M. *et al.* (1975). Chronic inflammatory polyradiculoneuropathy. *Mayo Clin. Proc.*, **50**, 621–651

Dyck, P. J., Lais, A. C., Hansen, S. M. *et al.* (1982a). Technique assessment of demyelination from endoneurial injection. *Exp. Neurol.*, **77**, 359–377

Dyck, P. J., O'Brien, P. C., Oviatt, K. F. *et al.* (1982b). Prednisone improves chronic inflammatory demyelinating polyradiculoneuropathy more than no treatment. *Ann. Neurol.*, **11**, 136–141

Dyck, P. J., O'Brien, P., Swanson, C. *et al.* (1985). Combined azathioprine and prednisone in chronic inflammatory demyelinating polyneuropathy. *Neurology*, **35**, 1173–1176

Dyck, P. J., Daube, J., O'Brien, P. *et al.* (1986). Plasma exchange in chronic inflammatory demyelinating polyradiculoneuropathy. *N. Engl. J. Med.*, **314**, 461–465

Enders, U., Karch, H., Toyka, K. V. *et al.* (1993). The spectrum of immune responses to *Campylobacter jejuni* and glycoconjugates in Guillain–Barré syndrome and in other neuroimmunological disorders. *Ann. Neurol.*, **34**, 136–144

Exley, A. R., Smith, N. and Winer, J. B. (1994). Tumour necrosis factor-alpha (TNF) and other cytokines in Guillain–Barré syndrome. *J. Neurol. Neurosurg. Psychiatry*, **57**, 1118–1120

Feasby, T. E., Gilbert, J. J., Brown, W. F. *et al.* (1986). An acute axonal form of Guillain–Barré polyneuropathy. *Brain*, **109**, 1115–1126

Feasby, T. E., Hahn, A. F., Koopman, W. J. and Lee, D. H. (1990). Central lesions in chronic inflammatory demyelinating polyneuropathy: an MRI study. *Neurology*, **40**, 476–478

Feasby, T. E., Hahn, A. F., Brown, W. F. *et al.* (1993). Severe axonal degeneration in acute Guillain–Barré syndrome: evidence of two different mechanisms. *J. Neurol. Sci.*, **116**, 185–192

Fisher, M. (1956). Syndrome of ophthalmoplegia, ataxia and areflexia. *N. Engl. J. Med.*, **255**, 57–65

French Cooperative Group on Plasma Exchange in Guillain–Barré Syndrome. (1987). Efficiency of plasma exchange in Guillain–Barré syndrome: role of replacement fluids. *Ann. Neurol.*, **22**, 753–761.

French Cooperative Group on plasma exchange in Guillain–Barré syndrome. (1992). Plasma exchange in Guillain–Barré syndrome: One-year follow-up. *Ann. Neurol.*, **32**, 94–97.

Fross, R. D. and Daube, J. (1987). Neuropathy in the Miller–Fisher syndrome: clinical and electrophysiologic findings. *Neurology*, **37**, 1493–1498

Fujii, H., Kondo, T., Yasuda, K. *et al.* (1993). An acute axonal form of Guillain–Barré syndrome with autoantibody against ganglioside GD1b – a case report. *No No Hattatsu*, **25**, 379–384

Gerard, A. (1981). Successful plasmapheresis in the Miller–Fisher syndrome. *Br. Med. J.*, **1**, 1627

Gherardi, R., Lebargy, F., Gaulard, P. *et al.* (1989). Necrotizing vasculitis and HIV replication in peripheral nerves. *N. Engl. J. Med.*, **321**, 685–686

Gibbels, E. and Giebisch, U. (1992). Natural course of acute and chronic monophasic inflammatory demyelinating polyneuropathies (IDP). *Acta Neurol. Scand.*, **85**, 282–291

Giegerich, G., Gengarol, C., Greiner, A. *et al.* (1994). Human T lymphocytes distinguish bovine from human P2 myelin protein: implications for immunological studies on inflammatory demyelinating neuropathy. *Neurology*, **44** (Suppl 2), A409

Grand'Maison, F., Feasby, T. E., Hahn, A. F. and Koopman, W. J. (1992). Recurrent Guillain–Barré syndrome. Clinical and laboratory features. *Brain*, **115**, 1093–1106

Gregson, N. A. and Leibowitz, S. (1985). IgM paraproteinaemia, polyneuropathy and MAG. *Neuropathol. Appl. Neurobiol.*, **11**, 329–347

Gregson, N. A., Koblar, S. and Hughes, R. A. C. (1993). Antibodies to gangliosides in Guillain–Barré syndrome: antigen specificity and relationship to clinical features. *Q. J. Med.*, **86**, 111–117

Grishaber, J. E., Cunningham, M. C., Rohret, P. A. and Strauss, R. G. (1992). Analysis of venous access for therapeutic plasma exchange in patients with neurological disease. *J. Clin. Apheresis*, **7**, 119–123

Gross, M. L. P. and Thomas, P. K. (1981). The treatment of chronic relapsing and chronic progressive idiopathic inflammatory polyneuropathy by plasma exchange, *J. Neurol. Sci.*, **52**, 69–78

Guillain, G., Barré, J. A. and Strohl, A. (1916). Sur un syndrome de radiculo-névrite avec hyperalbuminose du liquide céphalo-rachidien sans réaction cellulaire. Remarques sur les caractères cliniques et graphiques des réflexes tendineux. *Bull. Soc. Méd. Hôp. Paris*, **40**, 1462–1470

Guillain–Barré Syndrome Steroid Trial Group (1993). Double-blind trial of intravenous methylprednisolone in Guillain–Barré syndrome. *Lancet*, **341**, 586–590

Guiloff, R. J. (1977). Peripheral nerve conduction in Miller Fisher syndrome. *J. Neurol. Neurosurg. Psychiatry*, **40**, 801–807

Hahn, A. F., Feasby, T. E., Wilkie, L. and Lovgren, D. (1993). Antigalactocerebroside antibody increases demyelination in adoptive transfer experimental allergic neuritis. *Muscle Nerve*, **16**, 1174–1180

Hall, S. M., Hughes, R. A. C., Payan, J. *et al.* (1992). Motor nerve biopsy in severe Guillain–Barré syndrome, *Ann. Neurol.*, **31**, 441–444

Hallam, P. J., Harding, A. E., Berciano, J. *et al.* (1992). Duplication of part of chromosome 17 is commonly associated with hereditary motor and sensory neuropathy type I (Charcot–Marie–Tooth disease type 1). *Ann. Neurol.*, **31**, 570–572

Hartung, H.-P., Schwenke, C. Bitter-Suermann, D. and Toyka, K. V. (1987). Guillain–Barré syndrome: activated complement components C3a and C5a in CSF. *Neurology*, **37**, 1006–1009

Hartung, H.-P., Hughes, R. A. C., Taylor, W. A. *et al.* (1990). T cell activation in Guillain–Barré syndrome and in MS: elevated serum levels of soluble IL-2 receptors. *Neurology*, **40**, 215–218

Hartung, H.-P., Reiners, K., Michels, M *et al.* (1994). Serum levels of soluble E-Selectin (Elam-1) in immune mediated neuropathies *Neurology*, **44**, Suppl. 2, 409–410

Hawke, S. H. B., Hallinan, J. M. and McLeod, J. G. (1990). Cranial magnetic resonance imaging in chronic demyelinating polyneuropathy. *J. Neurol. Neurosurg. Psychiatry*, **53**, 794–796

Heininger, K., Liebert, U. G., Tokya, K. V. *et al.* (1984). Chronic inflammatory polyneuropathy – reduction of nerve conduction velocities in monkeys by systemic passive transfer of immunoglobulin. *J. Neurol. Sci.*, **66**, 1–14

Hodgkinson, S. J., Pollard, J. D. and McLeod, J. G. (1990). Cyclosporin A in the treatment of chronic demyelinating polyradiculoneuropathy. *J. Neurol. Neurosurg. Psychiatry*, **53**, 327–330

Honavar, M., Tharakan, J. K. J., Hughes, R. A. C. *et al.* (1991). A clinicopathological study of Guillain–Barré syndrome: nine cases and literature review. *Brain*, **114**, 1245–1270

Hoogendijk, J. E., Hensels, G., Gabreëls-Festen, A. A. W. M. *et al.* (1992). De-novo mutation in hereditary motor and sensory neuropathy type I. *Lancet*, **339**, 1081–1092

Hughes, R. A. C. (1990). *Guillain–Barré Syndrome*. Heidelberg: Springer-Verlag

Hughes, R. A. C. and Bihari, D. (1993). Acute neuromuscular respiratory paralysis. *J. Neurol. Neurosurg. Psychiatry*, **56**, 334–343

Hughes, R. A. C., Newsom-Davis, J. M., Perkin, G. D. and Pierce, J. M. (1978). Controlled trial of prednisolone in acute polyneuropathy. *Lancet*, **2**, 750–753

Hughes, R. A. C., Cameron, J. S., Hall, S. M. *et al.* (1982). Multiple mononeuropathy as the initial presentation of systemic lupus erythematosus – nerve biopsy and response to plasma exchange. *J. Neurol.*, **228**, 239–247

Hughes, R., Sanders, E., Hall, S. *et al.* (1992a). Subacute idiopathic demyelinating polyradiculoneuropathy. *Arch. Neurol.*, **49**, 612–616

Hughes, R. A. C., Atkinson, P., Coates, P. *et al.* (1992b). Sural nerve biopsies in Guillain–Barré syndrome: axonal degeneration and macrophage-mediated demyelination and absence of cytomegalovirus genome. *Muscle Nerve*, **15**, 568–575

Hund, E. F., Borel, C. O., Cornblath, D. R. *et al.* (1993). Intensive management and treatment of severe Guillain–Barré syndrome. *Crit. Care Med.*, **21**, 433–446

Irani, D. N., Cornblath, D. R., Chaudhry, V. *et al.* (1993). Relapse in Guillain–Barré syndrome after treatment with human immune globulin. *Neurology*, **43**, 872–875

Jackson, M. C., Godwin-Austen, R. B. and Whiteley, A. M. (1993). High-dose intravenous immunoglobulin in the treatment of Guillain–Barré syndrome: a preliminary open study. *J. Neurol.*, **240**, 51–53

Jacobs, B. C., Oomes, P. G., Hazenberg, M. P. *et al.* (1993). Epitopes on *Campylobacter jejuni/coli* can be recognised by anti-GM1 IgG antibodies in sera of Guillain–Barré patients. *Acta Gastro-Enterol. Belg.* **56**, Suppl: 9. (Abstract)

Jamieson, P. W., Giuliani, M. J. and Martinez, A. J. (1991). Necrotizing angiopathy presenting with multifocal conduction blocks. *Neurology*, **41**, 442–444

Kadlubowski, M. and Hughes, R. A. C. (1979). Identification of the neuritogen responsible for experimental allergic neuritis. *Nature*, **277**, 140–141

Kaji, R., Oka, N., Tsuji, T. *et al.* (1993). Pathological findings at the site of conduction block in multifocal motor neuropathy. *Ann. Neurol.*, **33**, 152–158

Kelly, J. J., Kyle, R. A., O'Brien, P. C. and Dyck, P. J. (1981). The prevalence of monoclonal gammopathy in peripheral neuropathy. *Neurology*, **31**, 1480–1483

Kermode, A. G., Laing, B. A., Carroll, W. M. and Mastaglia, F. L. (1992). Intravenous immunoglobulin for multifocal motor neuropathy. *Lancet*, **340**, 920–921

Khalili-Shirazi, A., Hughes, R. A. C., Brostoff, S. *et al.* (1992). T cell response to myelin proteins in Guillain–Barré syndrome. *J. Neurol. Sci.*, **111**, 200–203

Khalili-Shirazi, A., Atkinson, P., Gregson, N. and Hughes, R. A. C. (1993). Antibody responses to P_0 and P_2 myelin proteins in Guillain–Barré syndrome and chronic idiopathic demyelinating polyradiculoneuropathy. *J. Neuroimmunol.*, **46**, 245–252

Kinlen, L. J. (1985). Incidence of cancer in rheumatoid arthritis and other disorders after immunosuppressive treatment. *Am. J. Med.*, **78** (suppl A), 44–49

Kolkin, S., Nahman, N. S. and Mendell, J. R. (1987). Chronic nephrotoxicity complicating cyclosporin treatment of chronic inflammatory demyelinating polyradiculoneuropathy. *Neurology*, **37**, 147–148

Kornberg, A. J., and Pestronk, A. (1994). The clinical and diagnostic role of anti-GM_1 antibody testing. *Muscle Nerve*, **17**, 100–104

Koski, C. L., Humphrey, R. and Shin, M. L. (1985). Anti-peripheral myelin antibodies in patients with demyelinating neuropathy: quantitiative and kinetic determination of serum antibodies by complement component and fixation. *Proc Natl. Acad. Sci, USA*, **82**, 905–909

Koski, C. L., Gratz, E., Sutherland, J. and Mayer, R. F. (1986). Clinical correlation with anti-peripheral-nerve myelin antibodies in Guillain–Barré syndrome. *Ann. Neurol.*, **19**, 573–577

Koski, C. L., Chou, D. K. H. and Jungalwala, F. B. (1989). Anti-peripheral nerve myelin antibodies in Guillain–Barré syndrome bind a neutral glycolipid of peripheral myelin and cross-react with Forssman antigen. *J. Clin. Invest.*, **84**, 280–287

Krarup, C., Stewart, J. D., Sumner, A. J. *et al.* (1990). A syndrome of asymmetric limb weakness with motor conduction block. *Neurology*, **40**, 118–127

Kusonoki, S., Chiba, A. Kon, K. *et al.* (1994). N-acetylgalactosaminyl Guillain–Barré Syndrome. *Ann. Neurol.* **35**, 570–576

Lampert, P. W. (1969). Mechanism of demyelination in experimental allergic neuritis. Electron microscopic studies, *Lab. Invest.*, **20**, 127–138

Leger, J. M., Bouche, P., Bolgert, F. *et al.* (1989). The spectrum of polyneuropathies in patients infected with HIV. *J. Neurol. Neurosurg. Psychiatry*, **52**, 1369–1374

Lennon, S. M., Koblar, S., Hughes, R. A. C. *et al.* (1993). Reasons for persistent disability in Guillain–Barré syndrome. *Clin. Rehab.*, **7**, 1–8

Lewis, R. A., Sumner, A. J., Brown, M. J. and Asbury, A. K. (1982). Multifocal demyelinating neuropathy with persistent conduction block. *Neurology*, **32**, 958–964

Linington, C., Izumo, S., Suzuki, M. *et al.* (1984). A permanent rat T cell line that mediates experimental allergic neuritis in the rat *in vitro. J. Immunol.*, **133**, 1946–1950

Linington, C., Lassmann, H., Ozawa, K. *et al.* (1992). Cell adhesion molecules of the immunoglobulin supergene family as tissue-specific autoantigens: induction of experimental allergic neuritis (EAN) by P_O protein-specific T cell lines. *Eur. J. Immunol.*, **22**, 1813–1817

Lundkvist, I., van Doorn, P. A., Vermeulen, M. and Brand, A. (1993). Spontaneous recovery from the Guillain–Barré syndrome is associated with anti-idiotypic antibodies recognizing a cross-reactive idiotype on anti-neuroblastoma cell line antibodies. *Clin. Immunol. Immunopathol.*, **67**, 192–198

McCombe, P. A., McManis, P. G., Frith, J. A. *et al.* (1987a). Chronic inflammatory demyelinating polyradiculoneuropathy associated with pregnancy. *Ann. Neurol.*, **21**, 102–104

McCombe, P. A., Pollard, J. D. and McLeod, J. G. (1987b). Chronic inflammatory demyelinating polyradiculoneuropathy. *Brain*, **110**, 1617–1630

McGinnis, S., Kohriyama, T., Yu, R. K. *et al.* (1988). Antibodies to sulfated glucuronic acid containing glycosphingolipids in neuropathy associated with anti-MAG antibodies and in normal subjects. *J. Neuroimmunol.*, **17**, 119–126

McKhann, G. M., Griffin, J. W., Cornblath, D. R. *et al.* (1988). Plasmapheresis and Guillain–Barré Syndrome: analysis of prognostic factors and the effect of plasmapheresis. *Ann. Neurol.*, **23**, 347–353

McKhann, G. M., Cornblath, D. R., Ho, T. W. *et al.* (1991). Clinical and electrophysiological aspects of acute paralytic disease of children and young adults in northern China. *Lancet*, **338**, 593–597

McKhann, G. M., Cornblath, D. R., Griffin, J. W. *et al.* (1993). Acute motor axonal neuropathy: a frequent cause of acute flaccid paralysis in China. *Ann. Neurol.*, **33**, 333–342

Mendell, J. R., Kolkin, S., Kissel, J. T. *et al.* (1987). Evidence for central nervous system demyelination in chronic inflammatory demyelinating polyradiculoneuropathy. *Neurology*, **37**, 1291–1294

Miralles, F., Montero, J., Rene, R. and Martinez Matos, J. A. (1992a). Pure sensory Guillain–Barré syndrome. *J. Neurol. Neurosurg. Psychiatry*, **55**, 411–412

Miralles, G. D., O'Fallon, J. R. and Talley, N. J. (1992b). Plasma-cell dyscrasia with polyneuropathy – the spectrum of POEM syndrome. *N. Engl. J. Med.*, **327**, 1919–1923

Mishu, B., Ilyas, A. Koski, C. *et al.* (1993). Serologic evidence of previous *Campylobacter jejuni* infection in patients with Guillain–Barré syndrome. *Ann. Intern. Med.*, **118**, 947–953

Nobile-Orazio, E., Meucci, N., Barbieri, S. *et al.* (1993). High-dose intravenous immunoglobulin therapy in multifocal motor neuropathy. *Neurology*, **43**, 537–544

Oh, S. J., Joy, J. L. and Kuruoglu, R. (1992). "Chronic sensory demyelinating neuropathy": chronic inflammatory demyelinating polyneuropathy presenting as a pure sensory neuropathy. *J. Neurol. Neurosurg. Psychiatry*, **55**, 677–680

Oh, S. J., Kim, D. E. and Kuruoglu, R. (1994). What is the best diagnostic index of conduction block and temporal dispersion. *Muscle Nerve*, **17**, 489–493

Oka, N., Akiguchi, I., Kawasaki, T. *et al.* (1994). Elevated serum levels of Endothelial Leucocyte Adhesion Molecules in Guillain–Barré syndrome and Chronic Inflammatory Demyelinating Polyneuropathy. *Ann. Neurol.*, **35**, 621–624

Oomes, P. G., Van der Meché, F. G. A., Jacobs, B. C. *et al.* (1991). Antibodies to the ganglioside GM1 in sera of Guillain–Barré patients recognize epitopes on *Campylobacter* bacteria. Peripheral Nerve Study Group Meeting, Arden House, New York (Abstract)

Ormerod, I. E. C., Waddy, H. M., Kermode, A. G. *et al.* (1990). Involvement of the central nervous system in chronic inflammatory demyelinating polyneuropathy: a clinical, electrophysiological and magnetic resonance imaging study. *J. Neurol. Neurosurg. Psychiatry*, **53**, 789–793

Panayiotopoulos, C. P., Chroni, E. and Daskalopoulos, C. (1992). The significance of F-chronodispersion in the electrodiagnosis of Guillain–Barré syndrome and other motor neuropathies. *Arch. Neurol.*, **49**, 217–218

Parry, G. J. (1993). *Guillain–Barré Syndrome*. New York: Thieme.

Pestronk, A., Cornblath, D. R., Ilyas, A. A. *et al.* (1988). A treatable multifocal motor neuropathy with antibodies to GM1 ganglioside. *Ann. Neurol.*, **24**, 73–78

Pestronk, A., Chaudhry, V., Feldman, E. L. *et al.* (1990). Lower motor neuron syndromes defined by patterns of weakness, nerve conduction abnormalities and high titers of antiglycolipid antibodies, *Ann. Neurol.*, **27**, 316–326

Phillips, M. S., Stewart, S. and Anderson, J. R. (1984). Neuropathological findings in Miller–Fisher syndrome. *J. Neurol. Neurosurg. Psychiatry*, **47**, 492–495

Pollard, J. D. and Selby, G. (1978). Relapsing neuropathy due to tetanus toxoid. *J. Neurol. Sci.*, **37**, 113–125

Prineas, J. W. (1972). Acute idiopathic polyneuritis. An electronmicroscope study. *Lab. Invest.*, **26**, 133–147

Prineas, J. W. (1981). Pathology of the Guillain–Barré syndrome. *Ann. Neurol.*, **9** (suppl), 6–19

Prineas, J. W. and McLeod, J. G. (1976). Chronic relapsing polyneuritis. *J. Neurol. Sci.*, **27**, 427–458

Raphael, J. C., Masson, C., Morice, V. *et al.* (1984). Le syndrome de Guillain–Barré: étude retrospective de 233 observations. *Sem. Hôp. Paris*, **60**, 2543–2546

Rechthand, E., Cornblath, D. R. Stern, B. J. and Meyerhoff, J. O. (1984). Chronic demyelinating polyneuropathy in systematic lupus erythematosus. *Neurology*, **34**, 1375–1377

Roberts, M., Willison, H., Vincent, A. and Newsom-Davis, J. (1994). Serum factor in Miller–Fisher variant of Guillain–Barré syndrome and neurotransmitter release. *Lancet*, **343**, 454–455

Ronda, N., Hurez, V. and Kazatchkine, M. D. (1993). Intravenous immunoglobulin therapy of autoimmune and systemic inflammatory diseases. *Vox Sang.*, **64**, 65–72

Ropper, A. H. (1992). Current concepts: the Guillain–Barré syndrome. *N. Engl. J. Med.*, **326**, 1130–1136

Ropper, A. H. and Shahani, B. T. (1984). Diagnosis and management of acute areflexic paralysis with emphasis on Guillain–Barré syndrome. In *Peripheral Nerve Disorders. A Practical Approach* (A. K. Asbury and R. W. Gilliatt, eds), pp. 21–45, London: Butterworths.

Ropper, A. H., Wijdicks, E. F. M. and Truax, B. T. (1991). *Guillain–Barré Syndrome*. Philadelphia: F. A. Davis Company

Rosen, A. D. and Vastola, E. F. (1976). Clinical effects of cyclophosphamide in Guillain–Barré polyneuritis. *J. Neurol. Sci.*, **30**, 179–187

Rubin, M., Karpati, G. and Carpenter, S. (1987). Combined central and peripheral myelinopathy. *Neurology*, **37**, 1287–1290

Saida, T., Saida, K., Silberberg, D. H. and Brown, M. K. (1981). Experimental allergic neuritis induced by galactocerebroside. *Ann. Neurol.*, **9** (suppl), 87–101

Santoro, M., Uncini, A., Corbo, M. *et al.* (1992). Experimental conduction block induced by serum from a patient with anti-GM1 antibodies. *Ann. Neurol.*, **31**, 385–390

Server, A. C., Lefkowith, J., Braine, H. and McKhann, G. M. (1979). Treatment of chronic relapsing inflammatory polyradiculoneuropathy by plasma exchange. *Ann. Neurol.*, **6**, 258–261

Sharief, M. K., McLean, B. and Thompson, E. J. (1993). Elevated serum levels of tumor necrosis factor-α in Guillain–Barré syndrome. *Ann. Neurol.*, **33**, 591–596

Smith, G. D. P. and Hughes, R. A. C. (1992). Plasma exchange treatment and prognosis of Guillain–Barré syndrome. *Q. J. Med.*, **85**, 751–760

Sterman, A. B., Schaumburg, H. H. and Asbury, A. K. (1986). The acute sensory neuronopathy syndrome: a distinct clinical entity. *Ann. Neurol.*, **7**, 354–358

Stricker, R. B., Sanders, K. A., Owen, W. F. *et al.* (1992). Mononeuritis multiplex associated with cryoglobulinemia in HIV infection. *Neurology*, **42**, 2103–2105

Taylor, W. A. and Hughes, R. A. C. (1989). T lymphocyte activation antigens in Guillain–Barré syndrome and chronic idiopathic demyelinating polyradiculoneuropathy. *J. Neuroimmunol.*, **24**, 33–39

The Dutch Guillain–Barré Study Group (1994). Treatment of Guillain–Barré syndrome with high-dose imune globulins combined with methylpredrisolone: a pilot study. *Ann Neurol.*, **35**, 794–752

The Guillain–Barré Syndrome Study Group (1985). Plasmapheresis and acute Guillain–Barré syndrome. *Neurology*, **35**, 1096–1104

Thomas, P. K., Lascelles, R. G., Hallpike, J. F. and Hewer, R. L. (1969). Recurrent and chronic relapsing Guillain–Barré polyneuritis. *Brain*, **92**, 589–606

Thomas, P. K., Walker, R. W. H., Rudge, P. *et al.* (1987). Chronic demyelinating peripheral neuropathy associated with multifocal CNS demyelination. *Brain*, **110**, 53–76

Torvik, A. and Lundar, T. (1977). A case of chronic demyelinating polyneuropathy resembling the Guillain–Barré syndrome. *J. Neurol. Sci.*, **32**, 45–52

Toyka, K. V., Augspach, R., Paulus, W. *et al.* (1980). Plasma exchange in polyradiculoneuropathy. *Ann. Neurol.*, **8**, 205–206

Toyka, K. V., Augspach, R., Wietholter, H. *et al.* (1982). Plasma exchange in chronic inflammatory polyneuropathy: evidence suggestive of a pathogenic humoral factor. *Muscle Nerve*, **5**, 479–484

Toyka, K. V., Hartung, H.-P. and Steck, A. (1992). Plasmapheresis in chronic demyelinating polyneuropathy. *N. Eng. J. Med.*, **326**, 1089–1091

van der Hoop, R. G., Vecht, C. J., Van der Burg, M. E. L. *et al.* (1990). Prevention of cisplatin neurotoxicity with an ACTH (4-9) analogue in patients with ovarian cancer. *N. Eng. J. Med.*, **322**, 89–94

Van der Meché, F. G. A., Schmitz, P. I. M. and the Dutch Guillain–Barré Study Group (1992). A randomized trial comparing intravenous immune globulin and plasma exchange in Guillain–Barré syndrome. *N. Eng. J. Med.* **326**, 1123–1129

van Doorn, P. A., Brand, A., Strengers, P. F. W. *et al.* (1990). High-dose intravenous immunoglobulin treatment in chronic inflammatory demyelinating polyneuropathy: a double-blind, placebo-controlled, crossover study. *Neurology*, **40**, 209–212

Verma, A., Tandan, R., Adesina, A. M. *et al.* (1990). Focal neuropathy preceding chronic inflammatory demyelinating polyradiculoneuropathy by several years. *Acta Neurol. Scand.*, **81**, 516–521

Vermeulen, M., van Doorn, P. A., Brand, A. *et al.* (1993). Intravenous immunoglobulin treatment in patients with chronic inflammatory demyelinating polyneuropathy: a double blind, placebo controlled study. *J. Neurol. Neurosurg. Psychiatry*, **56**, 36–39

Vrethem, M., Larsson, B., von Schenck, H. and Ernerudh, J. (1993). Immunofixation superior to plasma agarose electrophoresis in detecting small M-components in patients with polyneuropathy. *J. Neurol. Sci.* **120**, 93–98

Vriesendorp, F. J., Mayer, R. F. and Koski, C. L. (1991). Kinetics of anti-peripheral nerve myelin antibody in patients with Guillain–Barré syndrome treated and not treated with plasmapheresis. *Arch. Neurol.*, **48**, 858–861

Vriesendorp, F. J., Mishu, B., Blaser, M. J. and Koski, C. L. (1993). Serum antibodies to GM1, GD1b, peripheral nerve myelin, and *Campylobacter jejuni* in patients with Guillain–Barré syndrome and controls: correlation and prognosis. *Ann. Neurol.*, **34**, 130–135

Waksman, B. H. and Adams, R. D. (1955). Allergic neuritis: experimental disease of rabbits induced by the injection of peripheral nervous tissue and adjuvants. *J. Exp. Med.*, **102**, 213–225

Waksman, B. H. and Adams, R. D. (1956). A comparative study of EAN in the rabbit, guinea-pig and mouse. *J. Neuropathol. Exp. Neurol.*, **15**, 293–310

Walsh, F. S., Cronin, M., Koblar, S. *et al.* (1991). Association between glycoconjugate antibodies and *Campylobacter* infection in patients with Guillain–Barré syndrome. *J. Neuroimmunol.*, **34**, 43–51

Willison, H. J., Veitch, J., Paterson, G. and Kennedy, P. G. E. (1993). Miller–Fisher syndrome is associated with serum antibodies to GQ1b ganglioside. *J. Neurol. Neurosurg. Psychiatry*, **56**, 204–206

Winer, J. B., Hughes, R. A. C. and Osmond, C. (1988a). A prospective study of acute idiopathic neuropathy. I. Clinical features and their prognostic value. *J. Neurol. Neurosurg. Psychiatry*, **51**, 605–612

Winer, J. B., Gray, I. A., Gregson,. N. A. *et al.* (1988b). A prospective study of acute idiopathic neuropathy. III. Immunologic studies *J. Neurol. Neurosurg. Psychiatry*, **51**, 619–625

Winer, J. B., Hughes, R. A. C., Anderson, M. J. *et al.* (1988c). A prospective study of acute idiopathic neuropathy. II. Antecedent events. *J. Neurol. Neurosurg. Psychiatry*, **51**, 613–618

Wrobel, C. J. and Watson, D. (1992). Plasmapheresis in chronic demyelinating polyneuropathy. *N. Engl. J. Med.*, **326**, 1089–1090

Young, R. R., Asbury, A. K., Corbett, J. L. and Adams, R. D. (1975). Pure pandysautonomia with recovery – description and discussion of diagnostic criteria. *Brain*, **98**, 613–636

Yuki, N., Yoshino, H., Sato, S. and Miyatake, T. (1990). Acute axonal neuropathy associated with anti-GM_1 antibodies following *Campylobacter* enteritis. *Neurology*, **40**, 1900–1902

Yuki, N., Sato, S., Fujimoto, S. *et al.* (1992a). Serotype of *Campylobacter jejuni*, HLA, and the Guillain–Barré syndrome. *Muscle Nerve*, **15**, 968–969

Yuki, N., Sato, S., Inuzuka, T. *et al.* (1992b). Axonal degeneration in the Guillain–Barré syndrome and anti-GM1 ganglioside antibodies. *Muscle Nerve*, **15**, 116

Yuki, N., Sato, S., Tsuji, S. *et al.* (1993a). Frequent presence of anti-G_{Q1b} antibody in Fisher's syndrome. *Neurology*, **43**, 414–417

Yuki, N., Taki, T., Inagaki, F. *et al.* (1993b). A bacterium lipopolysaccharide that elicits Guillain–Barré syndrome has a GM1 ganglioside-like structure. *J. Exp. Med.*, **178**, 1771–1775

Yuki, N., Yamada, M., Sato, S. *et al.* (1993c). Association of IgG anti-GD_{1a} antibody with severe Guillain–Barré syndrome. *Muscle Nerve*, **16**, 642–647

Yuki, N., Yamazaki, M., Kondo, H. *et al.* (1993d). Treatment of multifocal motor neuropathy with a high dosage of intravenous immunoglobulin. *Muscle Nerve*, **16**, 220–221

Yuki, N., Miyatake, T. and Ohsawa, T. (1993e). Beneficial effect of plasmapheresis on Fisher's syndrome. *Muscle Nerve*, **16**, 1267–1268

Zifko, U., Drlicek, M., Senautka, G. and Grisold, W. (1994). High dose immunoglobulin therapy is effective in the Miller–Fisher syndrome. *J. Neurol.*, **3**, 178–179

10
Neuropathies due to Lyme disease, leprosy and Chagas' disease
G. Said

INTRODUCTION

Neuropathies occur in infectious disorders due to a variety of agents that include viruses, especially retroviruses, bacteria (such as *Mycobacterium leprae*), spirochaetes, and parasites (such as *Trypanosoma cruzi*, the agent of Chagas' disease). This group of neuropathies affects the largest number of people in the world, and the neuropathies are often treatable or preventable. The mechanism of the nerve lesions that occur in this context may result both from the inflammatory reaction induced by the infective agent and from the immune reaction of the patient.

LYME DISEASE

First descriptions of the neurological complications associated with tick bite, namely paralysis and meningitis, were made in Europe (Afzelius, 1921; Garin and Bujadoux, 1922; Lipschütz, 1923; Bannwarth, 1944) but the recognition of Lyme disease as a separate entity occurred in the region of Old Lyme, Connecticut (USA) in the mid-1970s (Steere *et al.*, 1977), after an epidemic of arthritis, which led to convincing epidemiological evidence for a tick vector.

The manifestations of Lyme disease involve the skin, joints, heart and nervous system. The disease is caused by a tick-transmitted spirochaete, *Borrelia burgdorferi* (Burgdorfer *et al.*, 1982). Certain differences have been noted between American and European isolates of *B. burgdorferi* in morphology, outer surface proteins, plasmids and DNA homology (Wilson and Spielman, 1985).

Ticks of the genus *Ixodes* are the usual vectors. Ticks feed once during the three stages of their usual 2-year life. Larval ticks take one blood meal in late summer, nymphs feed during the following spring and early summer, and adults during that autumn (Steere, 1989). Most human infections with *B. burgdorferi* thus occur at that time of the year. In the United States, the preferred host for both the larval and nympheal stages of *I. dammini* is the white-footed mouse, while white-tailed deer are the preferred host of adult *I. dammini*. Transmission of *B. burgdorferi* by *I. scapularis* requires a minimum of a day-and-a-half of attachment (Piesman *et al.*, 1991).

In Europe, thousands of new cases of Lyme borreliosis occur each summer, particularly in Germany, Austria, Switzerland, France and Sweden. In the United States, more than 9600 cases were reported in 1992, and nearly 50 000 cases from 1982 to 1992, with more than 90% of cases in north-eastern coastal states, from Massachusetts to Maryland, Wisconsin and Minnesota in the mid-west, and California and Oregon in the west (Wilson and Spielman, 1985; Lane *et al*, 1991).

Clinical manifestations

After an incubation period of 7 to 10 days (range 3–31 days), the course of the disease follows three stages.

Stage 1

In 60–80% of cases, the patient first has **erythema migrans**, usually associated with mild constitutional symptoms including low-grade fever, headache, fatigue, arthralgias, myalgias and regional adenopathy. Localized erythema migrans results from local spreading of *B. burgdorferi* in the skin. It starts as a red macule or papule at the site of the bite and expands to form a large red ring with central clearing, more than 5 cm in diameter. Over days to weeks, the lesion usually expands and can reach a diameter of more than 30 cm. Untreated erythema migrans and associated symptoms typically resolve spontaneously in 3 to 4 weeks (Steere, 1989).

Stage 2

Within days or weeks after inoculation, the spirochaete may spread in the patient's blood to many sites and has been recovered from blood during this stage and from many organs. Secondary annular lesions, which resemble the primary erythema migrans, occur in about half of patients in association with migratory musculoskeletal and joint pain (Steere, 1989). The secondary lesions are of various shapes and size, generally smaller than the primary lesion. Widely disseminated symptoms seem to be more common in the United States than in Europe. By this time, the host starts to develop a strong immune response to *B. burgdorferi* antigens, the result being the destruction of spirochaetes by complement activation through immune complexes (Kochi and Johnson, 1988). Both polymorphonuclear leucocytes and monocytes readily phagocytose the spirochaete, and lymphocytic infiltration is observed histologically in all affected tissues with plentiful plasma cells, and in some sites, mild vasculitis.

After several weeks or months, 15–20% of patients develop neurological signs which usually start with radicular pain, often burning in character, associated or not with weakness, and little or no clinical signs of meningitis. Meningitis is the most common neurological abnormality in Lyme disease. It can be the first symptom, but is usually preceded by erythema migrans, and then begins after the skin lesions resolve. Papilloedema and increased cerebrospinal fluid (CSF) pressure can occur. CSF examination reveals a lymphocytic pleocytosis, usually a few tens or hundreds of cells/ml, with mild elevation of protein, a high proportion of immunoglobulins and oligoclonal bands. The CSF glucose level is usually normal but can be low

(Pachner and Steere, 1986: Reik *et al.*, 1985). The spirochaete has been cultured from the CSF on several occasions.

Multifocal spinal root or cranial nerve involvement often develop within a few days or weeks, with uni- or bilateral facial palsy and asymmetric sensorimotor radiculoneuropathy. Cranial neuropathy is present in 50% of patients with neurological abnormalities (Pachner and Steere, 1985; Reik *et al.*, 1986, 1971; Reik and Burgdorfer, 1986). Cranial nerve palsies resolve within weeks or months, sometimes incompletely, while sphincter disturbances also occur.

Peripheral neuropathy occurs in approximately half of patients with meningitis, focal or multifocal involvement being the most common presentation. Common patterns include painful thoracoabdominal sensory radiculitis associated with distal involvement. Both weakness and sensory loss improve within a few weeks, but recovery may take up to several months and often remains incomplete.

Electrophysiological testing of patients with peripheral neuropathy has shown evidence both of demyelination and of axonal degeneration, but axonal lesions usually predominate (Vallat *et al.*, 1987; Duray and Steere, 1988). Histologically, the nerve lesions are associated with lymphoplasmocytic inflammatory infiltrates that are maximal in nerve roots and produce mostly axonal lesions. The presence of *B. burgdorferi* has not been convincingly documented in the nerves. In a recent post-mortem study of one of our patients with multifocal peripheral nerve involvement and meningitis, who died from pulmonary embolism at this stage of the disease in spite of preventive treatment with low dose heparin, the peripheral nerves were normal, contrasting with the presence of an important inflammatory infiltration of the meninges, around spinal roots and cranial nerves, especially the facial nerves. The central nervous system (CNS) was not affected. Stage 2 neurological abnormalities usually last for weeks or months.

Cardiac involvement which includes fluctuating atrioventricular node block, mild left ventricular dysfunction, or, rarely, cardiomegaly or fatal pancarditis, occurs in 4–8% of the patients. The duration of cardiac abnormalities is usually brief and does not necessitate permanent insertion of a pacemaker (Steere *et al.*, 1980; Marcus *et al.*, 1985).

Stage 3

Arthritis occurs on average 6 months after the onset of the disease. It affects about 60% of the patients in the United States (Steere, 1989) and is characterized by asymmetric oligoarticular arthritis, especially of the knee; one or a few joints are also affected. The spirochaete has been occasionally cultured from joint fluid. Arthritis seems less common in Europe, the susceptibility to develop Lyme arthritis seeming to be genetically determined. The haplotype HLA-DR4 is commonly found in patients with chronic Lyme disease and is associated with poor response to antimicrobial treatment, suggesting the importance of immunogenetic factors.

A variety of late syndromes affecting the CNS has been described, including spastic paraparesis, ataxia, a relapsing multiple sclerosis like illness, bladder dysfunction, cognitive impairment, dementia and subacute encephalitis (Ackermann *et al.*, 1988; Halperin *et al.*, 1989; Pachner *et al.*, 1989). Although these patients had serological evidence of Lyme disease, they did not have intrathecal synthesis of antibody to *B. burgdorferi* or were not tested for it. Thus the evidence for chronic CNS complications of Lyme disease remains weak.

Diagnosis

From a neurological point of view, the presence of a subacute meningoradiculoneuritis with facial palsy and signs and symptoms suggesting a multifocal involvement of the peripheral nervous system is highly suggestive of Lyme borreliosis. The most frequently ordered test to screen for antibodies to *B. burgdorferi* is an enzyme-linked immunosorbent assay (ELISA), which has not yet been standardized. In addition its accuracy is unknown, with marked variability among laboratories, and common negative and, more often, false positive results (Steere, 1989; Bakken *et al.*, 1992). Titres should increase four-fold or more between the erythema migrans phase and subsequent neurological involvement. Many patients have asymptomatic *B. burgdorferi* infection, and in addition to that, false positive results, particularly with IgM, may occur both in healthy subjects and in patients with a variety of other diseases (Steere *et al.*, 1977). Refinements of serological methods may be helpful in the future to differentiate patients with residual positivity and false positive patients from those suffering from Lyme disease. Recently, criteria were proposed for positive Western immunoblotting that require the presence of bands at particular locations (Dressler *et al.*, 1993). Tests to detect genetic material, cell-mediated immune reaction to *B. burgdorferi* and antigens remain experimental (Spach *et al.*, 1993). The most specific diagnostic test for Lyme disease is the cultural isolation of *B. burgdorferi* from erythema migrans lesions but this procedure requires a special medium and is neither rapid nor widely available (Spach *et al.*, 1993).

Treatment

B. burgdorferi seems highly sensitive to tetracycline, ampicillin and ceftriaxone, but only moderately sensitive to penicillin. For early Lyme disease, localized stage 1 or disseminated stage 2 infection, oral tetracycline is generally an effective antibiotic (Steere *et al.*, 1983), though doxycycline, a long-acting tetracycline that achieves better tissue levels, may be preferable. The treatment should be administered for 10–30 days.

Although intravenous penicillin is generally considered effective in the treatment of neurological disease, ceftriaxone is now commonly used because it crosses the blood–brain barrier more readily and requires only once-a-day administration (Dattwyler *et al.*, 1988). Corticosteroids may be used with antibiotic treatment in some cases.

In view of the low risk of Lyme disease after a recognized deer-tick bite and uncertain effectiveness of prophylactic antimicrobial agents, routine antimicrobial prophylaxis for persons with a recognized deer-tick bite is not indicated (Shapiro *et al.*, 1992).

LEPROUS NEUROPATHY

Since the identification by Hansen, in Bergen (Norway), of a bacillus, *Mycobacterium leprae*, as the causative agent of leprosy in 1874, much has been learned about the natural history, the clinical and pathological manifestations, and the genetics of this organism, in addition to the treatment of leprosy. Subsequent improvements in the treatment, management and public health approach have all contributed to near eradication of the disease in industrialized countries. However, leprosy remains among the primary causes of neuropathy in the world even though the latest estimate of the number of leprosy cases world-wide is 5.5 million (Noordeen *et al.*, 1992). This is about half the number estimated in the early 1980s (World Health Organization, 1985), although some 2–3 million patients have residual deformity (Smith, 1992). This apparent decrease in the prevalence of leprosy results mainly from the shortening of the duration of treatment, on which this evaluation is based.

Leprosy is primarily found in tropical and subtropical developing countries. In some parts of Asia and Africa, the prevalence exceeds 10 per 1000 population and more than 0.5 million new cases are detected each year (Noordeen, 1991). Many of the neurological aspects of leprous neuropathies have been known for decades (Monrad-Krohn, 1923; Juliao and Rotberg, 1963; Dastur, 1978; Sabin and Swift, 1984), yet leprosy remains a challenge to immunologists because the form that the condition takes depends mainly on the immune reaction of the host to *M. Leprae* antigens. These range from the extremes of the lowest level cell-mediated immunity to *M. leprae*, the lepromatous pole, to that with the highest cell-mediated immunity, the tuberculoid pole (Ridley, 1974).

Mycobacterium leprae is an acid fast, Gram positive bacillus, and is an obligate intracellular parasite which has defied all attempts at cultivation *in vitro*. It exhibits the longest generation time of all bacteria, requiring 13 days to double in experimentally infected mice (Levy, 1976). Recent studies have led to identification of immunodeterminants that are limited in number (Engers *et al.*, 1986), with many also being components of the stress and oxidative responses and having primary sequences that have been remarkably well conserved throughout the biological kingdoms. Recent work has shown that the genome of *M. leprae* is represented by four contigs of overlapping clones, which together account for nearly 2.8 Mb of DNA. The current genome map of this uncultivable pathogen comprises 72 loci (Eigelmeier *et al.*, 1993). The major protein antigens of *M. leprae* include the 70- and 65-kDa heat shock proteins and the 12- and 18-kDa heat shock proteins. Another major antigen is represented by a 28-kDa protein, which is the superoxide dismutase of *M. leprae*. The genes which code for these antigens have been identified and detection of *M. leprae* made possible with polymerase chain reaction (PCR) amplification in skin and nerve biopsies of patients with paucibacillary leprosy (Chemouilli *et al.*, 1992).

Clinical manifestations

Specific cutaneous lesions

These include maculae and lepromatae, and reveal the disease in half or more of the patients, depending on the type of leprosy. In the others, small areas of sensory loss, circumscribed zones of anhidrosis or alopecia, paresis of facial muscles, hypochromic or atrophic cutaneous patches or painful enlargement of a nerve trunk are the presenting manifestations. Plantar ulcers and other trophic changes occur later in the course of the disease, as a consequence of sensory loss.

Sensory loss

Sensory loss, which is the most constant finding of leprous neuropathy, is due to mixed dermal nerve and nerve trunk damage, and is extremely variable in distribution, ranging from a small skin patch with impaired sensation to severe sensory loss over most of the body surface, avoiding only the body folds. Early cutaneous lesions show some preservation of sensation, with impairment of light touch, loss of thermal and pain sense, while proprioception is preserved, so patients can still use their largely anaesthetic limbs effectively, which leads to painless trauma and trophic changes. Loss of dermal pigment in the territory of affected cutaneous nerves leads to development of large depigmented anaesthetic patches in dark-skinned people, with loss of sweating in the corresponding areas. Cooler areas of the body seem more affected (Hastings *et al.*, 1968), but temperature-linked sensory loss, which is not observed in tuberculoid leprosy, cannot account for all the patterns of nerve lesions in leprosy. In some cases, complete loss of pain and temperature sensations in a certain area contrasts with preservation of tactile sensation. This classical dissociation of sensory loss is seldom complete in leprosy. In most cases all modalities of superficial sensations are affected. Sensory loss also occurs in the areas corresponding to maculae, demonstrating early involvement of sensory nerve terminals.

The topographical distribution of sensory disturbances is extremely variable. Sensory loss may effect an 'insular' pattern, in which anaesthetic areas of variable shape, size and number are found, and may or may not correspond to macular type of cutaneous lesions. These manifestations, which may last for years, are usually associated with other disturbances such as anhidrosis, alopecia and vasomotor areflexia (Juliao and Rotberg, 1963). They are also related to lesions of sensory nerve endings and/or to that of a limited number of nerve fascicles of a nerve trunk. Sensory loss may also take a nerve trunk pattern or, in some cases, a pseudo-radicular pattern, as a consequence of involvement of large nerve trunks. In cases of long-standing evolution, the distal parts of the limbs show the greatest sensory loss. This extends proximally to a greater or lesser extent, but rarely to the trunk. When the trunk is involved, sensory loss manifests as an insular pattern. Sensory loss does not affect the anterior aspect of the trunk in a length-dependent pattern, as in severe diabetic, amyloid or alcoholic polyneuropathy. In individual patients, dissociation between sensations may be found only in some areas. The large nerve trunks most commonly affected are the ulnar and the common peroneal nerves, followed by the median, posterior tibial, superficial radial, peroneal nerves and the greater auricular and facial nerves (Dastur *et al.*, 1966).

Nerve hypertrophy

Nerve trunks are palpably enlarged in one-third of the patients with leprosy (Said, 1980), sometimes before the occurrence of sensory loss in the corresponding territory. Superficial nerves, like the greater auricular nerve in the neck, the supraorbital branch of the trigeminal nerve or larger nerve trunks, especially the ulnar nerve above the elbow, the peroneal nerve, the radial cutaneous nerve at the lateral border of the wrist, are often enlarged. Nerve hypertrophy is sometimes associated with spontaneous tingling or with painful sensations. Nerve thickening is regular, cylindroid, or sometimes nodular. Palpation of the nerve itself is occasionally painful. It must be remembered that nerve hypertrophy is often difficult to ascertain clinically. On several occasions, we have found normal-sized nerves in patients referred for biopsy of palpably hypertrophic nerves. There are also other causes for nerve hypertrophy, including hypertrophic neuritis, neuromas, neurofibromatosis and amyloidosis. Isolated nerve hypertrophy is therefore not sufficient to establish the diagnosis of leprous neuropathy, even in endemic areas. In such cases, if the presence of *M. leprae* has not been demonstrated in skin, nerve biopsy is mandatory.

Motor disturbance and amyotrophy

Motor involvement is usually a late event in the course of the disease. Amyotrophy and motor weakness usually progress *pari passu*; in some cases however, amyotrophy is more marked than weakness, both of which predominate in the ulnar and median nerve territories, with characteristic claw hands. The peroneal nerve is predominantly affected in the lower limbs. Motor involvement and amyotrophy usually progress very slowly, in a roughly symmetrical way. Preservation of tendon reflexes in many cases of leprous neuropathy is characteristic of predominant involvement of the most distal part of the nerves and of cutaneous nerves.

Facial palsy with lagophthalmos

This occurs in one or both eyes, with sparing of the other muscles supplied by the facial nerve a classical feature of leprosy. Surgical exploration of the facial nerve showed involvement of one or several branches of division destined to the frontal muscles and to orbicularis oculi. This involvement is often associated with sensory loss in the malar region and in the cornea of the eye (Dastur *et al.*, 1966).

Trophic disturbances

Trophic ulcers that most often occur on the sole of the foot, are a common, non-specific, complication of loss of pain sensation. Severe sensory disturbances are always found in those areas where ulcers occur. Plantar ulcer is subsequent to microtrauma on skin that has lost sensation for pain. The absence of protective sensation of limb extremities leads to overuse, accidental self-injury, recurrent infections, and to gradual development of further deformities as observed in sensory neuropathy of different origin (Said, 1980), or in congenital indifference to pain (Landrieu *et al.*, 1990). Bone lesions and osteolysis are always distally located and often bilateral, and have a centripetal evolution, gradually affecting the phalanges, metacarpal and metatarsal bones, causing deformities of the limbs. Radiological examination reveals concentric progressive atrophy of phalanges and metatarsal and metacarpal bones. The process starts in the distal end of phalanges, destroys the joint surfaces and progresses without causing bone reaction.

The spectrum of clinical manifestations correlates well with the cellular immune responsiveness of the patient to *M. leprae* antigens which ranges from the extremity with the lowest cell-mediated immunity to *M. leprae*, the lepromatous pole, to that with the highest cell-mediated immunity, the tuberculoid pole (Sansonetti and Lagrange, 1981; Ridley and Jopling, 1966; Bloom *et al.*, 1983).

Immunological and morphological aspects

Lepromatous and borderline lepromatous leprosy

This represents the most common type of leprosy in many endemic areas of Africa. In nearly all cases there are associated characteristic skin lesions. They encompass the multibacillary forms of leprosy. Occasionally, there is no detectable skin lesion. Skin lesions are usually numerous consisting of macules, papules, nodules with infiltration and thickening of the skin, affecting predominantly the cooler areas of the body. At that stage, diffuse, bilateral and generally symmetrical nerve damage occurs. In such patients bacteria can be found in skin lesions, nasal smears, or even in the blood when sought. The majority of circulating bacilli are found intracellularly, in polymorphonuclear leucocytes, monocytes and large circulating histiocytes (Drutz *et al.*, 1972). In this form, the specific unresponsiveness of the host to antigens of the leprosy bacillus permits unchecked proliferation of bacilli (Pedley *et al.*, 1980; Van Voorhis *et al.*, 1982). This unresponsiveness is manifested by negative skin test to lepromin *in vivo* (Mitsuda reaction). In the inflammatory infiltrates of cutaneous lesions, most of the cells are of the monocyte-macrophage lineage and the remainder are predominantly suppressor T lymphocytes (Van Voorhis *et al.*, 1982). With respect to function, CD4+ T cells appeared to be strongly cytolytic for antigen presenting cells pulsed with antigens.

The more lepromatous the findings, in general the less marked are the symptoms (Pedley *et al.*, 1980). What appears 'early' clinically in leprosy is often extremely late on morphological examination of a nerve biopsy. Palpably enlarged nerves may be functioning well, but do eventually fail. In a combined clinical, electrophysiological and morphological study in seven patients with lepromatous leprosy, palpably enlarged cutaneous radial nerves, and with preservation of all modalities of sensations in the corresponding territory, we found that the conduction velocity of the radial cutaneous nerve did not significantly differ from those found in patients with lepromatous leprosy and hypertrophy of the cutaneous radial nerve with sensory deficit (Tzourio *et al.*, 1992). Conversely, the mean value of the action potential of the radial cutaneous nerve was significantly smaller in patients with sensory loss, suggesting that axon loss rather than demyelination of nerve fibres was responsible for sensory deficit. These findings also confirm that nerve conduction velocity may be decreased before any sensory deficit and can be used for detection of asymptomatic nerve involvement (Sebille, 1978).

Pathological aspects

Morphological study in patients with silent hypertrophy of the radial cutaneous nerve and lepromatous leprosy, multibacillary leprosy, showed preservation of the overall structure of the nerve, marked asymmetry of the inflammatory lesions between and within individual fascicles. Some fascicles were massively affected while others looked totally preserved, a feature which fits well with the occurrence of partial deficit in a nerve territory. Light microscopic examination of nerve cross-sections showed an extensive inflammatory reaction which affected the epineurium of all nerve specimens and the perineurium of most fascicles (Figure 10.1) and which was responsible for the nerve enlargement. Increase in nerve volume may lead to nerve compression in sites of physiological nerve entrapment and induce additional

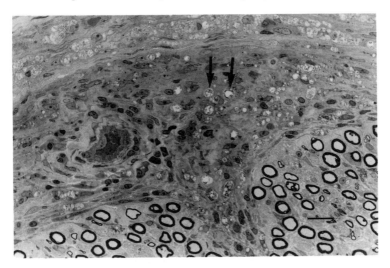

Figure 10.1 A 1-μm thick section of the superficial radial nerve from a patient with silent hypertrophy of the superficial radial nerve and lepromatous leprosy. Note that the density of nerve fibres is well preserved, in keeping with preservation of sensation in the corresponding territory. There is a marked hypertrophy of the perineurium which is invaded by inflammatory cells, many of which contain vacuoles (arrows) and *M. leprae*. Thionin blue staining. Bar = 20 μm.

damage of mechancial origin. Around some fascicles the perineurium had an 'onion-skin' hypertrophic appearance as noted by others (Figure 10.2) (Pearson and Weddell, 1975; Boddingius, 1977). Lymphocytic vasculitis affected nerve blood vessels in all nerve compartments. Vessels remained permeable to blood, making ischaemia an improbable factor of nerve damage at that stage. *M. leprae* are extremely numerous in lepromatous neuropathy, often being found in globoid clumps on Ziehl-stained, paraffin-embedded specimens. They are found in all nerve compartments and affect a large variety of cells, including perineurial cells, fibroblasts, cells of the macrophage–histiocyte lineage, Schwann cells and endothelial cells (Job, 1970; Barros *et al.*, 1987). *M. leprae* are easily identified on electron microscopic examination as dark, osmiophilic inclusions usually located in cytoplasmic vacuoles containing a phenolic glycolipid-I (PGL-I) and lipoarabinomannan, both produced in large amounts by *M. leprae* (Figure 10.3). In some nerve specimens from patients with nerve hypertrophy, the inflammatory infiltrates and infection of cells seem to follow connective tissue septa and vascular axes from the perineurium towards the endoneurium. In other cases, infection of endoneurial cells is observed without hypertrophic changes. Axons surrounded by a normal myelin sheath may contain occasional bacilli, but the likelihood that intra-axonal bacilli are responsible for nerve lesions is low.

On teased fibre preparations of nerve specimens from patients with silent hypertrophy of the superficial radial nerve in the setting of lepromatous leprosy (Tzourio *et al.*, 1992), segmental abnormalities of the myelin sheath, including segmental demyelination and/or the presence of short remyelinated internodes, predominate in some (Figure 10.4). The demyelinated fibres are often clustered and closely linked with debris-laden macrophages. Axonal degeneration of nerve fibres predominates in

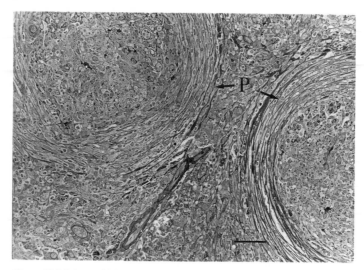

Figure 10.2 A 1-μm thick section of the superficial radial nerve from a patient with symptomatic hypertrophy of the superficial radial nerve and lepromatous leprosy. Note the enormous inflammatory infiltration that affects all nerve compartments, the onion-skin like hypertrophy of the perineurium (P) and the complete loss of nerve fibres. Thionin blue staining. Bar = 50 μm.

others. In many nerves, there is a marked proliferation of connective tissue surrounding and adhering to nerve fibres. All cases with symptomatic neuropathy are associated with severe axon loss, with average reduction of nerve fibre density to 5% of control values versus 25–30% in patients with silent hypertrophy of the radial nerve (Tzourio *et al.*, 1992) (Figures 10.2 and 10.4).

Another salient feature observed in nerves of patients with lepromatous leprosy is the intense proliferation of fibroblasts with increased synthesis of collagen leading to endo- and perineurial fibrosis. This degree of scarring is thought to hamper growth of regenerating fibres. Control of unwanted sclerosis would certainly improve the outcome of the neuropathy (Tzourio *et al.*, 1992).

Tuberculoid leprosy

At the other extreme of the spectrum, tuberculoid leprosy and borderline tuberculoid neuropathy, now often called paucibacillary forms of leprosy, are marked by complete nerve destruction. In this form patients develop high levels of specific cell-mediated immunity that ultimately kill and clear the bacilli in the tissues, inducing concurrent damage to the nerves that harbour the bacilli. Clinically tuberculoid lesions may be single or few, and are distributed asymmetrically in the vicinity of typical hypoaesthetic or anaesthetic hypopigmented skin lesions.

Histopathologically, the lesion is characterized by epithelioid-cell granulomata with intense lymphocytic infiltrations (Boddingius, 1977; Job, 1970). The nerve structure may no longer be identified in many cases and bacilli are not found in the lesions, but *M. leprae* antigens have been detected in nerves using anti-BCG anti-sera which cross-react with *M. leprae* antigens (Barros *et al.*, 1987). In skin lesions

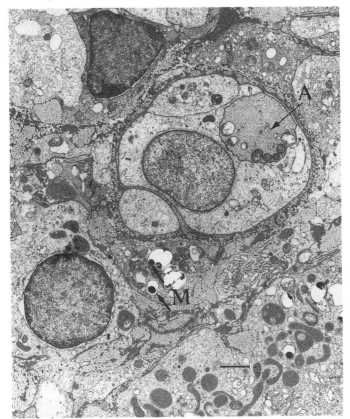

Figure 10.3 Electron micrograph of a biopsy specimen from a patient with lepromatous leprosy. The axon (A) is demyelinated and surrounded by Schwann cells and inflammatory infiltration. Note the presence of *M. leprae* (M) in vacuoles in the cytoplasm of a cell nearby. Uranyl acetate and lead citrate staining. Bar = 1 μm.

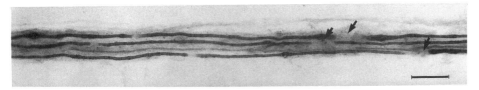

Figure 10.4 Teased osmicated fibres from a fascicular biopsy specimen of the superficial radial nerve. The patient had cutaneous signs of lepromatous leprosy, hypertrophy of the superficial radial nerve without sensory loss in the corresponding territory and slow conduction velocity of the superficial radial nerve. The photograph illustrates the demyelinative changes (arrows) often associated with early inflammatory lesions that accompany asymptomatic hypertrophy of the nerves in lepromatous leprosy. Bar = 100 μm.

the tuberculoid infiltrates predominantly contain helper T cells. The basis for the conspicuous destruction of nerve structure is thought to be a delayed type hypersensitivity reaction with specific helper T cells reacting with *M. leprae* antigens presented in the endoneurium by macrophages. Antigen may also be presented by

Schwann cells expressing the HLA-DR antigen induced by interferon γ released by helper T cells. Activation of macrophages in this context leads to release of a number of secretory products including neutral proteases, potent oxidizing agents which can oxidize thiol groups in enzymes, break bonds in proteins, lipids, and nucleic acids and initiate chain reactions involving free radicals that can propagate such damage (Nathan *et al.*, 1980). It is thus conceivable that when a delayed type hypersensitivity reaction occurs in the endoneurium it can lead to major damage, and even to necrosis and to intraneural abscesses (Said and Hontebeyrie, 1992).

Reactional states

One of the many concerns in patients under treatment for leprous neuropathy is the occurrence of a sudden alteration of the immunological status and the development of a reactional state.

The **reversal** or **upgrading reaction** is characterized by a heightened cell-mediated response occurring mainly in patients with the borderline lepromatous form of leprosy. It appears commonly during the first year of therapy, or later. During the first 6–12 months of therapy with dapsone alone, 50% of patients have this type of reaction. Patients who developed an upgrade reaction were found to have higher concentration of IgM anti-PGL-1 antibodies in the serum (Roche *et al.*, 1991). This reaction is identified by swelling and exacerbation of existing skin and nerve lesions in association with general malaise and fever. Painful swelling of nerve trunks is accompanied by sensory and motor deficit in the corresponding territory. In some cases, nerves which previously were apparently unaffected are heavily damaged. Endoneurial granulomata, multinucleated giant cells, lymphocytic infiltration, vasculitis and perineuritis are present on morphological examination. Necrosis of the endoneurial content may lead to nerve abscesses. No *M. leprae* are observed in this reaction. In summary, enhancement of the cell-mediated immune response in patients under treatment can itself lead to damage of nerve trunks.

Erythema nodosum leprosum (ENL) is almost exclusively seen at the lepromatous pole of the disease. If effective chemotherapy results in massive death of leprosy bacilli, ENL is common and affects an average 50% of patients by the end of the first year of treatment in some areas (Wemambu *et al.*, 1969). The multiple, acute, tender skin nodules that characterize ENL are frequently accompanied by fever, arthritis, oedema, muscle pains, iridocyclitis and acute peripheral nerve damage. ENL is considered a manifestation of the Arthus phenomenon with deposition of complement and immunoglobulin in a granular pattern around dermal vessels (Wenambu *et al.*, 1969). Tumour necrosis factor-alpha (TNFα) and interleukin-1 (IL1) serum concentrations are greatly increased in lepromatous leprosy and correlate with the severity of erythema nodosum leprosum (ENL) and with the incidence of reactions (Talamon *et al.*, 1994).

In a recent immunopathological study of nerve lesions in the different forms of leprous neuropathy, we found that the HLA-DR antigen was expressed by 72% of the endoneurial cells in lepromatous leprosy and in 95% in tuberculoid leprosy, versus 11% in control nerves (Talamon *et al.*, 1994). Schwann cells expressed HLA-DR antigens making them able to present foreign antigens to immunocompetent cells. It is also important to note that Schwann cells and many other nerve cells harbour many *M. leprae* in the multibacillary forms, and that the Schwann cells have a life expectancy which is as long as that of the patient under normal conditions. This long life of the Schwann cells allows *M. leprae* to survive intracellularly and proliferate. *M. leprae*, with its documented long generation time, can thus accumulate in the Schwann cells, usually without causing much damage. Immunolabelling of endoneurial cells showed that CD4 T cells markedly predominated in paucibacillary forms but were scarce in lepromatous leprosy and in ENL. Macrophages were also more numerous in the tuberculoid form. TNFα and urokinase, the activator of plasminogen, were secreted by approximately 2% of cells in the tuberculoid forms versus 0.2% in the lepromatous forms, and 0% in the controls (Talamon *et al.*, 1994). These findings support the concept of nerve lesions secondary to the action of products released by activated macrophages in the context of a delayed type hypersensitivity reaction in tuberculoid and in reversal reactions.

Investigators have tried to elucidate the mechanisms of immunoregulation in leprosy, that lead to the different patterns of leprous neuropathy. Sieling *et al.* (1993) found that the tuberculoid lesions are characterized by high levels of IL-2 and interferon-gamma (IFN-γ) mRNA. These authors suggest that the effect of these cytokines would promote cell-mediated immunity. In contrast, in lepromatous lesions, high levels of IL-4 and IL-10 mRNA would result in an augmentation of humoral response with concomitant suppression of cell-mediated immunity. However analysis of cytokine production by mycobacterium-reactive T cells by Mutis *et al.* (1993) showed that neither Il-4 nor IL-10 seemed to play a pivotal role in the specific unresponsiveness to *M. leprae*.

Diagnosis

Nerve biopsies are useful in the diagnosis and management of leprosy. In purely neuropathic forms which are seen in the tuberculoid form and, less often, in lepromatous leprosy, it is the only way to reach the diagnosis. It is especially useful in countries where leprosy is not common. In such countries, it must be kept in mind that leprous neuropathy may become symptomatic years or decades after an individual has moved from an endemic area. Where leprosy is endemic, nerve biopsy may be useful in differentiating leprous neuropathy from neuropathy of other origin, including diabetic neuropathy, hereditary sensory neuropathies or amyloid neuropathy which can lead to sensory and trophic manifestations and can be mistaken for leprous neuropathy. Ziehl staining of paraffin-embedded sections permits visualization of bacilli in the pluribacillary forms of the disease. Bacilli are scarce or absent from nerves with tuberculoid leprosy and in reactional states. In such forms, identification of *M. leprae* antigens using anti-BCG and MLO4 monoclonal antibodies in paraffin sections, with PAP immunoperoxidase, may be positive even when *M. leprae* cannot be found histologically. When there is no evidence of infection with *M. leprae*, it may be impossible to differentiate a neuropathy due to tuberculoid leprosy from sarcoid neuropathy. On the basis of cross-sectional studies, it appears that testing for PGL-I serum antibodies has high sensitivity for multibacillary cases but only moderate sensitivity for paucibacillary cases. Detection of sequences of *M. leprae* DNA by PCR techniques (Woods and Cole, 1990; Chemouilli *et al.*, 1992) may prove helpful in the diagnosis of paucibacillary leprous neuropathy and in the follow-up of patients under treatment, if such investigations become available in endemic areas.

Treatment

Enormous progress has been made in chemotherapy of leprosy thanks to control programmes of the WHO. The standard recommendation has been to treat patients with paucibacillary leprosy, which include the tuberculoid and borderline tuberculoid forms, for 6 months only, with daily unsupervised dapsone 100 mg, and monthly supervised rifampin 600 mg. All treatment is then stopped and the patient is kept under observation for 2 years. Multibacillary patients require treatment for a minimum of 2 years, but should preferably continue until skin smears are negative. The treatment consists of daily dapsone 100 mg, together with clofamizine 300 mg, both supervised. On completion, multibacillary patients should remain under observation for 5 years. Rifampin resistance emerged in some patients with lepromatous leprosy, who received only monotherapy. It stemmed from mutations in the *rpoB* gene, which encodes the β subunit of RNA polymerase of *M. leprae*. These findings will be of use for the development of a rapid screening procedure involving the PCR for monitoring the emergence of rifampin-resistant *M. leprae* strains (Honoré and Cole, 1993). Corticosteroids are useful in the treatment of reversal reaction and thalidomide in erythema nodosum leprosum. Contact tracing and disability prevention are other aspects of treatment of leprosy.

CHAGAS' DISEASE

In Chagas' disease, humans are infected with the trypomastigote form of *Trypanosoma cruzi* by blood-sucking bugs of the Triatoma subfamily, *Triatoma infestans*. The metacyclic trypanosome in insect faeces penetrates minute skin abrasions and mucous membranes of the conjunctiva. Other ways of transmission include congenital infection, laboratory accidents, organ transplantation and blood transfusion. Chagas' disease is widespread in Latin America where it affects an estimated 20 million people. After penetration into the host, the trypomastigote loses its flagellum, transforms into an amastigote and multiplies in pseudocysts. Some amastigotes may eventually transform back into trypomastigotes and circulate in the blood.

Initial local multiplication of the parasite may result in local inflammation with heat, redness and swelling (chagoma), and enlargement of satellite lymph nodes. During this phase of active parasite multiplication there is an intense interstitial inflammatory reaction with mononuclear cells. Later on, the parasite multiplication is suppressed by the cellular and humoral immune reaction of the host, and becomes increasingly difficult to detect in the tissues. Some 90% of patients survive the acute phase but it is doubtful whether the infection is ever eradicated. It remains asymptomatic throughout life in most of them, while others develop symptoms after a period of years.

The neurological manifestations are mainly characterized by the occurrence of the autonomic neuropathy in the chronic stage of the disease. There are some regional differences in Chagas' disease due to the existence of different strains of *T. cruzi*. The autonomic manifestations include cardiac and gastrointestinal involvement which are both associated with inflammatory lesions of muscle and autonomic ganglia and nerves (Fernandez *et al.*, 1992).

Peripheral neuropathy is not a prominent manifestation of Chagas' disease. It has been recognized in animal models (Barreira *et al.*, 1981; Said *et al.*, 1985; Gonzalez *et al.*, 1987; Molina *et al.*, 1987; Losavio *et al.*, 1989) before its identification in humans where it is rare (Nascimento *et al.*, 1991). Recently, Woodhouse (1993) compared 25 patients suffering from Chagas' disease with matched controls. Four of the chagasic patients provided histories of mild sensory neuropathy and on clinical examination were found to have impaired light touch sensation, vibration sense and two point discrimination. Peripheral neuropathy is much more common at a subclinical level in humans, especially upon electrophysiological examination both at the acute and at chronic phases of the disease (Sica *et al.*, 1986; Benavente *et al.*, 1989); the electromyographic abnormalities remain subtle. Experimental models of Chagas' disease have proven useful in understanding the pathophysiology of nerve and muscle lesions. In a series of investigations performed in the mouse model, we found that early localization of *T. cruzi* occurred in the acute phase, in the 3 weeks following inoculation, associated with mild lesions. At the chronic stage of the disease, the amastigotes were increasingly difficult to localize but immunostaining clearly showed the presence of *T. cruzi* antigens in nerve and muscle inflammatory infiltrates. Additionally, we have been able to show that endoneurial granulomas are due to a delayed type hypersensitivity reaction (Said *et al.*, 1985, Hontebeyrie-Joskowicz *et al.*, 1987; Ben Younes-Chennoufi *et al.*, 1988a,b). The question as to whether antibodies to *T. cruzi* cross-react with autoantigens or whether specific helper T lymphocytes are activated by such antigens remains a matter of controversy (Hontebeyrie-Joskowicz *et al.*, 1987; Ben Younes-Chennoufi *et al.*, 1988a,b).

Nifurtimox[R] and Benznidazole[R] are both used in the acute stage but are less active at the chronic stage. Only symptomatic treatment can be offered at the chronic stage.

REFERENCES

Ackermann, R., Rehse-Kupper, B., Gollmer, E. and Schmidt, R. (1988). Chronic neurologic manifestations of erythema migrans borreliosis. *Ann. N.Y. Acad. Sci.*, **539**, 16–23

Afzelius, A. (1921). Erythema chronicum migrans. *Acta Derm. Venerol. (Stockholm)*, **2**, 120–125

Bakken, L. L., Case, K. L., Callister, S. M. *et al.* (1992). Performance of 45 laboratories participating in a proficiency testing program for Lyme disease serology. *JAMA*, **268**, 891–895

Bannwarth, A. (1944). Zur Klinik und Pathogenese der "chronischen lymphocytaren Meningitis". *Arch. Psychiatr. Nervenkr.*, **117**, 161–185

Barreira, A., Said, G. and Kretti, A. (1981). Multifocal demyelinative lesions of peripheral nerves in experimental chronic Chagas disease. *Trans. R. Soc. Trop. Med. Hyg.*, **75**, 751

Barros, V. Shetty, V. P. and Antia, N. H. (1987). Demonstration of *Mycobacterium leprae* antigen in nerves of tuberculoid leprosy. *Acta Neuropathol.*, **73**, 387–392

Benavente, O. R., Patino Ledesma, O., Baez Pena, L. *et al.* (1989). Motor unit involvement in human Chagas' disease. *Arq. Neuro-Psiquiat. (Sao-Paolo)*, **47**, 283–286

Ben Younes-Chennoufi, A., Hontebeyrie-Joskowicz, M., Tricottet, V. *et al.* (1988a). Persistence of *Trypanosoma cruzi* antigens in the inflammatory lesions of chronically infected mice. *Trans. R. Soc. Trop. Med. Hyg.*, **82**, 77–83

Ben Younes-Chennoufi, A., Said, G., Eisen, H. *et al.* (1988b). Cellular immunity to *Trypanosoma cruzi* is mediated by helper T cells (CD4+). *Trans. R. Soc. Trop. Med. Hyg.*, **82**, 84–89

Bloom, B. R. and Godal, T. (1983). Selective primary health care: strategies for control of disease in the developing world. V. Leprosy. *Rev. Infect. Dis.*, **5**, 765–780

Boddingius, J. (1977) Ultrastructural changes in blood vessels of peripheral nerves in leprosy neuropathy. II Borderline, borderline lepromatous and lepromatous patients. *Acta Neuropath.*, **40**, 21–39

Burgdorfer, W., Barbour, A. G., Hayes, S. F. *et al.* (1982). Lyme disease – a tick borne spirochetosis? *Science*, **216**, 1317–1319

Chemouilli, P., Woods, C., Cole, S. and Said, G. (1992). Diagnostic value of PCR in paucibacillary leprous neuropathy, (abstract). *J. Neurol.*, **239**, S125

Dastur, D. K. (1978). Leprosy. In *Handbook of Clinical Neurology*, Vol. 33 (P. J. Vinken and G. W. Bruyn, eds), pp. 421–468, Amsterdam: North Holland Publishing Company

Dastur,D. K., Antia, N. H. and Divekar, S. C. (1966). The facial nerve in leprosy. II Pathology, pathogenesis, electromyography and clinical correlation. *Int. J. Leprosy*, **34**, 118–138

Dattwyler, R. J., Halperin, J. J., Volkman, D. J. and Luft, B. J. (1988). Treatment of late Lyme borreliosis – randomized comparison of ceftriaxone and penicillin. *Lancet*, **1**, 1191–1194

Dressler, F., Whalen, J. A., Reinhardt, B. N. and Steere, A. C. (1993). Western blotting in the serodiagnosis of Lyme disease. *J. Infect. Dis.*, **167**, 392–400

Drutz D. J., Chen, T. S. N. and Weng-Hsiang, L. (1972). The continuous bacteremia of lepromatous leprosy. *N. Engl. J. Med.*, **287**, 159–164

Duray, P. H. and Steere, A. C. (1988). Clinical pathologic correlations of Lyme disease by stage. *Ann. N.Y. Acad, Sci.*, **539**, 65–79

Eigelmeier, K., Honoré, N., Woods, S. A. *et al.* (1993). Use of an ordered cosmid library to deduce genomic organization of *Mycobacterium leprae*. *Mol. Microbiol.*, **7**, 197–206

Engers, H. D., Houba. V., Bennedsen, J. *et al.* (1986). Results of a World Health Organization in full-sponsored workshop to characterize antigens recognised by mycobacterium specific monoclonal antibodies. *Infect. Immunol.*, **51**, 718–720

Fernandez, A., Hontebeyrie, M. and Said, G. (1992). Autonomic neuropathy and immunological abnormalities in Chagas' disease. *Clin. Autonom. Res.*, **2**, 409–412

Garin, C. and Bujadoux, C. (1922). Paralysie par les tiques. *J. Méd. Lyon*, **3**, 765–767

Gonzalez Cappa, S. M., Sanz, O. P., Müller, L. A. *et al.* (1987). Peripheral nervous system damage in experimental Chagas' disease. *Am. J. Trop. Med. Hyg.*, **36**, 41–45

Halperin, J. J., Luft, B. J., Anand, A. K. *et al.* (1989). Lyme neuroborreliosis: central nervous system manifestations. *Neurology*, **39**, 753–759

Hastings, R. C., Brand, P. W., Mansfield, E. R. and Elner, T. D. (1968). Bacterial density in the skin in lepromatous leprosy as related to temperature. *Leprosy Rev.*, **39**, 71–74

Honoré, N. and Cole, S. (1993). Molecular basis of rifampin resistance in *Mycobacterium leprae*. *Antimicrob. Agents Chemother.*, **37**, 414–418

Hontebeyrie-Joskowicz, M., Said, G., Milon, G. *et al.* (1987). L3T4+ T cells able to mediate parasite-specific delayed type hypersensitivity play a role in the pathology of experimental Chagas' disease. *Eur. J. Immunol.*, **17**, 1027–1033

Job, C. K. (1970). *Mycobacterium leprae* in nerve lesions in lepromatous leprosy. An electron microscopic study. *Arch. Pathol.*, **89**, 195–207

Juliao, O. F. and Rotberg, A. (1963). Neural involvement in leprosy. In *Tropical Neurology* (L. Van Bogaert, L. Pereyra Kafer and G. F. Poch, eds), pp. 43–80, Buenos Aires: Lopez Libreros Editores

Kochi, S. K. and Johnson, R. C. (1988). Role of immunoglobulin G in killing of *Borrelia burgdorferi* by the classical complement pathway. *Infect. Immun.*, **56**, 314–321

Landrieu, P., Said, G. and Alaire, C. (1990). Dominantly transmitted congenital indifference to pain. *Ann. Neurol.*, **27**, 574–578

Lane, R. S., Piesman, J. and Burgdorfer, W. (1991). Lyme borreliosis: relation of its causative agent to its vectors and hosts in North America and Europe. *Annu. Rev. Entomol.*, **36**, 587–609

Levy, L. (1986). Studies of the mouse footpad technique for cultivation of *Mycobacterium leprae*. III. Doubling time during logarithmic multiplication. *Leprosy Rev.*, **57**, 103–106

Lipschütz, B. (1923). Weiterer Beitrag zur Kenntis des "Erythema chronicum migrans". *Arch. Dermatol. Syph.*, **143**, 365–374

Losavio, A., Jones, M. C., Sanz, O. P. *et al.* (1989). A sequential study of the peripheral nervous system involvement in experimental Chagas' disease. *Am. J. Trop. Med. Hyg.*, **41**, 539–547

Marcus, L. C., Steere, A. C., Duray, P. H. *et al.* (1985). Fatal pancarditis in a patient with coexistent Lyme disease and babesiosis: demonstration of spirochetes in the myocardium. *Ann. Intern. Med.*, **103**, 374–376

Molina, H. A., Cardoni, R. L. and Rimoldi, M. T. (1987). The neuromuscular pathology of experimental Chagas' disease. *J. Neurol. Sci.*, **81**, 287–300

Monrad-Krohn, G. H. (1923). The neurological aspect of leprosy. Videnskapsselskapets Skrifter. I. *Mat-Naturv. Klasse*, **16**, 1–78

Mutis, T., Kraakman, E. M., Cornelisse, Y. E. *et al.* (1993). Analysis of cytokine production by *Mycobacterium*-reactive T cells. *J. Immunol.*, **150**, 4641–4651

Nascimento, O. J. M., De Freitas, M. R. G. and Chimelli, L. (1991). Polyneuropathie axonale dans la maladie de Chagas. *Rev. Neurol.*, **147**, 679–681

Nathan, C. F., Murray, H. W. and Cohn, Z. A. (1980). The macrophage as an effector cell. *N. Engl. J. Med.*, **303**, 622–626

Noordeen, S. K. (1991). A look at world leprosy. *Leprosy Rev.*, **62**, 72–86

Noordeen, S. K., Lopez Bravo, L. and Sundaresan, T. K. (1992). Estimated number of leprosy cases in the world. *Bull. WHO*, **70**, 7–10

Pachner, A. R. and Steere, A. C. (1985). The triad of neurologic manifestations of Lyme disease: meningitis, cranial neuritis, and radiculoneuritis. *Neurology*, **35**, 47–53

Pachner, A. R., Duray, P. and Steere, A. C. (1989). Central nervous system manifestations of Lyme disease. *Arch. Neurol.*, **46**, 790–795

Pearson, J. M. H. and Weddell, A. G. M. (1975). Perineurial changes in untreated leprosy. *Leprosy Rev.*, **46**, 51–67

Pedley, J. C., Harman, D. J., Waudby, H. and McDougall, A. C. (1980). Leprosy in peripheral nerves: histopathological findings in 119 untreated patients in Nepal. *J. Neurol. Neurosurg. Psychiatry*, **43**, 198–204

Piesman, J., Maupin, G. O., Campos, E. G. and Happ, C. M. (1991). Duration of adult female *Ixodes dammini* attachment and transmission of *Borrelia burgdorferi*, with description of a needle aspiration isolation method. *J. Infect. Dis.*, **163**, 895–897

Reik, L., Steere, A. C., Bartenhagen,. N. H. *et al.* (1979). Neurologic abnormalities of Lyme disease. *Medicine (Baltimore)*, **58**, 281–294

Reik, L. Jr., Burgdorfer, W. and Donaldson, J. O. (1986). Neurologic abnormalities in Lyme disease without erythema chronicum migrans. *Am. J. Med.*, **81**, 73–78

Ridley, D. S. (1974). Histological classification and the immunological spectrum of leprosy. *Bull. WHO*, **51**, 451–465

Ridley, D. S. and Jopling, W. H. (1966). Classification of leprosy according to immunity. A five group system. *Int. J. Leprosy*, **34**, 255–273

Roche, P., Theuvenet, W. J. and Britton, W. J. (1991). Risk factors for type-1 reactions in borderline leprosy patients. *Lancet*, **338**, 654–657

Sabin, T. D. and Swift, T. R. (1984). Leprosy, *In Peripheral Neuropathy*, Vol. 2 (P. J. Dyck, P. K. Thomas, E. H. Lambert and R. Bunge, eds), pp. 1955–1987, Philadelphia: W. B. Saunders

Said, G. (1980). A clinicopathologic study of acrodystrophic neuropathies. *Muscle Nerve*, **3**, 491–501

Said, G. and Hontebeyrie, M. (1992). Nerve lesions induced by macrophage activation. *Res. Immunol.*, **143**, 589–599

Said, G., Joskowicz, M., Barreira, A. *et al.* (1985). Neuropathy associated with experimental Chagas' disease. *Ann. Neurol.*, **18**, 676–683

Sansonetti, P. and Lagrange, P. H. (1981). The immunology of leprosy: speculations on the leprosy spectrum. *Rev. Infect. Dis.*, **3**, 422–469

Sebille A. (1978). Respective importance of different nerve conduction velocities in leprosy. *J. Neurol. Sci.*, **38**, 89–95

Shapiro, E. D., Gerber, M. A., Holabird, N. B. *et al.* (1992). A controlled trial of antimicrobial prophylaxis for Lyme disease after deer-tick bites. *N. Engl. J. Med.*, **237**, 1769–1773

Sica, R. E. P., Filipini, D., Panizza, M. *et al.* (1986). Involvement of the peripheral sensory nervous system in human chronic Chagas' disease. *Medicina (Buenos Aires)*, **46**, 662–668

Sieling, P. A., Abrams, J. S., Yamamura, M. *et al.* (1993). Immunosuppressive roles for IL-10 and IL-4 in human infection. In vitro modulation of T cell responses in leprosy. *J. Immunol.*, **150**, 5501–5510

Smith, W. C. S. (1992). The epidemiology of disability in leprosy including risk factors. *Leprosy Rev.*, **63** (suppl), 23–30

Spach, D. H., Liles, W. C., Campbell, G. L. *et al.* (1993). Tick-borne diseases in the United States. *N. Engl. J. Med.*, **329**, 934–947

Steere, A. C. (1989). Lyme disease. *N. Engl. J. Med.*, **321**, 586–596

Steere, A. C., Batsford, W. P., Weinberg, M. *et al.* (1980). Lyme carditis: cardiac abnormalities of Lyme disease. *Ann. Intern. Med.*, **93**, 8–16

Steere, A. C., Hutchinson, G. J., Rahn, D. W. *et al.* (1983). Treatment of early manifestations of Lyme disease. *Ann. Intern. Med.*, **99**, 22–26

Steere, A. C., Malawista, S. E., Snydman, D. R. *et al.* (1977). Lyme arthritis: an epidemic of oligoarticular arthritis in children and adults in three Connecticut communities. *Arthritis Rheum.*, **20**, 7–17

Talamon, C., Tzourio, C., Said, G. (1994). Immunolabeling of cells and secretory products of macrophages in different patterns of leprous neuropathy. *J. Neurol.*, **241**, (suppl 1), S16–S17

Tzourio, C., Said, G., Milan, J. (1992). Asymptomatic nerve hypertrophy in lepromatous leprosy: A clinical, electrophysiological and morphological study. *J. Neurol.*, **239**, 367–374

Vallat, J. M., Hugon, J., Lubeau, M. *et al.* (1987). Tick-bite meningoradiculoneuritis: clinical electrophysiologic, and histologic findings in 10 cases. *Neurology*, **37**, 749–753

Van Voorhis, W. C., Kaplan, G., Sarno, E. N. *et al.* (1982). The cutaneous infiltrates of leprosy. *N. Engl. J. Med.*, **307**, 1593–1597

Wenambu, S. N. C., Turk, J. L., Walters, M. F. R. and Rees R. J. W. (1969). Erythema nodosum leprosum: a clinical manifestation of Arthus phenomenon. *Lancet*, **ii**, 933–935

Wilson, M. L. and Spielman, A. (1985). Seasonal activity of immature *Ixodes dammini*. *J. Med. Entomol.*, **22**, 408–414

Woodhouse, J. I. (1993). The prevalence of clinical peripheral neuropathies in human chronic Chagas' disease. *J. R. Army Med. Corps*, **139**, 54–55

Woods, S. A. and Cole, S. (1990). A family of dispersed repeats in *Mycobacterium leprae*. *Mol. Microbiol.*, **4**, 1745–1751

World Health Organization (1985). Epidemiology of leprosy in relation to control: report of a WHO study group. *WHO Technical Report Series*, 716

11
Peripheral neuropathies in human immunodeficiency virus type 1 infection

D. R. Cornblath and J. C. McArthur

INTRODUCTION

This chapter concerns the spectrum of peripheral neuropathies seen in individuals with human immunodeficiency virus type 1 (HIV) infection. It is important to remember that acquired immunodeficiency syndrome (AIDS) was described in 1981 (Gottlieb et al., 1981; Masur et al., 1981), that description of the central nervous system (CNS) complications first appeared in 1983 (Pitlik et al., 1983), and that the first report to concentrate on peripheral neuropathy appeared in 1985 (Levy et al., 1985). While many peripheral nervous system (PNS) disorders occurring in individuals with HIV infection have been described, including acute and chronic inflammatory demyelinating polyneuropathy, syndromes of mono-neuropathies, multiple mononeuropathies or polyradiculopathies, distal symmetric polyneuropathy, and toxic neuropathies due to retroviral therapies (Table 11.1), only some are unique to the HIV-infected population. Thus, the clinician must be alert to other causes of these syndromes, before ascribing them to HIV infection alone.

An association of specific neuropathic syndromes with specific stages of HIV infection is known (Table 11.2) (Cornblath and McArthur, 1989). For example, the inflammatory demyelinating polyneuropathies, both Guillain–Barré syndrome (GBS) and chronic inflammatory demyelinating polyneuropathy (CIDP), are most frequently seen at the time of seroconversion or during the phase of early infection when the patient has no constitutional symptoms (CDC Category A). By contrast, the distal symmetric polyneuropathy syndrome is seen exclusively in those with immunodeficiency, whose CD4 counts have dropped below $300/\mu l$ and may have already developed AIDS. We have previously speculated that these associations provide clues to pathogenesis (Cornblath and McArthur, 1989). For example, the early neuropathic syndromes may result from immune dysregulation, while the latter ones may be a consequence of immune failure.

EPIDEMIOLOGY OF PERIPHERAL NEUROPATHY IN HIV INFECTION

Multiple studies have been undertaken to investigate the incidence of peripheral neuropathy in HIV-infected individuals (Chavanet et al., 1987, 1988; Levy et al.,

Table 11.1 Peripheral neuropathies in HIV infection

Neuropathies with seroconversion
   Guillain–Barré syndrome
   Facial or brachial neuropathies
   Bilateral hearing dysfunction
Distal symmetric polyneuropathy
Inflammatory demyelinating polyneuropathies
   Guillain–Barré syndrome
   Chronic inflammatory demyelinating polyneuropathy
Mononeuropathies
Multiple mononeuropathies
   Vasculitis
   Cytomegalovirus
   Polyradiculopathies
     Cytomegalovirus
     Lymphomatous
     Syphilitic
Toxic neuropathies

Table 11.2 Neuropathies and HIV infection

Neuropathy	*Stage of infection most commonly associated*
GBS	CDC category A
CIDP	CDC category A
Mononeuropathies	CDC categories B, C
DSPN	CDC category C
Polyradiculopathies	CDC category C

GBS, Guillain–Barré syndrome; CIDP, chronic inflammatory demyelinating polyneuropathy; DSPN, distal symmetric polyneuropathy. CDC category A, asymptomatic or persistent generalized lymphadenopathy; CDC category B, symptomatic, not A or C conditions; CDC category C, AIDS-indicator conditions. (From Centers for Disease Control, 1993.)

1988; So *et al.*, 1988; Gastaut *et al.*, 1989; Koch *et al.*, 1989; McArthur *et al.*, 1989; Hall *et al.*, 1991; Gulevich *et al.*, 1992; Winer *et al.*, 1992; Barohn *et al.*,1993; Fuller *et al.*, 1993). While some have looked at individuals at specific stages of disease, others have looked at entire populations of HIV-infected persons across the spectrum of disease severity. Fortunately, these studies have come to similar conclusions. In otherwise asymptomatic HIV-infected individuals, symptomatic peripheral neuropathy without known cause, and therefore presumably related to HIV infection, is rare, occuring in <1% of individuals (McArthur *et al.*, 1989; Winer *et al.*, 1992; Barohn *et al.*, 1993; Fuller *et al.*, 1993). However, as the disease progresses, up to 30% of those with AIDS will develop symptomatic peripheral neuropathy (So *et al.*, 1988). A recent epidemiological survey in a large cohort of homosexual men found that the incidence rate of sensory neuropathy was 1.7% annually. The incidence was much higher in men with lower CD4 counts, 8% for CD4 counts <100/μl and showed a significant rise over time. Part of this rise was the consequence of exposure to potentially toxic antiretrovirals, but even after adjusting for this, a significant temporal increase in the incidence of sensory neuropathy was apparent (Bacellar *et al.*, 1993). By the time of autopsy, almost all (>95%) those dying with AIDS will have pathological evidence of peripheral nerve damage (de la Monte *et al.*, 1988; Mah *et al*; 1988; Henin *et al.*, 1990; Griffin *et al.*, 1994). Two recent studies (Winer *et al.*, 1992; Husstedt *et al.*, 1993) suggest that with time up to 60% of AIDS patients develop symptomatic neuropathy. Several caveats should be mentioned concerning these conclusions. First, the definition of 'peripheral neuropathy' is not standardized across these studies, and these working definitions have not undergone validation. Second, among the various series, the ancillary studies performed to look for other causes of neuropathy have varied considerably. In most series, if 'no obvious cause is present,' then the neuropathy is assumed to be due to HIV infection. This may or may not be valid. Third, the risk factors in the cohorts studied vary, which may explain some of the variability in the results. For example, the incidence of peripheral neuropathy is highest in cohorts of intravenous drug users, most likely due to concomitant alcohol use.

NEUROPATHIES ASSOCIATED WITH HIV SEROCONVERSION AND EARLY HIV INFECTION

In 5–10% of individuals recently infected with HIV, seroconversion manifests as a 'mononucleosis-type' illness (Cooper *et al.*, 1985). Initially, HIV ELISA serology is negative but Western blot testing may reveal one or two 'suggestive' bands. As time passes, more bands develop on Western blot testing, and later the ELISA serology is positive. In rare cases, this sequence of serological events has accompanied the development of specific neuropathic syndromes. The most dramatic is Guillain–Barré syndrome (GBS) (Hagberg *et al.*, 1986; Vendrell *et al.*, 1987; Persuy *et al.*, 1988). In some parts of the world, seroconversion is frequently associated with GBS (Conlon, 1989); in North America and Europe, this is a rare association. In all respects, the clinical disorder is identical to other cases of GBS, both the clinical features and the response to therapy. The differentiating feature is the occurrence of a transient cerebrospinal fluid (CSF) pleocytosis (Raphael *et al.*, 1991) differing from the usual albumino–cytological dissociation seen in HIV-seronegative GBS. Other authors have described cases of uni- or bilateral facial palsy (Piette *et al.*, 1986; Wiselka *et al.*, 1987; Belec *et al.*, 1989; Wechsler and Ho, 1989), bi-brachial palsy (Calabrese *et al.*, 1987), and bilateral hearing dysfunction (Grimaldi *et al.*, 1993) in association with HIV seroconversion or early HIV infection. These disorders are indistinguishable from those that occur in association with other viral diseases. Thus, HIV testing should be considered in individuals with these specific, acute, neurological illnesses **and** appropriate risk factors. If initial serology is negative, follow-up testing may be appropriate.

DISTAL SYMMETRIC POLYNEUROPATHY (DSPN)

The most common neuropathy associated with HIV infection occurs in the late stages of disease (Snider *et al.*, 1983; McArthur, 1987; Cornblath and McArthur, 1988; Leger *et al.*, 1988; 1989, Miller *et al.*, 1988a,b; Parry, 1988; So *et al.*, 1988; Gastaut *et al.*, 1989; Winer *et al.*, 1992; Fuller *et al.*, 1993; Winer, 1993). Various names have been used to describe this syndrome, including 'predominantly sensory neuropathy' (PSN) (Cornblath and McArthur 1988) and 'distal sensory polyneuro-pathy' (DSPN) (Miller *et al.*, 1988a,b). All describe the predominantly distal and mainly sensory features of this illness. As stated above, the frequency of this late-stage neuropathy ranges from 30% in clinical studies to 100% of autopsied cases.

Clinical features

The clinical features are stereotypic. Patients complain of numbness or pain, initially confined to the soles. Onset is frequently relatively abrupt, and many patients develop symptoms over a few days or weeks after a systemic illness such as pneumocystis pneumonia. Shortly thereafter, the abnormal sensation ascends but rarely goes above the ankles. These symptoms, if painful, can be quite disabling. Occasionally, sensory symptoms progress further, but rarely involve the hands. In most series, weakness is not symptomatic. On examination, reduced or absent ankle reflexes are virtually universal. Sensory thresholds to all modalities are raised in the feet, and may be slightly so in the hands. Hyperpathia and hyperalgesia can be detected in some patients. Weakness, usually involving the foot muscles, is minimal. Frequently, knee reflexes are increased, reflecting a degree of concurrent encephalopathy or myelopathy. In some cases, the neuropathy is progressive and continues to be troublesome until death. In others, symptoms remain relatively quiescent or may even improve over time.

Spinal fluid evaluation demonstrates a mildly elevated protein content in 40–50% of patients, but this is not helpful diagnostically because of the frequency of CSF abnormalities in HIV infection. In the majority of patients with this syndrome, the CSF is acellular; the presence of CSF pleocytosis should raise the possibility of concurrent CNS infection (McArthur *et al.*, 1988).

Nerve conduction studies reflect axonal loss and document a more widespread motor–sensory polyneuropathy than detected clinically. Evidence of axonal loss is most severe in the legs, frequently with absent sural sensory responses. In addition, motor conduction abnormalities are frequent and include reduced distal evoked amplitudes and minimally reduced conduction velocities in the legs, and prolonged F-wave latencies in both arms and legs. Needle electromyography demonstrates denervation potentials and evidence of chronic partial denervation and reinnervation usually confined to leg and foot muscles.

Pathological features

Pathological studies, both biopsy (Figure 11.1) and autopsy, have shown that the main features are Wallerian-like degeneration of myelinated and unmyelinated axons in the distal regions of sensory nerves (de la Monte *et al.*, 1988; Mah *et al.*, 1988; Rance *et al.*, 1988; Grafe and Wiley, 1989; Henin *et al.*, 1990; Griffin *et al.*, 1995). A more modest and variable degree of demyelination and remyelination and of epineurial perivascular lymphocytic infiltration has also been noted in most studies.

In the autopsy series from Johns Hopkins (Griffin *et al.*, 1995), all lower-extremity peripheral nerves were abnormal to some degree. Most contained abnormal numbers of myelinated fibres undergoing Wallerian-like degeneration. In the most severely involved nerves, there was extensive fibre loss with most of the remaining fibres in the distal sural nerve undergoing Wallerian-like degeneration. In all cases, fibre loss and Wallerian-like degeneration were much more marked in distal than in proximal regions. In a few cases the distal accentuation could be seen in proximal and distal

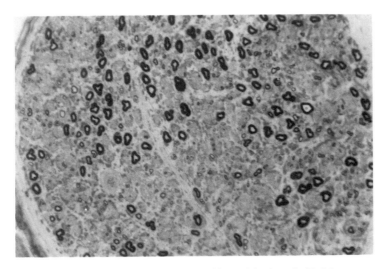

Figure 11.1 Low-power image of sural nerve biopsy (plastic-embedded 1-μm section stained with toluidine blue) from a patient with AIDS and distal symmetric polyneuropathy showing loss of nerve fibres without inflammation.

portions of the sural nerve. The dorsal root ganglia frequently contained small numbers of neurons undergoing degeneration, with excessive numbers of macrophages and variable numbers of lymphocytes. However, in none was the degree of neuronal loss comparable with the degree of axonal loss seen in the sural nerves in severely affected cases. This distribution of pathology conforms to distal axonal degeneration. This is supported by the presence of degeneration of the rostral gracile tract in the spinal cord in some cases (Rance *et al.*, 1988). In most nerves, there was also degeneration of unmyelinated axons. In two cases from the Johns Hopkins series (Griffin *et al.*, 1995), only small numbers of myelinated fibres were degenerating, and unmyelinated fibre loss was the most prominent finding. Both patients had severely painful sensory neuropathies. These cases suggest that, as in other painful neuropathies, disease of the unmyelinated fibres may underlie the development of spontaneous pain.

In this series, there was also variable but frequently prominent demyelination of peripheral nerves. It is possible that the demyelination and fibre degeneration are separable, and that the demyelination was not simply 'secondary' demyelination in response to chronic axonal disease.

When occurring in the late stages of HIV infection, this syndrome is distinctive and evaluation for other causes of neuropathy reveals none. Thus, the illness is presumably a consequence of advanced HIV infection and the resulting immunological failure.

Pathogenesis

The pathogenesis of predominantly sensory neuropathy is unknown. The clinical and autopsy studies suggest that DSPN is extraordinarily common among patients dying with AIDS. Although some workers have suggested that the disease is caused either by systemic cytomegalovirus (CMV) infection (Fuller *et al.*, 1989; Grafe and Wiley, 1989) or by infection of dorsal root ganglia by HIV (Grafe and Wiley, 1989), both of these remain hypotheses without firm support. Our own data show that the mean CD4 count within 9 months of onset of DSPN is 203/μl ($\pm$219) compared with 110/μl ($\pm$108) for CMV retinitis. This suggests that the temporal sequence is for neuropathy to predate retinitis. In another series, DSPN was identified in 17% of patients with CMV retinitis, and in 21% of those without CMV retinitis. These data tend to contradict any direct association between CMV disease and DSPN (unpublished data). More likely, multiple potential factors are present in patients with AIDS that contribute to the development of DSPN, including HIV infection itself, macrophage activation with local cytokine release, progressive immunosuppression, co-existent CMV infection, and nutritional inadequacy. Further studies are needed.

Treatment

There is no known treatment for this neuropathy. Therapy of the pain follows that used for other painful neuropathies, including tricyclic antidepressants, carbamazepine, phenytoin, mexilitine, and lastly, narcotic analgesics (Casey, 1988; Cornblath and Glass, 1994). In our experience, the most successful narcotic regimens are methadone 10–20 mg three times daily or transdermal fentanyl (Duragesic, 25–100 μg/h). None of these symptomatic therapies is ideal. AIDS patients are frequently intolerant of the psychoactive side effects of many of these drugs, so that potentially effective doses cannot be given. From a practical standpoint, it is best to start therapy with the lowest possible dose of an agent, increasing gradually so as to allow for the development of tolerance to the side effects. Even with this strategy, only limited numbers of individuals with DSPN achieve symptomatic relief.

INFLAMMATORY DEMYELINATING POLYNEUROPATHY (IDP)

Several reports have suggested an association between HIV infection and the inflammatory demyelinating polyneuropathies (Miller *et al.*, 1985, 1988a,b; Cornblath *et al.*, 1987; Dalakas and Pezeshkpour, 1988; Parry, 1988), both GBS and CIDP. Since those early reports, few epidemiological series have documented these types of neuropathies in cohorts of HIV-seropositive individuals (Hall *et al.*, 1991; Winer *et al.*, 1992; Barohn *et al.*, 1993; Fuller *et al.*, 1993). This most likely reflects both referral bias – that is, since the initial reports clinicians are less likely to refer these cases to tertiary centres – and the uncommonness of the cases. In any case, it is important to know that HIV infection is one of the possible associations with both GBS and CIDP, and should be included in the differential diagnosis in individuals presenting with these syndromes. GBS and CIDP share many features. In both, motor findings predominate; sensory symptoms and signs are usually minor. Electrophysiological studies demonstrate a demyelinating polyneuropathy with variable degrees of axonal loss. Pathologically, both disorders show macrophage-mediated demyelination and lymphocytic infiltrates, and superimposed axonal loss. In most cases, CSF protein is elevated. Both disorders are presumably immune-mediated (Hartung *et al.*, 1988; Toyka *et al.*, 1988) and are treated with a variety of immunosuppressive or immunomodulatory methods, including plasmapheresis, human immune globulin, and prednisone.

Most cases of GBS and CIDP occur in HIV-infected patients who are otherwise asymptomatic; that is, there are no systemic features of HIV infection such as weight loss, oral thrush, fevers, diarrhoea, zoster, or AIDS-defining illness. As mentioned above, GBS may be a manifestation of seroconversion. Both GBS and CIDP may be the first manifestation of illness that leads to the identification of concurrent HIV infection (Cornblath *et al.*, 1987).

Clinical features

The clinical features of HIV-infected individuals with GBS or CIDP do not differ from those of patients who are HIV uninfected. There are, however, several features that distinguish HIV-seronegative from HIV-seropositive individuals with IDP. The first is the finding of HIV infection which, as discussed above, may be associated with a seroconversion illness. Second, in HIV seropositives circulating CD4+/ CD8+ T cell ratios are inverted, reflecting loss of CD4 (T helper) lymphocytes. Third, patients with HIV-seropositive GBS or CIDP frequently have CSF pleocytosis (Cornblath *et al.*, 1987), a feature useful in suggesting the association of HIV infection and IDP. Fourth, many patients have polyclonal elevations of serum immunoglobulins.

The electrophysiological features of HIV-seropositive individuals with GBS or CIDP do not differ from those in HIV-seronegative patients. The primary electrophysiological finding is usually widespread demyelination. On occasion, only evidence of axonal degeneration is found.

In active cases, pathological evidence of ongoing demyelination characterized by myelin stripping by macrophages is present. Both the extent of axonal degeneration and the extent of lymphocytic infiltration vary. These findings are typical of IDP in seronegative cases.

Treatment

There are no clinical trials to guide decisions about therapy in HIV-seropositive patients with GBS or CIDP. Since the clinical diseases are similar to HIV-seronegative patients, studies of presumably HIV-seronegative populations apply to the HIV-seropositive patient. In GBS, both plasmapheresis (Osterman *et al.*, 1984; Guillain–Barré Study Group, 1985; French Cooperative Group on Plasma Exchange and Guillain–Barré Syndrome, 1987) and infusions of human immune globulin (van der Meché *et al.*, 1992) are effective. In CIDP, both corticosteroids (Dyck *et al.*, 1982) and plasmapheresis (Dyck *et al.*, 1991) have been used successfully. However, not all cases require therapy (Berger *et al.*, 1987). If symptoms are mild or do not interfere with patient function, watchful monitoring may be more prudent than active immunosuppression.

It is likely that GBS and CIDP in HIV-seropositive individuals occur on an immunopathogenic basis (Mishra *et al.*, 1985; Toyka and Heininger, 1987), perhaps analogous to other immune-mediated phenomena such as idiopathic thrombocytopenic purpura, which also occurs at this stage of HIV infection. One could postulate that the sequence of events that occurs in patients with other virus infections that result in GBS or CIDP also occurs in those with HIV infection.

MONONEUROPATHY AND MULTIPLE MONONEUROPATHY

Individual cranial or limb mononeuropathies occur not infrequently during the course of HIV infection (Lipkin *et al.*, 1985). These include the facial and lateral femoral cutaneous nerves among others (Winer *et al.*, 1992; Fuller *et al.*, 1993). In addition, occasional isolated or multifocal mononeuropathies may be due to *Herpes zoster*, infiltration from systemic lymphoma, or syphilis (see below). In patients with advanced HIV infection with wasting syndrome, entrapment neuropathies are common.

Rare reports have described individuals with multiple mononeuropathies due to vasculitis in a setting of symptomatic HIV infection (Said *et al.*, 1987, 1988; Estes *et al.*, 1989; Gherardi *et al.*, 1989; Cornblath *et al.*, 1992). These individuals present with typical vasculitic-type multiple mononeuropathy syndromes that show multifocal axon loss lesions physiologically. Some may also have hepatitis-B infection, and the neuropathy may be related to immune complex deposition (Cupps and Fauci, 1981). Pathologically, vasculitis involves small- to medium-sized vessels. Many of these cases appear to have 'isolated PNS vasculitis'. The rarity of these cases does not allow definitive statements about therapy.

CYTOMEGALOVIRUS (CMV)

CMV is an opportunistic viral infection that occurs frequently in individuals with advanced HIV infection who have CD4 counts $< 100/\mu$l. A distinctive neurological syndrome, CMV polyradiculoneuropathy, occurs in those with AIDS (Tucker *et al.*, 1985; Eidelberg *et al.*, 1986; Behar *et al.*, 1987; Mahieux *et al.*, 1989; Fuller *et al.*, 1990a; Miller *et al.*, 1990).

Clinical features

The clinical features are noteworthy. Over days to weeks, an asymmetric cauda equina syndrome that is predominantly motor develops. Low back pain with radiation into one leg may be the earliest symptom, followed by urinary incontinence. Shortly thereafter, asymmetric leg weakness and saddle sensory disturbance develop. If untreated, the syndrome usually advances rapidly to a flaccid paraplegia with bowel and bladder disturbance. In most cases, the disease remains at this stage for some period of time. Occasionally, arm weakness or cranial nerve involvement may occur. The majority of affected individuals die unless treated.

Spinal fluid analysis reveals a typical picture of polymorphonuclear pleocytosis, hypoglycorrhachia, and elevated protein content. This CSF profile is frequent enough in this syndrome, and so unusual otherwise in advanced HIV infection to be almost diagnostic. In about 50% of cases, CSF viral cultures will reveal CMV, but positive culture results may take up to 1 week after the lumbar puncture. Evidence of CMV can be found elsewhere, including in the retina, blood and urine, more promptly. A recent letter suggested that cytological examination of a spun specimen of CSF can be used for diagnostic purposes. This is a potential advancement in the rapid diagnosis of this syndrome (Glass and Erozan, 1993). Electrodiagnostic studies reveal primarily evidence of axon loss in lumbosacral roots with denervation potentials (fibrillations and positive sharp waves) in leg muscles. There is little or no evidence of demyelination. Lumbar MRI scans may show enhancing nerve roots and thickening of the dura (Talpos *et al.*, 1991).

Treatment

Recognition of this clinically distinct entity has led to therapeutic intervention in several reported cases. Ganciclovir, an antiviral agent effective against CMV, has been used in those instances, and treatment resulted in either stabilization or improvement (Graveleau *et al.*, 1989; Fuller *et al.*, 1990a; Miller *et al.*, 1990). An alternative agent, phosphonoformate (Foscarnet), can be used if CMV resistance is suspected (Cohen *et al.*, 1993) or if the patient develops polyradiculitis while already receiving ganciclovir for CMV disease.

In AIDS patients polyradiculopathy may have causes other than CMV (So and Olney, 1994). Lymphomatous meningitis (Fuller *et al.*, 1993), syphilis (Lanska *et al.*, 1988), or even a more benign syndrome may present similarly. Spinal fluid studies, with special attention to syphilis serology, cytopathology, and cultures, are most helpful in distinguishing these syndromes.

Pathological features

CMV has also been reported as causing a multifocal neuropathy, predominantly affecting the arms (Fuller *et al.*, 1990b; Cornblath *et al.*, 1992; Simpson and Olney, 1994). In our two cases, electrodiagnostic studies suggested that the primary pathological process was demyelination. Sural nerve biopsies revealed positive CMV immunostaining (Figure 11.2), inflammation, cytomegalic cells and prominent demyelination (Figure 11.3). CMV was cultured from other sites, and both patients were treated with ganciclovir, with stabilization of the neuropathy.

TOXIC NEUROPATHY

Like HIV-seronegative individuals, HIV-infected individuals may develop peripheral neuropathy from exposure to neurotoxins. These may include potentially neurotoxic medications that any patient might receive, such as vincristine, isoniazid, dapsone, metronidazole, nitrofurantoin, or, more importantly, potentially neurotoxic antiretrovirals such as dideoxycytidine (ddC, zalcitabine) (Dubinsky *et al.*, 1988; Yarchoan *et al.*, 1988; Merigan *et al.*, 1989; Berger *et al.*, 1993), dideoxyinosine (ddI, didanosine) (Lambert *et al.*, 1990), and stavudine (d4T) (Petersen *et al.*, 1992).

In Phase 1 studies of ddC, a dose-dependent peripheral neuropathy developed in the majority of individuals (Dubinsky *et al.*, 1988; Yarchoan *et al.*, 1988; Merigan *et al.*, 1989). Symptomatically, there were painful dysaesthesias in the feet; similar symptoms were noted in the hands in 50% of patients. Clinically, there were elevations in sensory thresholds at distal sites and loss of ankle reflexes. Sensory evoked potential amplitudes were reduced, suggesting either neuropathy or neuronopathy. If

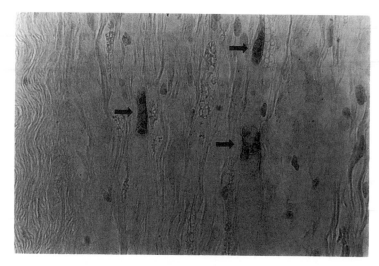

Figure 11.2 Low-power image of sural nerve biopsy from a patient with AIDS and CMV-associated polyradiculopathy. The biopsy has been immunostained for CMV and positively-stained cells are indicated by arrows.

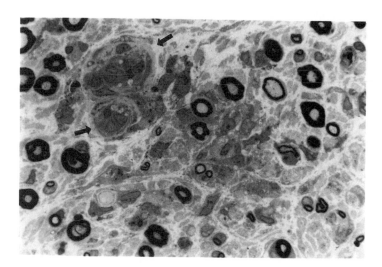

Figure 11.3 Low-power image of sural nerve biopsy from a patient with AIDS and CMV-associated polyradiculopathy (plastic-embedded 1-μm section stained with toluidine blue) showing loss of nerve fibres, occasional demyeli-nated fibres, and megalic cells, representing both macrophages and endothelial cells (arrows).

the neuropathy was not severe and the drug was stopped, then symptoms, signs, and electrophysiological findings improved in the majority of individuals. The neuropa-thy was dose dependent. All individuals receiving either 0.06 or 0.03 mg/kg orally every 4 hours developed neuropathy, with a time of onset of 52 and 60 days, respec-tively. Some 80% of patients receiving 0.01 mg/kg developed neuropathy, but the time to onset was longer, 83 days. Only two of 12 patients (17%) receiving 0.005 mg/ kg developed neuropathy, and this was after 123 days. Recovery was related to the dose of drug received. All patients taking the two lower doses recovered in 6 months. Patients receiving 0.03 mg/kg recovered in 1 year, but some patients at the higher doses were reported to have persisting neurological disability. A recent report of patients receiving lower doses of ddC (1–2.25 mg/day) showed that 34% developed symptomatic neuropathy within 6 months (Blum *et al.*, 1993); thus, even at currently used doses, toxic neuropathy can be anticipated to occur frequently with ddC.

Like ddC, ddI and d4T cause a dose-related peripheral neuropathy. The frequency of symptomatic peripheral neuropathy is not as well studied as with ddC, but the incidence appears to be higher in patients with more advanced HIV disease and lower CD4 counts. Apparently 10–20% of those receiving current doses of ddI (200 mg twice daily) or d4T (20–40 mg twice daily) develop symptomatic peripheral neuropathy. As with other neurotoxins, neuropathy is more likely to develop in the setting of a pre-existing neuropathy. The clinical features of the neuropathies are strikingly similar to those seen with ddC and suggest that further studies are needed to determine the appropriate dose regimen that minimizes toxicity.

Most reviews of peripheral neuropathy and HIV infection (Cornblath *et al.*, 1992; Simpson and Olney, 1994) contain a section on autonomic neuropathy. This association, if it exists at all, is very tenuous. Stimulated by an early report in *The Lancet* describing 'abnormal' cardiac reflexes in five AIDS patients undergoing invasive procedures (Craddock *et al.*, 1987), other investigators reported selected similar cases, or the results of autonomic testing in individuals with HIV infection (Evenhouse *et al.*, 1987; Lin-Greenberg and Taneja-Uppal, 1987; Miller and Semple, 1987; Mulhall and Jennens, 1987; Villa, 1987; Cohen and Laudenslager, 1989). These studies were poorly controlled (Lohmoller *et al.*, 1987), and little has been written on this subject since 1990 (Freeman *et al.*, 1990). Whether autonomic dysfunction is a result of HIV infection itself or of the multiple systemic abnormalities present in these individuals is currently unknown and awaits further study.

REFERENCES

Bacellar, H., Munoz, A., Miller, E. N. *et al.* (1994). Temporal trends in the incidence of HIV-1 related neurologic diseases: Multicenter AIDS Cohort Study, 1985–1992. *Neurology*, **44**, 1892–1900

Barohn, R. J., Gronseth, G. S., LeForce, B. R. *et al.* (1993). Peripheral nervous system involvement in a large cohort of human immunodeficiency virus-infected individuals. *Arch. Neurol.*, **50**, 167–171

Behar, R., Wiley, C. and McCutchan, J. A. (1987). Cytomegalovirus polyradiculoneuropathy in acquired immune deficiency syndrome. *Neurology*, **37**, 557–561

Belec, L., Gherardi, R., Georges, A. J. *et al.* (1989). Peripheral facial paralysis and HIV infection: report of four African cases and review of the literature. *J. Neurol.*, **236**, 411–414

Berger, A. R., Arezzo, J. C., Schaumburg, H. H. *et al.* (1993). 2′,3′-Dideoxycytidine (ddC) toxic neuropathy: a study of 52 patients. *Neurology*, **43**, 358–362

Berger, J. R., Difini, J. A., Swerdloff, M. A. and Ayyar, D. R. (1987). HIV seropositivity in Guillain–Barré syndrome (letter). *Ann. Neurol.*, **22**, 395–396

Blum, A., Dal Pan, G., Raines, C. *et al.* (1993). ddC-related toxic neuropathy: risk factors and natural history. *Neurology*, **43**, A190–191 (abstract)

Calabrese, L. H., Profitt, M. R., Levin, K. H. *et al.* (1987). Acute infection with the human immunodeficiency virus (HIV) associated with acute brachial neuritis and exanthematous rash. *Ann. Intern. Med.*, **107**, 849–851

Casey, K. L. (1988). Toward a rationale for the treatment of painful neuropathies. In *Proceedings of the Vth World Congress on Pain* (R. Dubner, G. F. Gebhart and M. R. Bond, eds), pp. 165–174, Amsterdam: Elsevier

Centers for Disease Control (1993). 1993 revised classification system for HIV infection and expanded surveillance case definition for AIDS among adolescents and adults. *MMWR*, **41**, 1–19

Chavanet, P., Giroud, M., Lancon, J. P. *et al.* (1987). Neuropathies infracliniques chez les malades HIV + (Subclinical neuropathies in HIV-positive patients) (letter). *Presse Méd.*, **16**, 1764

Chavanet, P. Y., Giroud, M., Lancon, J. -P. *et al.* (1988). Altered peripheral nerve conduction in HIV-patients. *Cancer Detect. Prev.*, **12**, 249–255

Cohen, B. A., McArthur, J. C., Grohman, S. *et al.* (1993). Neurologic prognosis of CMV polyradiculo-myelopathy in AIDS. *Neurology*, **43**, 493–499

Cohen, J. A. and Laudenslager, M. (1989). Autonomic nervous system involvement in patients with human immunodeficiency virus infection. *Neurology*, **39**, 1111–1112

Conlon, C. P. (1989). HIV infection presenting as Guillain–Barré syndrome in Lusaka, Zambia. *Trans. R. Soc. Trop. Med. Hyg.*, **83**, 109

Cooper, D. A., Gold, J., Maclean, P. *et al.* (1985). Acute AIDS retrovirus infection: definition of a clinical illness associated with seroconversion. *Lancet*, **1**, 537–540

Cornblath, D. R. and Glass, J. D. (1994). Peripheral neuropathy. In *Handbook of Pain Management*, 2nd edn (C. D. Tollison, J. R. Satterthwaite and J. W. Tollison, eds), pp. 463–469, Baltimore: Williams & Wilkins

Cornblath, D. R. and McArthur, J. C. (1988). Predominantly sensory neuropathy in patients with AIDS and AIDS-related complex. *Neurology*, **38**, 794–796

Cornblath, D. R. and McArthur J. C. (1989). Pathogenesis of peripheral neuropathies associated with human immunodeficiency virus infection: hypotheses. In *AIDS 89–90: News and Views on Research and Control* (G. de-The, ed.), pp. 69–73, Paris: McGraw-Hill

Cornblath, D. R., McArthur, J. C., Kennedy, P. G. E. *et al.* (1987). Inflammatory demyelinating peripheral neuopathies associated with human T-cell lymphotropic virus type III infection. *Ann. Neurol.*, **21**, 32–40

Cornblath, D. R., McArthur, J. C., Parry, G. and Griffin, J. W. (1992). Peripheral neuropathies in human immunodeficiency virus infection. In *Peripheral Neuropathy* (P. J. Dyck, P. K. Thomas, J. W. Griffin, P. A. Low and J. Poduslo, eds), Philadelphia: W.B. Saunders

Craddock, C., Pasvor, G., Bull, R. *et al.* (1987). Cardiorespiratory arrest and autonomic neuropathy in AIDS. *Lancet*, **2**, 16–18

Cupps, T. R. and Fauci, A. S. (1981). *The Vasculitides*. Philadelphia: W. B. Saunders

Dalakas, M. C. and Pezeshkpour, G. H. (1988). Neuromuscular diseases associated with human immunodeficiency virus infection. *Ann. Neurol.*, **23**(suppl), S38–48

de la Monte, S. M., Gabuzda, D. H., Ho, D. D. *et al.* (1988). Peripheral neuropathy in the acquired immunodeficiency syndrome. *Ann. Neurol.*, **23**, 485–492

Dubinsky, R. M., Dalakas, M., Yarchoan, R. and Broder, S. (1988). Follow-up of neuropathy from 2′,3′-dideoxycytidine. *Lancet*, **1**, 832

Dyck, P. J., O'Brien, P. C., Oviatt, K. F. *et al.* (1982). Prednisone improves chronic inflammatory demyelinating polyradiculoneuropathy more than no treatment. *Ann. Neurol.*, **11**, 136–141

Dyck, P. J., Low, P. A., Windebank, A. J. *et al.* (1991). Plasma exchange in polyneuropathy associated with monoclonal gammopathy of undetermined significance. *N. Engl. J. Med.*, **325**, 1482–1486

Eidelberg, D., Sotrel, A., Vogel, H. *et al.* (1986). Progressive polyradiculopathy in acquired deficiency syndrome. *Neurology*, **36**, 912–916

Estes, M. L., Calabrese, L. H., Yen-Lieberman, B. *et al.* (1989). Human immunodeficiency virus (HIV) and necrotizing peripheral nerve vasculitis: an autoimmune phenomenon? *Neurology*, **39** (suppl 1), 293 (abstract)

Evenhouse, M., Haas, E., Snell, E. *et al.* (1987). Hypotension in infection with the human immunodeficiency virus. *Ann. Intern. Med.*, **107**, 598–599

Freeman, R., Roberts, M. S., Friedman, L. S. and Broadbridge, C. (1990). Autonomic function and human immunodeficiency virus infection. *Neurology*, **40**, 575–580

French Cooperative Group on Plasma Exchange and Guillain-Barré Syndrome (1987). Efficacy of plasma exchange in Guillain–Barré syndrome: role of replacement fluids. *Ann. Neurol.*, **22**, 753–761

Fuller, G. N., Jacobs, J. M. and Guiloff, R. J. (1989). Association of painful peripheral neuropathy in AIDS with cytomegalovirus infection. *Lancet*, **2**, 937–941

Fuller, G. N., Gill, S. K., Guiloff, R. J. *et al.* (1990a). Ganciclovir for lumbosacral polyradiculopathy in AIDS. *Lancet*, **1**, 48–49

Fuller, G. N., Greco, C. and Miller, R. G. (1990b). Cytomegalovirus and mononeuropathy multiplex in AIDS. *Neurology*, **40**(Suppl 1), 301 (abstract)

Fuller, G. N., Jacobs, J. M. and Guiloff, R. J. (1993). Nature and incidence of peripheral nerve syndromes in HIV infection. *J. Neurol. Neurosurg. Psychiatry*, **56**, 372–381

Gastaut, J. L., Gastaut, J. A., Pellissier, J. F. *et al.* (1989). Neuropathies with HIV infection. Prospective study of 56 cases. *Rev. Neurol. (Paris)*, **145**, 451–459

Gherardi, R., Lebargy, F., Gaulard, P. *et al.* (1989). Necrotizing vasculitis and HIV replication in peripheral nerves. *N. Engl. J. Med.*, **321**, 685–686

Glass, J. D. and Erozan, Y. S. (1993). Rapid diagnosis of cytomegalovirus polyradiculitis in a patient with acquired immunodeficiency syndrome. *Ann. Neurol.*, **34**, 239

Gottlieb, M. S., Schroff, R., Schanker, H. M. *et al.* (1981). *Pneumocystis carinii* pneumonia and mucosal candidiasis in previously healthy homosexual men. *N. Engl. J. Med.*, **305**, 1425–1431

Grafe, M. R. and Wiley, C. A. (1989). Spinal cord and peripheral nerve pathology in AIDS: the roles of cytomegalovirus and human immunodeficiency virus. *Ann. Neurol.*, **25**, 561–566

Graveleau, P., Perol, R. and Chapman, A. (1989). Regression of cauda equina syndrome in AIDS patients being treated with ganciclovir. *Lancet*, **2**, 511–512

Griffin, J. W., Crawford, T. O., Taylor, W. R. *et al.* (1995). Sensory neuropathy in AIDS. I. Neuropathology. *Brain* (in press)

Grimaldi, L. M. E., Luzi, L., Martino, G. V. *et al.* (1993). Bilateral eighth cranial nerve neuropathy in human immunodeficiency virus infection. *J. Neurol.*, **240**, 363–366

Guillain–Barré Study Group (1985). Plasmapheresis and acute Guillain–Barré syndrome. *Neurology*, **35**, 1096–1104

Gulevich, S. J., Kalmijn, J. A., Thal, L. J. *et al.* (1992). Sensory testing in human immunodeficiency virus type 1-infected men. *Arch. Neurol.*, **49**, 1281–1284

Hagberg, L., Malmvall, B.-E., Svennerholm, L. *et al.* (1986). Guillain–Barré syndrome as an early manifestation of HIV central nervous system infection. *Scand. J. Infect. Dis.*, **18**, 591–592

Hall, C. D., Snyder, C. R., Messenheimer, J. A. *et al.* (1991). Peripheral neuropathy in a cohort of human immunodeficiency virus-infected patients: incidence and relationship to other nervous system dysfunction. *Arch. Neurol.*, **48**, 1273–1274

Hartung, H.-P., Heininger, K., Schafer, B. *et al.* (1988). Immune mechanisms in inflammatory polyneuropathy. *Ann. N.Y. Acad. Sci.*, **540**, 122–161

Henin, D., Masson, C., Ratinahirana, H. *et al.* (1990). Morphometric and immunohistochemical study of the L5 posterior root ganglia. Correlation with superficial peroneal nerve abnormalities in 26 cases of AIDS. *J. Neurol. Sci.*, **98**(suppl), 158 (abstract)

Husstedt, I. W., Grotemeyer, K. H., Busch, H. and Zidek, W. (1993). Progression of distal–symmetric polyneuropathy in HIV infection: a prospective study. *AIDS*, **7**, 1069–1073

Koch, T. K., Koerper, M. A., Wesley, A. M. *et al.* (1989). Absence of an AIDS-related peripheral neuropathy in children and young adult hemophiliacs. *Ann. Neurol.*, **26**, 476–477

Lambert, J. S., Seidlin, M., Reichman, R. C. *et al.* (1990). 2′,3′-Dideoxyinosine (ddI) in patients with the acquired immunodeficiency syndrome or AIDS-related complex. A phase I trial. *N. Engl. J. Med.*, **322**, 1333–1340

Lanska, M. J., Lanska, D. J. and Schmidley, J. W. (1988). Syphilitic polyradiculopathy in an HIV-positive man. *Neurology*, **38**, 1297–1301

Leger, J. M., Bolgert, F., Bouche, P. *et al.* (1988). Peripheral nervous system and HIV infection. 13 cases. *Rev. Neurol.*, **144**, 789–796.

Leger, J. M., Bouche, P., Bolgert, F. *et al.* (1989). The spectrum of polyneuropathies in patients infected with HIV. *J. Neurol. Neurosurg. Psychiatry*, **52**, 1369–1374.

Levy, R. M., Bredesen, D. E. and Rosenblum, M. L. (1985). Neurological manifestations of the acquired immunodeficiency syndrome (AIDS): experience at UCSF and review of the literature. *J. Neurosurg.*, **62**, 475–495

Levy, R., Janssen, R., Bush, T. and Rosenblum, M. (1988). Neuroepidemiology of acquired immunodeficiency syndrome. *J. AIDS*, **1**, 31–40

Lin-Greenberg, A. and Taneja-Uppal, N. (1987). Dysautonomia and infection with the human immunodeficiency virus. *Ann. Intern. Med.*, **106**, 167

Lipkin, W. I., Parry, G., Kiprov, D. and Abrams, D. (1985). Inflammatory neuropathy in homosexual men with lymphadenopathy. *Neurology*, **35**, 1479–1483

Lohmoller, G., Matuschke, A. and Goebel, F. D. (1987). Testing for neurological involvement in HIV infection. *Lancet*, **2**, 1532

Mah, V., Vartavarian, L. M., Akers, M.-A. and Vinters, H. V. (1988). Abnormalities of peripheral nerve in patients with human immunodeficiency virus infection. *Ann. Neurol.*, **24**, 713–717

Mahieux, F., Gray, F., Fenelon, G. *et al.* (1989). Acute myeloradiculitis due to cytomegalovirus as the initial manifestation of AIDS. *J. Neurol. Neurosurg. Psychiatry*, **52**, 270–274

Masur, H., Michelis, M. A., Greene, J. B. *et al.* (1981). An outbreak of community-acquired *Pneumocystis carinii* pneumonia. Initial manifestations of cellular immune dysfunction. *N. Engl. J. Med.*, **305**, 1431–1438

McArthur, J. C. (1987). Neurologic manifestations of AIDS. *Medicine*, **66**, 407–437

McArthur, J. C., Cohen, B. A., Farzedegan, H. *et al.* (1988). Cerebrospinal fluid abnormalities in homosexual men with and without neuropsychiatric findings. *Ann. Neurol.*, **23**(suppl), S34–37

McArthur, J. C., Cohen, B. A., Selnes, O. A. *et al.* (1989). Low prevalence of neurological and neuropsychological abnormalities in otherwise healthy HIV-1 infected individuals: results from the Multicenter AIDS Cohort Study. *Ann. Neurol.*, **26**, 601–611

Merigan, T. C., Skowron, G., Bozzette, S. A. *et al.* (1989). Circulating p24 antigen levels and responses to dideoxycytidine in human immunodeficiency virus (HIV) infections: A phase I and II study. *Ann. Intern. Med.*, **110**, 189–195

Miller, R. F. and Semple, S. J. G. (1987). Autonomic neuropathy in AIDS. *Lancet*, **2**, 343–344

Miller, R. G., Parry, G., Lang, W. *et al.* (1985). AIDS-related inflammatory polyradiculoneuropathy: prediction of response to plasma exchange with electrophysiologic testing. *Muscle Nerve*, **8**, 626 (abstract)

Miller, R. G., Kiprov, D. D., Parry, G. and Bredesen, D. E. (1988a). Peripheral nervous system dysfunction in acquired immunodeficiency syndrome. In *AIDS and the Nervous System* (M. L. Rosenblum, R. M. Levy and D. E. Bredesen, eds), pp. 65–78, New York: Raven Press

Miller, R. G., Parry, G., Pfaeffl, W. *et al.* (1988b). The spectrum of peripheral neuropathy associated with ARC and AIDS. *Muscle Nerve*, **11**, 857–863

Miller, R. G., Storey, J. R. and Greco, C. M. (1990). Ganciclovir in the treatment of progressive AIDS-related polyradiculopathy. *Neurology*, **40**, 569–574

Mishra, B. B., Sommers, W., Koski, C. K. and Greenstein, J. I. (1985). Acute inflammatory demyelinating polyneuropathy in the acquired immune deficiency syndrome. *Ann. Neurol.*, **17**, 131–132

Mulhall, B. P. and Jennens, I. (1987). Testing for neurological involvement in HIV infection. *Lancet*, **2**, 1531–1532

Osterman, P. O., Lundemo, G., Pirskanen, R. *et al.* (1984). Beneficial effects of plasma exchange in acute inflammatory polyradiculoneuropathy. *Lancet*, **2**, 1296–1298

Parry, G. J. (1988). Peripheral neuropathies associated with human immunodeficiency virus infection. *Ann. Neurol.*, **23**(suppl), S49–53

Persuy, P. H., Arnott, G., Fortier, B. *et al.* (1988). Favorable issue of a Guillain-Barré's syndrome in a case with recent infection by the human immunodeficiency virus. *Rev. Neurol.*, **144**, 32–35

Petersen, E., Ramirez-Ronda, C., Schwartz, R. *et al.* (1992). Findings from a phase II study of stavudine (d4T). *VIII International Conference on AIDS//III STD World Congress, Amsterdam*, p. B60, Amsterdam: Congrex Holland B.V.

Piette, A. M., Tusseau, F., Vignon, D. *et al.* (1986). Acute neuropathy coincident with seroconversion for anti-LAV/HTLV-III. *Lancet*, **1**, 852

Pitlik, S. D., Fainstein, V., Bolivar, R. *et al.* (1983). Spectrum of central nervous system complications in homosexual men with acquired immune deficiency syndrome. *J. Infect. Dis.*, **148**, 771–772

Rance, N., McArthur, J. C., Cornblath, D. R. *et al.* (1988). Gracile tract degeneration in patients with sensory neuropathy and AIDS. *Neurology*, **38**, 265–271

Raphael, S. A., Price, M. L., Lischner, H. W. *et al.* (1991). Inflammatory demyelinating polyneuropathy in a child with symptomatic human immunodeficiency virus infection. *J. Pediatr.*, **118**, 242–245

Said, G., Lacroix, C., Andrieu, J. N. *et al.* (1987). Necrotizing arteritis in patients with inflammatory neuropathy and human immunodeficiency virus (HIV-III) infection. *Neurology*, **37**(suppl 1), 176

Said, G., Lacroix-Ciaudo, C., Fujimura, H. *et al.* (1988). The peripheral neuropathy of necrotizing arteritis: a clinicopathological study. *Ann. Neurol.*, **23**, 461–465

Simpson, D. M. and Olney, R. K. (1994). Peripheral neuropathies associated with human immunodeficiency virus infection. *Neurol. Clin.*, **10**, 685–711

Snider, W. D., Simpson, D. M., Nielsen, S. *et al.* (1983). Neurological complications of acquired immune deficiency syndrome: analysis of 50 patients. *Ann. Neurol.*, **14**, 403–418

So, Y. T. and Olney, R. K. (1994). Acute lumbosacral polyradiculopathy in acquired immunodeficiency syndrome: experience in 23 patients. *Neurology*, **35**, 53–58

So, Y. T., Holtzman, D. M., Abrams, D. I. and Olney, R. K. (1988). Peripheral neuropathy associated with acquired immunodeficiency syndrome: prevalence and clinical features from a population-based survey. *Arch. Neurol.*, **45**, 945–948

Talpos, D., Tien, R. D. and Hesselink, J. R. (1991). Magnetic resonance imaging of AIDS-related polyradiculopathy. *Neurology*, **41**, 1996–1997

Toyka, K. V. and Heininger, K. (1987). Humoral factors in peripheral nerve disease. *Muscle Nerve*, **10**, 222–232

Toyka, K. V., Hartung, H.-P., Schafer, B. *et al.* (1988). Immune mechanisms in acute and chronic inflammatory polyneuropathies. *J. Neuroimmunol.*, **20**, 277–283

Tucker, T., Dix, R. D., Katzen, C. *et al.* (1985). Cytomegalovirus and herpes simplex virus ascending myelitis in a patient with acquired immune deficiency syndrome. *Ann. Neurol.*, **18**, 74–79

van der Meché, F. G. A., Schmitz, P. I. M. and Dutch Guillain–Barré Study Group (1992). A randomized trial comparing intravenous immune globulin and plasma exchange in Guillain–Barré syndrome. *N. Engl. J. Med.*, **326**, 1123–1129

Vendrell, J., Heredia, C., Pujol, M. *et al.* (1987). Guillain–Barré syndrome associated with seroconversion for anti-HTLV-III. *Neurology*, **37**, 544

Villa, A. (1987). Autonomic neuropathy and HIV infection (letter). *Lancet*, **2**, 915

Wechsler, A. F. and Ho, D. D. (1989). Bilateral Bell's palsy at the time of HIV seroconversion. *Neurology*, **39**, 747–748

Winer, J. B. (1993). Neuropathies and HIV infection [editorial]. *J. Neurol. Neurosurg. Psychiatry*, **56**, 739–741

Winer, J. B., Bang, B., Clarke, J. R. *et al.* (1992). A study of neuropathy in HIV infection. *Q. J. Med.*, **302**, 473–488

Wiselka, M. J., Nicholson, K. G., Ward, S. C. and Flower, A. J. E. (1987). Acute infection with human immunodeficiency virus associated with facial nerve palsy and neuralgia. *J. Infect.*, **15**, 189–190

Yarchoan, R., Thomas, R. V., Allain, J.-P. *et al.* (1988). Phase 1 studies of 2'3'-dideoxycytidine in severe human immunodeficiency virus infection as a single agent and alternating with zidovudine (AZT). *Lancet*, **1**, 76–81

12
Toxic peripheral neuropathies

H. H. Schaumburg and J. G. Kaplan

INTRODUCTION

Peripheral neuropathy is an undesired side effect of a wide variety of pharmaceutical, occupational and environmental agents. Epidemic outbreaks of environmental/occupational toxic-neuropathy may follow from exposure to potent neurotoxins and from improper use of compounds with limited neurotoxicity; isolated pharmaceutically related instances are usually iatrogenic.

Interest in clinical neurotoxicology has increased as research in neuroscience has helped identify the pathogenesis of conditions arising from exposure to certain pharmaceutical and industrial agents. Conversely, increased understanding of the mechanisms of toxic injury to nerves has afforded insight into mechanisms of naturally occurring peripheral neuropathies.

Basic principles

There are few specific therapies for toxic neuropathies; the most important step in treatment is recognition of the offending neurotoxin, since improvement usually follows removal (Schaumburg and Berger, 1993). In massive industrial exposure this is usually simple. In cases of insidious environmental exposure, careful history of working conditions, similar symptoms in co-workers, and improvement while away from work help identify the offending agent.

Pharmaceutical-induced neuropathies develop with variable latency following initiation of therapy or changes in dosage (Schaumburg, 1991). Although toxic neuropathies generally improve after removal of the agent, commencement of recovery may be delayed and symptoms may worsen for weeks following removal from exposures, the 'coasting' phenomenon (Schaumburg, 1991).

The clinical features of toxic neuropathy depend on the pharmacokinetics and site of action of the neurotoxin as well as individual susceptibility factors. Prominent factors are: underlying illness, metabolic dysfunction influencing drug metabolism, and the simultaneous use of other medications which may also be neurotoxic (LeQuesne, 1993).

Distal axonopathy is the most common form of toxic neuropathy; most are sensory–motor or purely sensory in onset, with eventual diminution of nerve action potential amplitude detected by nerve conduction studies and loss of large myelinated fibres in nerve biopsy. Many agents are lipid soluble and readily cross into the central nervous system (CNS) or peripheral nervous system (PNS). Others gain access through fenestrated capillaries in the dorsal root ganglia, some cause a diffuse sensory neuronopathy syndrome following massive exposure (e.g. pyridoxine). The distal ends of dorsal column central projections of sensory neurons are also affected in toxic distal axonopathy; this contributes to delayed or incomplete recovery (Schaumburg and Spencer, 1979). Toxins that have long half-lives (suramin) or that affect biosynthetic Schwann cell pathways (diphtheria toxin), may have a delayed onset and recover slowly even though their primary effect is on myelin (Kaplan, 1980; La Rocca *et al.*, 1990). Autonomic dysfunction is rearely a prominent feature of toxic neuropathy; exceptions include acrylamide (LeQuesne, 1993) and vinca alkaloids (Bradley *et al.*, 1970). Agents such as *n*-hexane (Korobkin *et al.*, 1975) and organophosphates (Cavanagh, 1954) which cause simultaneous degeneration of CNS motor pathways may cause spasticity that is manifested only after recovery from the peripheral axonopathy. Pure or predominantly motor toxic neuropathy is extremely rare; the sole exceptions are dapsone (Gutmann *et al.*, 1976) and lead (Buchthal and Behse, 1979).

Improved understanding of neurotoxic mechanisms should lead to prevention by limiting exposure in industrial and pharmacological applications, identifying individuals at particular risk and by developing means, e.g. neuronotrophic rescue agents, to blunt or prevent peripheral neuronal dysfunction.

Neurologists must not only be able to identify toxic neuropathy, but must also recognize situations in which trivial coincidental exposure or slight increases in body burdens falsely implicate a toxic cause in a patient with a neuropathy of different cause. This chapter represents a condensed summary of recognized biological, industrial and pharmaceutical neurotoxins. Newly identified agents and recent insights into the pathogenesis of known neurotoxins are emphasized.

Pathogenesis

The biochemical pathogeneses of toxic neuropathies remain, in many instances, poorly understood despite great efforts towards their elucidation. This is especially true in the case of central-peripheral distal axonopathies, which comprise the majority of toxic neuropathies. In these disorders of obscure pathogenesis, there is symmetrical **axonal degeneration** beginning in the distal elements of long, large CNS and PNS fibres which eventually spread proximally with time (Schaumburg and Spencer, 1979). It is not clear whether cytoskeletal elements, the neural soma, axonal transport or other elements are involved in these disorders (Thomas, 1980), although several neurotoxins are known to disrupt the function of microtubules, elements necessary for axonal transport. Colchicine and the vinca alkaloids cause microtubules in dividing cells to disassemble and block axonal transport. Taxol, on the other hand, has a unique mechanism of action; it binds to tubulin and promotes microtubule assembly thereby disrupting normal cell functions including mitosis, cell proliferation, neurite initiation and branching. The precise link between these *in vitro* effects and clincial neuropathy remains uncertain, but suggests mechanisms involving axonal transport or cell division.

Chemically unrelated compounds may cause neuropathies which have morphological similarities, among these, carbon disulphide (Seppalainen and Haltia, 1980), acrylamide (Gold *et al.*, 1985) and 2,5-hexanedione (2,5-HD), a metabolite of methyl *n*-butyl ketone (M*n*BK) (Altenkirch *et al.*, 1977) have been shown to induce the accumulation of neurofilaments distally before axonal breakdown. Several mechanisms, including interference with metabolic pathways or the function of neurofilaments, have been offered to explain this phenomenon. It is not clear that these morphological similarities reflect a common pathogenesis (Schaumburg and Spencer, 1979; Schaumburg, 1991).

The neurotoxicity of organophosphate (OP) compounds has received great scrutiny, although even with these agents, details regarding pathogenesis remain unclear. Several weeks after high exposure to OPs, a severe sensory–motor neuropathy called organophosphate-induced delayed polyneuropathy (OPIDP) may ensue (Kaplan *et al.*, 1993b). It has long been held that only OPs which can inactivate the enzyme system known as neuropathy target esterase (NTE), a hydrolase independent from acetyl choline esterase (AChE), cause OPIDP. The prevailing theory states that only OPs that can inactivate NTE by covalently binding to the active site, cleaving a lateral side chain from the phosphorylated NTE and leaving a charged monosubstituted phosphate residue at the active site, cause OPIDP. This cleaving is referred to as 'aging' of NTE (Kaplan *et al.*, 1993b). According to this view, OPs which competitively inhibit NTE without aging it, do not cause OPIDP. OPs have been assessed *in vitro* by NTE assays to predict their neurotoxicity. Agents which have little or no aging activity or which have a high therapeutic index (ratio of AChE activity/NTE aging) are presumed not to be neurotoxic in industrial and environmental applications. Traditional theory held that pretreatment with OPs that inhibit but do not age NTE would protect from OPIDP. In fact, when given before agers, these compounds do protect experimental animals from OPIDP.

Recent studies suggest that the role of NTE aging in OPIDP may be more complex than previously recognized; the dosing sequence of agers and non-agers is apparently critical in the development of OPIDP. It is now known that non-agers, which protect from OPIDP when given before agers (*vide supra*), actually enhance the neurotoxic potential of agers when administered immediately afterwards (promotion). Further, OPIDP has now been described following exposure to two non-agers, and the non-ager, methamidophos, has been reported to cause neuropathy in a form of self-promoted OPIDP. These studies suggest the NTE aging may not be the critical step in the genesis of OPIDP. Finally, it has been shown that lymphocyte NTE is markedly depressed in patients with alcoholic neuropathy, suggesting that other neurotoxins may affect the NTE system and possibly interact with OP compounds (Richardson, 1992; Kaplan *et al.*, 1993b).

Recent evidence demonstrates that chlorpyrifos, an OP with moderate aging potential, causes reversible sensory neuropathy and cognitive deficits when improperly used as a fumigant with exposure to far less OP than is necessary to produce OPIDP (see chlorpyrifos). This observation, taken in concert with recent observations regarding the mechanism of organophosphate neuropathy, suggests that caution be used in the prediction of the neurotoxic potential of newly developed OPs, and that the NTE assay alone may be inadequate (Kaplan *et al.*, 1993b).

Demyelination is a less important mechanism than axonal degeneration in toxic neuropathies, and when it does occur it is usually a secondary phenomenon. Diphtheria toxin, one of the rare agents which causes a toxic demelinating neuropathy probably acts by inhibiting Schwann cell protein synthesis, thereby giving rise to the delayed onset of weakness as myelin restoration is impaired following its normal turnover (Kaplan, 1980). Perhexilene (Pollet *et al.*, 1977), amiodarone (Martinez-Arizala. *et al.*, 1983) and chloroquine (Whisnant, *et al.*, 1963) give rise to novel morphologic features of prominent demyelination and Schwann cell lamellar inclusions from inactivation of the lysosomal enzyme sphingomyelinase (Schaumburg, 1991). In the case of perhexilene, there is a genetically determined vulnerability; individuals at risk cannot hydroxylate debrisoquine. Administration of perhexilene to the Dark Agouti rat, a poor hydroxylator of debrisoquine, causes lipid inclusions similar to those described in human neuropathy (Schaumburg, 1991).

INDUSTRIAL, ENVIRONMENTAL AND BIOLOGICAL AGENTS

Acrylamide

Acrylamide monomer is an important industrial agent used for grouting or flocculation and is a potent neurotoxin; the polymer is not. The monomer is a white, water-soluble powder, readily absorbed by inhalation or ingestion. Most instances of neuropathy occur following cutaneous exposure; exfoliative dermatitis with erythema and desquamation of the hands often precedes neuropathy (Spencer and Schaumburg, 1974).

Acrylamide neuropathy is characterized by acral sensory loss with minimal paraesthesias (Garland and Patterson, 1967). Vibration sense is affected out of proportion to other sensory modalities. Gait ataxia is a prominent feature, possibly reflecting selective involvement of muscle spindle afferents or cerebellar pathways. Diffuse areflexia is common, in contrast to most toxic neuropathies which are characterized by selective loss of the Achilles reflexes. Most eventually develop distal weakness; autonomic dysfunction is variable, many sweat profusely (Garland and Patterson, 1967; Spencer and Schaumburg, 1974).

Central nervous system dysfunction may occur after high-level acrylamide exposure. Cerebellar ataxia with broad-based unstable gait, incoordination and intention tremor have been reported, as have encephalopathy with hallucinations and memory loss.

Removal from exposure in the early stages results in recovery, although subtle weakness or sensory loss may remain (Spencer and Schaumburg, 1974). Prolonged exposure may eventuate in permanent severe weakness, sensory loss, memory loss and ataxia (Garland and Patterson, 1967). We suggest that the combined use of quantitative assessment of distal limb vibration sense (QST) and nerve conduction studies are sufficiently sensitive to allow screening of asymptomatic acrylamide workers for signs of subclinical neuropathy (Schaumburg, 1991).

The biochemical mechanism underlying neurotoxicity is unclear. Experimental studies have shown early defects in retrograde axonal transport in distal regions of sensory nerves after acrylamide exposure (Gold *et al.*, 1985). Human sural nerve biopsies display large-fibre axonal degeneration; clinical electrophysiology studies show significant decrease in amplitude of sensory and motor nerve action potentials and denervational changes in distal muscles (Fullerton, 1969; Sumner and Asbury, 1975).

Allyl chloride

Allyl chloride (3-chloropropene) is a liquid used primarily in the manufacture of epoxy resins. Distal symmetric sensorimotor axonal polyneuropathy follows prolonged high-level atmosphere exposure. Electrodiagnostic abnormalities include distal nerve conduction abnormalities and spontaneous activity on needle electromyography. Recovery is excellent after removal from exposure. Experimental animal studies show multifocal neurofilament accumulation and degeneration of large myelinated axons (He *et al.*, 1985).

Arsenic

Arsenic neurotoxicity usually results from ingestion of the trivalent (arsenite) form in murder or suicide attempts. Smelters and miners may be exposed to the less toxic pentavalent (arsenate) form, a contaminant of copper and lead ores.

Two types of arsenic neuropathy exist. Massive, single overdose (usually arsenite) in homicide or suicide attempts produces immediate vomiting and circulatory collapse. Survivors develop neuropathy within 1 to 3 weeks, characterized by **subacute** onset of sensory loss and variable weakness. In severe cases, an acute paralytic syndrome may occur which eventually evolves into a distal axonopathy pattern. Systemic signs of arsenic intoxication (skin changes, anaemia) appear later and are often not present at the onset of neuropathy. Recovery largely depends on the severity of neuropathy (LeQuesne and McLeod, 1977).

Chronic low-level exposure to inorganic arsenic causes a consistent three-stage illness. Malaise characterizes stage one, followed by hyperkeratosis, skin darkening and characteristic white transverse striations of the nails (Mees' lines); the third stage is peripheral neuropathy. In this form of arsenic exposure, sensory abnormalities predominate with prominent vibration and position sense loss and burning paraesthesias. Weakness is variable, and usually mild. Recovery is generally excellent after exposure is terminated (Schaumburg, 1991).

Treatment of both forms entail chelation with either British antilewisite (BAL) or penicillamine. There is no convincing evidence that chelation is effective in the later stages of arsenic neuropathy (Schaumburg, 1991).

In chronic exposure, assay of hair is preferable. Pubic hair is suggested because of coincidental environmental exposure of scalp, hair and nails. In acute cases, urine assay may be helpful (LeQuesne, 1993).

There is no animal model of arsenic neuropathy. Electrophysiological and pathological studies of humans suggest distal axonopathy (LeQuesne and McLeod, 1977).

Buckthorn

The fruit of the buckthorn shrub *Karwinska humboldtiana* is neurotoxic and produces rapid, painless ascending quadriparesis 1 to 3 weeks after ingestion. Sensory loss is minimal and buckthorn intoxication may be confused with Guillain–Barré syndrome or poliomyelitis. No electrodiagnostic studies are available and a single sural biopsy showed segmental demyelination and axonal swelling. Experimental studies suggest both axonal degeneration and segmental demyelination (Weller *et al.*, 1980).

Carbon disulphide

Carbon disulphide (CS_2) is a solvent used in the manufacture of rayon fibre and cellophane film. High-level inhalation exposure leads to cognitive and extrapyramidal dysfunction. Peripheral neuropathy results from prolonged low-level exposure with paraesthesias, sensory loss and hyperreflexia in the lower limbs. Continued exposure causes distal weakness, and eventually, hand numbness. Nerve conduction studies show distal slowing. Recovery is slow and incomplete, which may reflect involvement of central sensory axons. Experimental animal studies show focal swelling with accumulations of neurofilaments in spinal cord and peripheral axons. Paranodal myelin sheaths are thinned and retracted from the node at the site of swellings, possibly accounting for slow nerve conduction in this primary distal axonopathy (Seppalainen and Haltia, 1980).

Cyanide and derivatives

Acute, massive cyanide poisoning is usually fatal. Chronic cyanide exposure is not associated with peripheral neuropathy. Chronic thiocyanate exposure, which occurs primarily from the consumption of cassava leads to dysfunction in both the PNS and CNS. Initial complaints of acral paraesthesias are followed by distal weakness, proprioceptive loss and ataxia. Optic atrophy, sensorineural hearing loss and corticospinal tract degeneration with resultant spasticity are common. The pathogenesis of chronic thiocyanate poisoning is unknown and there are no reports describing the results of deleting cassava from the diet. Sodium cyanate neuropathy is described under Pharmaceutical agents (see below). The relationship between thiocyanate, sodium cyanate and cyanide toxicity is unclear (Osuntokun *et al.*, 1970).

Dimethylaminopropionitrile (DMAPN)

DMAPN, a catalyst which causes an unusual axonopathy accompanied by urinary retention and sexual dysfunction, is of historical interest only as it has been withdrawn from use (Schaumburg, 1991).

Diphtheria

Infection of the upper airway or skin with *Corynebacterium diphtheriae* leads to cardiomyopathy and diffuse polyneuropathy in one-fifth of cases. Vaccination has virtually eliminated this disease from North America.

    C. diphtheriae secretes a protein exotoxin which inhibits myelin synthesis and may also activate cytotoxic mechanisms. Release of exotoxin leads to two stages of neuropathy. Local neuropathy occurs 3 weeks after infection, due to local spread of toxin. Oropharyngeal infection is followed by: palatal paralysis, pharyngeal numbness, difficulty mobilizing secretions and, eventually, paralysis of accommodation; local limb paralysis follows dermal wound infection. Generalized sensorimotor neuropathy begins 8 to 12 weeks after infection, is primarily distal and may cause sensory ataxia. Improvement is usually rapid and complete. The pathology of diphtheritic neuropathy is widespread non-inflammatory demyelination confined to fibres in the spinal nerve roots. It is thought that lesions correspond to areas where the blood–nerve barrier is permeable, allowing access of the large exotoxin molecules to the radicular Schwann cells. The toxin inhibits myelin protein biosynthesis (Kaplan, 1980).

Chlorpyrifos (see also organophosphates)

Chlorpyrifos (O,O-dimethyl-o-3,5,6-trichloro-2-pyridyl-phosphorothioate) is an organophosphate (OP) insecticide effective against a broad spectrum of agricultural and household pest species (Kaplan et al., 1986). When used properly, chlorpyrifos has been considered safe. Reversible sensory axonopathy and cognitive dysfunction have been recently ascribed to exterminator applied chlorpyrifos (Kaplan et al., 1992). Patients experienced symptoms of peripheral neuropathy with paraesthesias and numbness after repeated exposure to this agent in enclosed, commercially fumigated sites (Kaplan et al., 1986).

The common syndrome of organophosphate-induced delayed peripheral neuropathy (OPIDP) has been reported once following massive monophasic exposure to chlorpyrifos (Kaplan et al., 1986). This two-stage illness is characterized by an initial cholinergic reaction with varying degrees of diarrhoea, gastrointestinal distress, bradycardia and lacrimation followed in several weeks by distal, symmetrical, sensorimotor, peripheral neuropathy characterized by paraesthesias, numbness, sensory loss, ataxia and significant weakness. OPIDP is discussed in detail in the sections relating to organophosphates and pathogenesis. Another case report claims transient bulbar and respiratory difficulties in a child found playing next to a bottle of chlorpyrifos, although the suggested cause and effect relationship is unconvincing (Kaplan et al., 1986).

Ethylene oxide

Ethylene oxide is a gas used in the sterilization of heat-sensitive medical instruments and biomedical materials. Chronic low-level exposure can cause distal axonopathy with numbness, sensory loss and prominent reflex loss (Gross et al., 1979). In some cases, cognitive impairment (Crystal et al., 1988) may accompany neuropathy and experimental animal studies confirm that this is a distal axonopathy (Ohnishi et al., 1986). Improvement follows termination of exposure. Typically, ethylene oxide exposure occurs via inhalation; however, excess ethylene oxide in dialysis tubing has recently been postulated to contribute to peripheral neuropathy in chronic haemodialysis patients (Windebank and Blexrud, 1989).

Hexacarbons (*n*-hexane and methyl *n*-butyl ketone)

n-Hexane and methyl *n*-butyl ketone (M*n*BK) are described together as both act through a common intermediary, 2,5-hexanedione (2,5-HD) to produce peripheral neuropathy. *n*-Hexane is a solvent with wide industrial application in glues, thinners and lacquers. Intoxication occurs with accidental occupational exposure or following inhalation abuse (glue sniffing) (Altenkirch *et al.*, 1977). M*n*BK is inherently more neurotoxic than *n*-hexane but its use has been curtailed since it was implicated in a massive outbreak of toxic neuropathy in a fabric plant (Allen *et al.*, 1975). Methyl ethyl ketone (MEK) was erroneously alleged to cause peripheral neuropathy in humans; however, the case reports were unconvincing and neurotoxicity could not be duplicated in animal experiments. Its sole neurotoxic function is its ability to potentiate the effects of *n*-hexane or M*n*BK (Schaumburg, 1991).

Peripheral neuropathy develops insidiously after exposure to either agent (Allen *et al.*, 1975; Altenkirch *et al.*, 1977). Distal sensory loss predominates early, but is eventually overshadowed by severe weakness. Subacute onset of severe ascending weakness following high-level exposure in glue sniffers may suggest Guillain–Barré syndrome (Altenkirch *et al.*, 1977). Tendon reflexes are minimally affected; even in severe cases usually only the Achilles reflex is lost. Improvement correlates with severity of neuropathy, permanent deficits frequently result from prolonged high-level exposure (Cianchetti *et al.*, 1976). Coasting may last for 2–4 months following removal (Schaumburg, 1991). Spasticity and hyperreflexia, reflecting corticospinal tract degeneration, may appear following recovery from neuropathy (Allen *et al.*, 1975). Nerve biopsy reveals multifocal paranodal, giant axonal swellings accompanied by myelin retraction (Altenkirch *et al.*, 1977). Paranodal demyelination with secondary myelin changes is likely responsible for markedly slowed nerve conduction. Needle electromyography (EMG) shows prominent abnormal spontaneous activity in established cases. Abnormalities of human visual, somatosensory and brainstem auditory evoked potentials reflect the widespread involvement of CNS axons displayed by experimental animals (Chang, 1987). The mechanism of neurotoxicity is dependent upon the 1,4-gamma diketone structure. Other gamma diketones such as 2,5-heptanedione and 3,6-octanedione also cause neuropathy. The pathophysiology of neurofilament accumulation is unclear; it is suggested that it results from local cross-linking of neurofilaments by the circulating gamma diketone (Schaumburg, 1991).

Lead

Lead neuropathy is rare in North America. Its nature is unclear; lead produces demyelinating neuropathy in experimental animals, while axonal degeneration is the only abnormality encountered in human nerve biopsies (Schaumburg, 1991). A plethora of clinical findings is ascribed to adult lead intoxication. Older reports describe distinct patterns of clinical involvement including wrist drop, shoulder girdle weakness, intrinsic hand muscle atrophy, foot drop and laryngeal paralysis; contemporary reports usually describe generalized weakness. Subclinical neuropathy, as evidenced by nerve conduction abnormalities in workers exposed to lead, has been suggested, but recent studies challenge this notion. Lead neuropathy, in all reports, is characterized by weakness with minimal if any sensory dysfunction (Buchthal and Behse, 1979).

The diagnosis of plumbism can be supported by an elevated urinary lead level, especially when promoted by prior dosing with chelating agents (Akari and Honma, 1976).

Treatment includes removal from exposure and excretion of the mobilizable body burden by the chelating agents penicillamine or EDTA. Lead storage occurs in bone; illnesses associated with bone demineralization may evoke or reactivate plumbism (Seppalainen *et al.*, 1979).

Mercury

Metallic mercury and mercury vapour may cause subacute, predominantly motor axonal, neuropathy which clinically mimics Guillain–Barré syndrome and is reversible. There are few studies of this very rare entity and its pathogenesis is uncertain. Tremor and emotional lability, without evidence of peripheral nerve dysfunction, is the most common neurotoxic syndrome associated with metallic mercury and mercury vapour (Windebank, 1993).

Organophosphates (see also chlorpyrifos and Introduction)

Organophosphorus esters (OPs) have three major industrial applications: insecticides, petroleum additives and modifiers of plastics. Inhibition of acetylcholinesterase (AChE) is common to all OPs and is the basis for their use as insecticides; some OPs also cause a widespread central and peripheral distal axonopathy. Axonal dysfunction begins several weeks following exposure, a process referred to as organophosphate-induced delayed peripheral neuropathy (OPIDP). OPIDP occurs independently from and is not related to the initial AChE inhibition.

Considerable variability in nervous system cholinergic reactions occurs with OPs due to differences in dose, absorption and inherent neurotoxicity of the individual compounds. Inhalation exposure to potent AChE inhibitors causes rapid onset of muscarinic and nicotinic dysfunction; death results from pulmonary compromise, a consequence of bronchoconstriction (muscarinic) and muscle paralysis (nicotinic) (Richardson, 1992).

Lower-level exposure causes a sequence of muscarinic and nicotinic inhibition. Immediate (type I muscarinic) cholinergic symptoms include gastrointestinal distress, miosis, lacrimation and diarrhoea. Type II (nicotinic) effects occur after a variable interval and include limb and bulbar weakness, respiratory difficulties and behavioural changes (Namba *et al.*, 1971). The nicotinic reaction, if delayed more than 12 hours, is called the 'intermediate syndrome' (Senanayake and Karalliedde, 1987). OP intoxication may be fatal in this stage due to respiratory or cardiac failure. Atropine and pralidoxine, a cholinesterase reactivator, may blunt the initial muscarinic effects, and are dangerous during the intermediate (type II) phase. Atropine and pralidoxine may exacerbate cardiac arrhythmia in the presence of nicotinic respiratory compromise, and are best withheld until adequate ventilation is ensured. Neither of these agents affects OPIDP (Schaumburg, 1991).

OPIDP follows OP exposure by 10–20 days. The onset of OPIDP is heralded by cramping of calves, acral paraesthesias and distal weakness (Namba *et al.*, 1971). The course is subacute and maximal involvement occurs within 14 days of onset. In severe cases, there may be mild proximal weakness. OPIDP is predominantly motor; however, sensory loss is invariably present on careful clinical examination. Distal weakness and atrophy are accompanied by ataxia and loss of Achilles reflexes (Schaumburg, 1991). One report claims that reversible, rapid onset, demyelinating neuropathy indistinguishable from Guillain–Barré syndrome may occur in children following OP intoxication (Kaplan *et al.*, 1993b) (see also chlorpyrifos). The biochemical pathogenesis of OPIDP is discussed in the chapter Introduction.

Signs of myelopathy eventually appear in many cases. These signs may be initially obscured by peripheral neuropathy; in the ensuing months, lower-limb spasticity appears and position sense loss persists (Smith and Spalding, 1959).

Laboratory studies are of limited use in the diagnosis of any of the stages of OP-induced neurotoxicity. Depressed red cell AChE levels, which eventually normalize, may be helpful in documenting exposure. In the intermediate syndrome, electrophysiological studies may demonstrate abnormalities of neuromuscular transmission. In OPIDP, neurophysiological studies show diminished action potential amplitude, indicative of distal axonopathy.

Polychlorinated biphenyls (PCBs)

PCBs, extensively used as plasticizers, have achieved notoriety as waterway pollutants. Outbreaks of PCB neuropathy have been confined to ingestion of food cooked in oil contaminated with tetrachlorobiphenyl (TCBP). Affected individuals develop acne, brown nails and distal peripheral neuropathy with sensory loss, areflexia and slowing of nerve conduction (Murai and Kuroiwa, 1971). The nature and pathogenesis of this neuropathy is unclear; nerve conduction slowing has been shown in rats intoxicated with PCB (Ogawa, 1971).

Spanish toxic oil syndrome

The Spanish toxic oil syndrome (STOS) is a multisystem disorder characterized by respiratory insufficiency, headache and eosinophilia; it may be rapidly fatal. STOS occurred as an epidemic resulting from ingestion of adulterated rapeseed oil. The nature of the adulterant is not known. The neuromuscular syndrome, which occurs in over 90% of survivors, is characterized by sensory loss, diffuse weakness and myalgias (Ricoy *et al.*, 1983). Sural nerve biopsy shows lymphocytic infiltration of peri- and epineurium; endoneurial inflammation is rare and vasculopathy is not described in the biopsies (Martinez *et al.*, 1984). The exact pathogenesis is unclear, although vasculitis and eosinophil-bound toxins have been suggested (Martinez *et al.*, 1984).

Thallium

Thallium salts cause severe neuropathy and diffuse CNS degeneration, which has led to discontinuation of their use as depilatories and rodenticides. Three types of neuropathy occur with thallium ingestion, related to dosage and tempo of intoxication (Cavanagh *et al.*, 1974).

Acute, massive intoxication, usually accompanied by acute gastrointestinal distress, causes neuropathy within 1 week, heralded by severe burning paraesthesias. Varying degrees of weakness occur, but sensory involvement usually predominates. Tendon reflexes are often preserved, which, together with cranial nerve sparing, helps distinguish cases with severe involvement from Guillain–Barré syndrome. Death may follow from ventilatory or cardiac failure. CNS dysfunction may result from anoxia. Hair loss, which appears weeks after thallium intoxication, only provides retrospective evidence of acute intoxication (Bank *et al.*, 1972).

A subacute, slowly progressive, painful, mainly sensory polyneuropathy occurs with more prolonged, low-level exposure. In this form, alopecia is a helpful clue (Schaumburg, 1991). Chronic thallium exposure rarely causes neuropathy, and when it occurs it is overshadowed by extrapyramidal dysfunction (Prick, 1979). Experimental animal studies show accumulation of swollen mitochondria in distal axons before degeneration of nerve fibres (Spencer *et al.*, 1973). Human electrodiagnostic studies show mainly diminution of amplitude of compound nerve action potentials, suggesting distal axonopathy. Treatment with potassium chloride or Prussian blue is suggested, although its efficacy is unproven (Schaumburg, 1991).

Trichlorethylene

Trichlorethylene (TCE) is a solvent in widespread industrial use; it formerly served as a general anaesthetic. TCE probably is not neurotoxic; cranial neuropathy likely results from dichloracetylene (DCA) generated by the interaction of TCE with alkali. Neurotoxicity of TCE is confined to the cranial nerves, primarily the trigeminal, which led to its past usage in intractable cases of trigeminal neuralgia. High-level exposure results in additional involvement of the facial, oculomotor and optic nerves (Buxton and Hayward, 1967). The pathogenesis is unclear; no animal model exists. The frequent association between orofacial herpes simplex and TCE exposure may indicate that the pathogenesis of trigeminal neuropathy involves reactivation by TCE of latent virus in the ganglia (Cavanagh and Buxton, 1989).

Vacor (PNU)

Vacor, *N*-3-pyridylmethyl-*N*-p-nitrophenyl urea (PNU), is a structural analogue of nicotinamide which is used as a rodenticide. Ingestion of PNU leads to acute, severe distal axonopathy with prominent autonomic dysfunction. Massive ingestion leads to rapid-onset limb weakness, cranial nerve dysfunction, urinary retention and loss of postural reflexes (LeWitt, 1980). Neuropathy is accompanied by acute diabetes from destruction of pancreatic islet cells (Pont *et al.*, 1979). Survivors have diabetes and autonomic dysfunction with variable weakness. Post-mortem studies suggest Wallerian degeneration of peripheral nerves, nerve roots and ganglia (LeWitt, 1980).

Administration of single doses of PNU to experimental animals results in terminal axonopathy accompanied by selective impairment of fast anterograde axonal transport. Experimental PNU neuropathy can be prevented by pretreatment with nicotinamide. This suggest that an NAD-dependent enzyme is inhibited by PNU, leading to disruption of energy-dependent fast anterograde axon transport in somatic and autonomic nerves (Watson and Griffin, 1987).

PHARMACEUTICAL AGENTS

Amiodarone

Amiodarone, a potent ventricular antiarrhythmic, causes tremor, optic neuropathy and peripheral neuropathy. Peripheral neuropathy occurs with a prolonged serum concentration exceeding 2.4 mg/l. Absorption is variable following oral administration; usually dosages of less than 400 mg/day are safe, although neuropathy has been reported with standard doses of 200 mg/day (Meier *et al.*, 1979; Martinez-Arizala *et al.*, 1983). Lower-limb weakness appears early, followed by generalized sensorimotor neuropathy with chronic exposure. The degree of recovery depends on dose and chronicity of administration. Nerve biopsy findings include prominent demyelination and Schwann cell lamellar inclusions. Severe slowing of nerve conduction velocity is characteristic of the advanced stage. The likely mechanism of amiodarone neuropathy is inhibition of phospholipase, reflected by the Schwann cell lamellar inclusions (Schaumburg, 1991). Amiodarone neuropathy shares many features with perhexilene maleate neuropathy (*vide infra*) which results from inactivation of the lysosomal enzyme sphingomyelinase (Said, 1978).

Chloramphenicol

Chloramphenicol produces peripheral and optic neuropathy following high-dose, long-term administration. This is now rare because of the limited use of chloramphenicol. Chloramphenicol neuropathy produces numbness of the feet and calf tenderness; it is reversible after withdrawal (Joy *et al.*, 1960).

Chloroquine

Chloroquine is an antimalarial, occasionally used for dermatological conditions. Its principal toxicity is myopathy which affects cardiac and skeletal muscle. Chloroquine produces only a mild neuropathy. Sural biopsy studies show segmental demyelination and dense laminar inclusions similar to those associated with perhexilene and amiodarone toxicity (Whisnant *et al.*, 1963).

Colchicine

Neuromyopathy occurs with chronic high level dosage of colchicine or in individuals whose gouty nephropathy allows the accumulation of toxic levels with the usual treatment of 0.6 mg twice daily (Kuncl *et al.*, 1987). Neuropathy is usually overshadowed by clinical and laboratory evidence of myopathy. Patients develop proximal weakness with elevated serum creatine kinase and signs of myopathy on needle EMG. Most display mild sensory loss and acral paraesthesias. Sensory nerve conduction studies show decreased amplitude with normal conduction velocity, in accord with sural biopsy findings of axonal loss with secondary myelin changes. Patients generally improve when colchicine is stopped. Colchicine neuropathy may result from defective axonal transport due to impaired microtubule assembly, a mechanism similar to that proposed for vincristine (Kuncl *et al.*, 1987).

Dapsone

Dapsone is a sulphone used to treat leprosy, pneumocystis pneumonia and some dermatological conditions. Motor neuropathy occasionally follows long-term, high-level treatment, usually for dermatological disease. Weakness, the predominant feature of dapsone neuropathy, may be diffuse but frequently affects the arms disproportionately; the median nerve is particularly vulnerable (Gutmann *et al.*, 1976). The appearance of hand weakness without sensory symptoms may lead to an erroneous diagnosis of motor neuron disease (Helander and Partanen, 1978). Electrodiagnostic studies show slowing of motor nerve conduction and signs of denervation with needle EMG (Gutmann *et al.*, 1976). Sural biopsy studies have shown mild, non-specific changes in sensory axons (Koller *et al.*, 1977).

The mechanism of neuropathy is unclear. Dapsone is metabolized by acetylation. It has been suggested that its sporadic occurrence may reflect variable acetylation, as with isoniazid, although one report describes neuropathy in a fast acetylator (Gutmann *et al.*, 1976; Koller *et al.*, 1977; Helander and Partanen, 1978).

Nucleoside neuropathies (ddC, ddI, d4T)

The nucleosides dideoxycytidine (ddC), dideoxyinosine (ddI) and d4T are inhibitors of reverse transcriptase and are used to treat HIV infection. Peripheral neuropathy is a dose-limiting side effect of these agents. High doses (> 0.03 mg/kg six times per day for 8 weeks) which were given in initial studies caused subacute, painful neuropathy in all. At current low doses of ddI (5 mg/kg) less than 10% of patients develop a mild, readily reversible, sensory neuropathy. History of prior neuropathy or exposure to other neurotoxins predispose to nucleoside neuropathy.

In the original high-dose study, neuropathy was heralded by intense acral paraesthesias; burning and lancinating leg pain appeared before objective sensory loss or electrodiagnostic abnormalities developed. Later, signs of distal axonopathy predominated with sensory loss exceeding weakness. Withdrawal of drug was followed by a coasting period lasting up to 6 weeks during which neuropathy continued to worsen. The degree of recovery depended on the severity of neuropathy, overall state of the patient, and concomitant AIDS neuropathy. The mechanism of nucleoside neuropathy is unclear. Experimental studies in primates have produced slowed nerve conduction but no convincing morphological evidence of nerve fibre degeneration (Hirsch and D'Aquila, 1993).

Disulfiram

Disulfiram (Antabuse) is used in the treatment of alcoholism. The principal toxicity of disulfiram is peripheral neuropathy, which frequently must be distinguished clinically from that of alcoholism. Most instances occur at standard therapeutic doses (250–500 mg daily) and commence months to years after onset of treatment; they generally improve following drug withdrawal. Clinical, electrodiagnostic and sural biopsy findings are those of distal axonopathy. In two reported biopsies, axonal swellings filled with intermediate filaments are described. It has been suggested that carbon disulphide, a metabolite of disulfiram, may be responsible (Gardner-Thorpe and Benjamin, 1971; Moddel *et al.*, 1978; Mokri *et al.*, 1981).

Doxorubicin

Doxorubicin is a chemotherapeutic agent which, in laboratory animals, causes widespread degeneration of sensory and gasserian ganglia eventuating in a sensory neuronopathy syndrome. No human instances are reported; this may reflect species differences, lower human dosage, or erroneous attribution of neurotoxic effects to other chemotherapeutic agents or underlying neoplasia (Cho *et al.*, 1980).

Ethambutol

Ethambutol (EMB) is an antituberculous agent which causes peripheral and optic neuropathy following prolonged dosing above 20 mg/kg per day. Sensory neuropathy is usually mild and generally improves after EMB is discontinued. Studies in the mouse suggest that EMB produces a distal axonopathy (Nair *et al.*, 1980).

Ethionamide

Ethionamide is a rarely used antituberculous agent which causes sensory neuropathy of unclear pathogenesis (Leggat, 1962).

Gold

Organic gold compounds, used to treat rheumatoid arthritis, cause many idiosyncratic reactions, commonly dermatological or renal; peripheral neuropathy is rare. A painful, dysaesthetic neuropathy with prominent muscle pain and myokymia has been ascribed to gold. Slowing of nerve conduction reflects the segmental demyelination seen on nerve biopsies. Axonal degeneration is also present in biopsies. The pathogenesis of gold-induced neuropathy is unclear. Fever, rash and renal abnormalities suggest an immunological mechanism, although vasculitis has not been documented in biopsies. This toxic neuropathy may be difficult to distinguish from the neuropathy of rheumatoid arthritis or rheumatoid vasculitis; the latter is frequently accompanied by nodules, greatly elevated rheumatoid factor and long duration of arthritis. Isolated case reports suggest that gold therapy may precipitate Guillain–Barré syndrome (Walsh, 1970; Katrak *et al.*, 1980).

Hydralazine

The antihypertensive agent, hydralazine, rarely may cause a mild distal axonopathy, probably due to pyridoxine deficiency in a mechanism similar to that of isoniazid (*vide infra*) (Raskin and Fishman, 1965).

Isoniazid (INH)

Isoniazid (INH) is a widely used antituberculous agent which causes peripheral neuropathy by inhibition of pyridoxal phosphokinase, the enzyme which catalyses pyridoxine phosphorylation (Ochoa, 1970). INH is deactivated by acetylation; individuals unable to acetylate normally (slow acetylators) develop higher levels of INH and are more susceptible to neuropathy (Paulsen and Nilsson, 1985).

INH neuropathy is dose dependent; doubling the usual dose of 3 mg/kg per day results in an eightfold increase in neuropathy. Distal paraesthesias, calf pain and numbness begin from 3 weeks to 6 months after onset of therapy, depending on dose and individual susceptibility. Neuropathy can be avoided by co-administration of 100 mg of pyridoxine/day without affecting the antituberculous action of INH (Ochoa, 1970).

Metronidazole

Metronidazole, an antimicrobial used in treatment of Gram negative infections and Crohn's disease, causes distal axonopathy, usually with cumulative doses exceeding 30 g. The resulting large-fibre sensory neuropathy is reversible if metronidazole is immediately discontinued. Sural nerve biopsies demonstrated loss of large myelinated fibres. There is no experimental animal model (Coxon and Pallis, 1976; Bradley *et al.*, 1977).

Misonidazole

Misonidazole, a congener of metronidazole, is a cell sensitizer for radiotherapy. It causes dose-limiting subacute peripheral neuropathy after administration of 11 g/m^2 given at a rate exceeding 6 g/m^2 weekly. Biopsy and electrophysiological studies suggest distal axonopathy (Urtasun *et al.*, 1978). Experimental animal intoxication produces widespread multifocal necrosis of the CNS, but not peripheral neuropathy. A metabolite, desmethylmisonidazole, also causes peripheral neuropathy (Urtasun *et al.*, 1978; Mamoli *et al.*, 1979).

Nitrofurantoin

Nitrofurantoin, a broad-spectrum antibiotic used to treat urinary tract infections, causes a rapidly progressive distal axonopathy. The fulminant onset of weakness may erroneously suggest a diagnosis of Guillain–Barré syndrome. Patients with underlying diabetes or renal failure appear to be at greater risk, presumably from underlying peripheral neuropathy, although it is also suggested that toxic levels occur with normal dosage in patients with renal failure because of failure to excrete nitrofurantoin (Toole *et al.*, 1968).

Experimental animal and human sural nerve biopsy studies suggest distal axonopathy, although one report describes dorsal root degeneration and chromatolysis of sensory ganglia and anterior horn cells. The mechanism of action is unclear (Schaumburg, 1991).

Nitrous oxide

Nitrous oxide, a dental anaesthetic and aerosol food propellant, can cause megaloblastic anaemia and myelopathy indistinguishable from pernicious anaemia. Neurological dysfunction usually occurs following abusive self-administration. Moderate levels of self-administration cause peripheral neuropathy. Prolonged high doses also result in myelopathy and optic atrophy. Acral paraesthesias, numbness of the hands and feet and ataxia are common initial features. At this stage, reflexes are attenuated and nerve conduction studies show mild slowing. Continued self-administration results in spasticity, hyperreflexia, and severe acral sensory loss (Layzer *et al.*, 1978; Sahenk *et al.*, 1978).

Nitrous oxide interferes with vitamin B_{12} metabolism. In primates intoxicated with nitrous oxide the resemblance to vitamin B_{12} deficiency is striking; both conditions display megaloblastic anaemia, myeloneuropathy, and pathological evidence of spongy degeneration in the spinal cord dorsal and lateral columns and axonal degeneration in peripheral nerves (Amess *et al.*, 1978; Layzer *et al.*, 1978; Schaumburg, 1991). Experimental evidence suggests that nitrous oxide produces megaloblastic anaemia by inhibition of methionine synthetase; co-administration of methionine prevents myelopathy in the primate model (Frasca *et al.*, 1986).

Perhexiline maleate

Perhexiline maleate, an agent previously used to treat angina pectoris, causes severe peripheral neuropathy with prominent weakness, cranial nerve involvement and dysautonomia following treatment with 300–400 mg/day for 4–12 months.

The clinical profile, electrodiagnosis and nerve biopsy indicate a combination of primary segmental demyelination and axonal degeneration (Said, 1978).

Phenytoin

Phenytoin (diphenylhydantoin) is an anticonvulsant which causes cerebellar degeneration and peripheral neuropathy with chronic usage. Phenytoin-induced neuropathy is rare, deficits are usually confined to diminution of tendon reflexes and mild nerve conduction abnormalities, although on occasion patients may develop significant sensory loss. Recovery usually follows drug withdrawal (Lovelace and Horwitz, 1968). A single report of a sural biopsy describes axonal degeneration with secondary demyelination (Ramirez *et al.*, 1986). Short-term administration of phenytoin to experimental animals produces nerve conduction abnormalities; in humans, mild neuropathy is encountered with long-term, high-level dosage (Lovelace and Horwitz, 1968).

Platinum (cisplatin)

Cisplatin (*cis*-diamine-dichlorplatinum) is a widely used chemotherapeutic agent effective against a wide spectrum of malignancies. If cumulative dosage exceeds 225–500 mg/m^2, cisplatin causes a large-fibre, progressive sensory distal axonopathy or neuronopathy which spares motor nerves. Large-fibre sensory loss is uniformly encountered, causing position and vibration sense loss with occasional pseudoathetosis; pain and thermal sensation is frequently normal (Roelofs *et al.*, 1984). Autonomic dysfunction, especially gastroparesis and vomiting, is frequent. Neuropathy from low-dose exposure (500 mg/m^2) usually is reversible (Roelofs *et al.*, 1984). Prolonged high-dose exposure may result in permanent, severe large-fibre sensory loss with ataxia and loss of manual dexterity. Occasionally, the onset of cisplatin neuropathy is delayed and patients experience initial symptoms up to 4 months after drug withdrawal; it is then difficult to distinguish between cisplatin toxicity and sensory neuronopathy associated with the underlying malignancy (Roelofs *et al.*, 1984). Isolated limb neuropathy can result from intra-arterial injection of cisplatin (Pomes *et al.*, 1986).

The mechanism of cisplatin neuropathy is unclear. Axonal loss is described in sural nerve biopsies and in dorsal columns in necropsy studies (Clark *et al.*, 1980). A recent meticulous human electrophysiological study suggests that neuronal dysfunction is the initial event (Schaumburg, 1991).

Pyridoxine

Pyridoxine (vitamin B_6), an essential, water-soluble micronutrient is a co-enzyme in decarboxylation and transamination reactions. When the recommended daily requirement of 2.5 mg is greatly exceeded, sensory neuronopathy may ensue. The rapidity of onset, severity and reversibility of neuropathy depends largely on the dose and method of administration of pyridoxine (Schaumburg *et al.*, 1983). An irreversible sensory neuronopathy syndrome with explosive onset of profound generalized ataxia has been described following massive intravenous dosage (Albin *et al.*, 1987), while a gradual sensory distal sensory axonopathy usually follows prolonged oral consumption of lower doses (Schaumburg *et al.*, 1983).

Acute sensory neuronopathy was reported in two individuals given 180 g of pyridoxine intravenously in the treatment of mushroom poisoning. One week later, they developed profound permanent sensory ataxia and transient autonomic neuropathy. Sensory action potentials were normal while motor nerve conduction studies showed slight diminution of amplitude (Albin *et al.*, 1987).

Reversible distal sensory neuropathy of gradual onset is associated with high-dose oral pyridoxine (Schaumburg *et al.*, 1983). The natural history of pyridoxine-induced neuropathy is stereotyped. The onset of symptoms varies with dose; daily intake of less than 1 g requires more than a year to produce neuropathy while greater exposure produces neuropathy in months (Parry and Bredesen, 1985). Neuropathy is heralded by unsteady gait and numb feet followed by loss of manual dexterity (Schaumburg *et al.*, 1983). The distal symmetrical sensory neuropathy which ensues affects mainly the large-fibre functions of vibration and position sense; limb ataxia may mimic weakness as movements are misdirected and poorly controlled. Nerve conduction studies show widespread severe attenuation of sensory nerve action potentials with normal conduction velocity. Sural nerve biopsy studies reveal axonal degeneration. Most patients recover following withdrawal of pyridoxine (Schaumburg *et al.*, 1983). Controlled administration to volunteers has demonstrated that quantitatively measured sensory thresholds become elevated before neuropathy is symptomatic (Berger *et al.*, 1989).

The pathogenesis and biochemical basis of pyridoxine neurotoxicity are unknown. The exclusively sensory involvement and the presence of neuronopathy after high-dose exposure probably reflect the anatomical vulnerability of dorsal root ganglia cells. A tissue culture study suggests that its effects are related to its co-enzyme activity. Both the acute and chronic syndrome are readily produced in laboratory animals (Schaumburg *et al.*, 1983).

Sodium cyanate

Sodium cyanate was formerly used to treat sickle cell anaemia. Sensorimotor neuropathy occurred following conventional dosages. Approximately one-third of volunteers developed neuropathy in a random, prospective study. Most patients develop distal axonopathy (Petersen *et al.*, 1974). Experimental animals develop demyelination in spinal roots in addition to distal axonopathy (Tellez-Nagel *et al.*, 1977).

Suramin

Suramin, a polysulphonated, naphthylurea antiparasitic agent, has recently been used in chemotherapy against a number of refractory malignancies. Significant neuropathy occured in four of the first 38 patients treated. In two of these patients, neuropathy progressed to generalized flaccid paralysis with respiratory and bulbar dysfunction, resembling Guillain–Barré syndrome. The other two developed reversible neuropathy with flaccid limb paralysis. Cerebrospinal fluid (CSF) protein was elevated in all. Nerve conduction studies show features of demyelination with conduction block and slowing of conduction in concert with signs of axonal degeneration including decreased amplitude and evidence of degeneration on needle EMG testing. The onset of neuropathy correlates with the maximal plasma suramin level; 40% develop neuropathy with levels above 350 mg/ml. There is no correlation with total suramin dose or duration of treatment. Suramin has a long plasma half-life (44–54 days), which probably accounts for the fact that patients may continue to worsen for several weeks after suramin is withdrawn.

The pathogenesis of suramin neuropathy is unclear. Suramin is known to displace several growth factors from their receptors, including fibroblast growth factor, which has been found to exert a marked trophic effect on peripheral neurons *in vitro*. Suramin also inhibits DNA polymerase and lysosomal enzymes, allowing the accumulation of glycosaminoglycans and gangliosides. In experimental animals, suramin exposure leads to the formation of cytoplasmic inclusions of concentric arrays of closely packed membranes in both neurons and glia (La Rocca *et al.*, 1990).

Taxol

Taxol is a chemotherapeutic plant alkaloid used against solid tumours. It is administered in a series of intravenous courses at 3-week intervals. Doses above 200 mg/m^2 are associated with neuropathy. Symptoms of neuropathy begin suddenly soon after administration and abate gradually. Continued treatment causes intensification of symptoms as neuropathy ensues. Initial symptoms of acral paraesthesias and dysaesthesias herald the onset of distal sensory loss accompanied by tendon reflex loss. With low dosage, sensory symptoms predominate; motor dysfunction has only been reported following prolonged high doses (Lipton *et al.*, 1989). Myopathy may occur with co-administration of other chemotherapeutic agents (Chaudhry *et al.*, 1994). Nerve conduction studies indicate both axonal degeneration and demyelination, which may be secondary. Neuropathy has become the limiting factor in taxol usage (Kaplan *et al.*, 1993a).

Taxol binds to tubulin and promotes microtubule assembly. Neuronal tissue cultures treated with taxol display bundles of microtubules throughout the cytoplasm that disrupt mitosis, neurite initiation and branching (Lipton *et al.*, 1989). Nerve growth factor (NGF) can blunt these *in vitro* effects and can delay the onset of neuropathy in experimental animals (Apfel *et al.*, 1991).

Thalidomide

Thalidomide, the sedative–hypnotic which received publicity in the early 1960s due to its teratogenicity, is also a potent neurotoxin. Currently it is in limited use mainly for dermatological conditions such as erythema nodosum leprosum, discoid lupus and prurigo holdolaris.

Initial symptoms are always sensory; usually numbness and tingling occur in the feet, then in the hands. Insensitivity to pain and touch is profound; vibration and position senses are less affected. Weakness is variable, occurs later and may involve proximal muscles. Long tract involvement with Babinski signs and hyperreflexia may occur. Signs of systemic involvement including brittle nails and palmar erythema are prominent. Neuropathy occurs after approximately 1 year at doses of 25–50 mg, but more rapidly with higher doses. Recovery is variable following thalidomide withdrawal; sensory function often recovers incompletely and slowly. Nerve conduction studies show severe attenuation of sensory nerve action potential amplitudes with sparing of motor nerve conduction velocity. It has been suggested that frequent assessment of sural nerve amplitude is effective in detecting early neuropathy in asymptomatic individuals receiving thalidomide (Fullerton and Kremer, 1961; Fullerton and O'Sullivan, 1968).

L-Tryptophan

Ingestion of L-tryptophan has been implicated in over 1000 cases of the eosinophilia–myalgia syndrome (EMS), which is characterized by myositis, muscle pain, tenderness and elevated eosinophil counts. Peripheral neuropathy has been described in several series; it usually is an axonopathy which may be multifocal in the pattern of multiple mononeuropathy. Theories of pathogenesis include vasculitis from an immunologically mediated reaction to contaminants, and also direct local effects of eosinophil-borne toxins or toxic metabolities of L-Tryptophan, including the kynurenine quinolinic acid which can act at the *N*-methyl-D-aspartate receptor. Treatment with immunosuppressives may supress eosinophilia but does not appear to affect the clinical course of EMS or neuropathy. This condition shares many features with the Spanish toxic oil syndrome (Burns *et al.*, 1994).

Vincristine

Vincristine is a plant alkaloid in chemotherapeutic use against a wide spectrum of malignancies. Neurotoxicity is a dose-limiting factor. Vincristine neuropathy usually occurs in a stereotyped manner with sensory symptoms at onset. Paraesthesias of the fingers usually herald neuropathy; later they appear in the feet followed by variable degrees of distal sensory loss. Weakness, cramps and clumsiness soon follow and are often severe. Weakness dominates vincristine neuropathy and is frequently disabling. Reflexes are lost early, probably reflecting muscle spindle afferent dysfunction.

Autonomic neuropathy with gastroparesis, constipation and urinary retention is frequent. Trigeminal sensory loss develops in 5-10% of cases.

Vincristine neuropathy is usually reversible even when there is significant weakness. In some patients, neuropathy abates following dose reduction, thus allowing continued use (Bradley *et al.*, 1970; Casey *et al.*, 1973).

Sural nerve biopsy studies show axonal degeneration as the prominent feature; biopsy of proximal muscles demonstrates myopathic changes. CNS changes develop in experimental animals exposed to vincristine (Bradley *et al.*, 1970; Casey *et al.*, 1973).

Vincristine binds to tubulin, the microtubule subunit protein, thereby inhibiting mitotic spindle formation. It is widely held that tubulin binding impairs axonal transport producing nerve fibre breakdown. Experimental studies that demonstrate abnormalities in fast axonal transport and cystoskeletal architecture support this notion (Sahenk *et al.*, 1987).

Putative neurotoxins

Many compounds have been implicated as neurotoxins in single case reports. Included in this category are amitriptyline (LeWitt and Forno, 1985), cytosine arabinoside (AraC) (Russell and Powles, 1974), lithium (Vanhooren *et al.*, 1990), methyl bromide (Kantarijian and Shaheen, 1963), glutethimide (Nover, 1967), phenylzine (Heller and Friedman, 1983) and phenobarbital (Taylor and Posner, 1989). Further studies will be necessary to determine whether these compounds can be confirmed as neurotoxins.

REFERENCES

Albin, R. L., Greenberg, H. S., Townsend, J. B. *et al.* (1987). Acute sensory neuropathy – neuronopathy from pyridoxine overdose. *Neurology*, **37**, 1729–1732

Allen, N., Mendel, J. R., Billmaier, J. *et al.* (1975). Toxic polyneuropathy due to methyl *n*-butyl ketone. *Arch. Neurol.*, **32**, 209–218

Altenkirch, H., Mager, J., Stoltenburg, G. and Helmbrecht, J. (1977). Toxic polyneuropathies after sniffing a glue thinner. *J. Neurol.*, **214**, 137–152

Amess, J. A. C., Rees, C. M., Burman, J. F. Nancekivilli, D. G. (1978). Megaloblastic hemopoiesis in patients receiving nitrous oxide. *Lancet*, **1**, 339–342

Apfel, S. C., Lipton, R. B., Arezzo, J. C. and Kessler, J. A. (1991). Nerve growth factor prevents toxic neuropathy in mice. *Ann. Neurol.*, **29**, 87

Araki, S. and Honma, T. (1976). Relationships between lead absorption and peripheral nerve conduction velocities in lead workers. *Scand. J. Work Environ. Health*, **4**, 225–231

Bank, W. J., Pleasure, D. E., Suzuki, K. *et al.* (1972). Thallium poisoning. *Arch. Neurol.*, **26**, 456–464

Berger, A., Schaumburg, H. H., Arezzo, J. *et al.* (1989). A prospective study of pyridoxine intoxication. *Ann. Neurol.*, **26**, 167

Bradley, W. G., Lassman, L. P., Pearce, G. W. and Walton, J. N. (1970). The neuromyopathy of vincristine in man. Clinical, electrophysiological and pathological studies. *J. Neurol. Sci.*, **10**, 107–131

Bradley, W. G., Karlsson, I. J. and Rassol, C. G. (1977). Metronidazole neuropathy. *Br. Med. J.*, **2**, 610–611

Buchthal, F. and Behse, F. (1979). Electrophysiology and nerve biopsy in men exposed to lead. *Br. J. Ind. Med.*, **36**, 135–147

Burns, S. M., Lange, D. J., Jaffe, I. *et al.* (1994). Axonal neuropathy in eosinophilia myalgia syndrome. *Muscle Nerve*, **17**, 293–298

Buxton, P. H. and Hayward, M. (1967). Polyneuritis cranialis associated with industrial trichlorethylene poisoning. *J. Neurol. Neurosurg. Psychiatry*, **30**, 511–518

Casey, E. B., Jelliffe, A. M., LeQuesne, P. M. and Millett, Y. L. (1973). Vincristine neuropathy – clinical and electrophysiological observations. *Brain*, **96**, 69–86

Cavanagh, J. B. (1954). The toxic effects of tri-ortho-cresyl phosphate on the nervous system. *J. Neurol. Neurosurg. Psychiatry*, **17**, 163–172

Cavanagh, J. B. and Buxton, P. H. (1989). Trichlorethylene cranial neuropathy: Is it really a toxic neuropathy or does it activate latent herpes virus? *J. Neurol. Neurosurg. Psychiatry*, **52**, 297–303

Cavanagh, J. B., Fuller, N. H., Johnson, H.R. M. and Rudge, P. (1974). The effects of thallium salts, with particular reference to the nervous system changes. *Q. J. Med.*, **43**, 293–319

Chang, Y. C. (1987). Neurotoxic effects of *n*-hexane on the human central nervous system: evoked potential abnormalities in *n*-hexane polyneuropathy. *J. Neurol. Neurosurg. Psychiatry*, **50**, 269–274

Chaudhry, V., Rowinsky, E. K., Sartorius, S. E. *et al.* (1994). Peripheral neuropathy from taxol and cisplatin combination chemotherapy: clinical and electrophysiological studies. *Ann. Neurol.*, **35**, 304–311

Cho, E. S., Spencer, P. S., Jortner, B. S. and Schaumburg, H. H. (1980). A single intravenous injection of doxorubicin (adriamycin) induces sensory neuropathy in rats. *Neurotoxicology*, **1**, 583–591

Cianchetti, C., Abbritti, G., Perticoni, G. *et al.* (1976). Toxic polyneuropathy of shoe-industry workers. *J. Neurol. Neurosurg. Psychiatry*, **39**, 1151–1161

Clark, A. W., Parhad, I. M., Griffin, J. W. and Price, D. L. (1980). Neurotoxicity of cis-platinum: pathology of the central and peripheral nervous systems. *Neurology*, **30**, 429

Coxon, A. and Pallis, C. A. (1976). Metronidazole neuropathy. *J. Neurol. Neurosurg. Psychiatry*, **39**, 403–405

Crystal, H. A., Schaumburg, H. H., Grober, E. *et al.* (1988). Cognitive impairment and sensory loss associated with chronic low-level ethylene oxide exposure. *Neurology*, **38**, 567–569

Frasca, V., Riazza, B. S. and Matthews, R. G. (1986). *In vitro* inactivation of methionine synthase by nitrous oxide. *J. Biol. Chem.*, **261**, 257–263

Fullerton, P. M. (1969). Electrophysiological and histological observations on peripheral nerves in acrylamide poisoning in man. *J. Neurol. Neurosurg. Psychiatry*, **32**, 186–192

Fullerton, P. M. and Kremer, M. (1961). Neuropathy after intake of thalidomide (Distaval). *Br. Med. J.*, **2**, 855–858

Fullerton, P. M. and O'Sullivan, D. J. (1968). Thalidomide neuropathy: a clinical, electrophysiological and histological follow-up. *J. Neurol. Neurosurg. Psychiatry*, **31**, 543–551

Gardner-Thorpe, C. and Benjamin, S. (1971). Peripheral neuropathy after disulfiram administration. *J. Neurol. Neurosurg. Psychiatry*, **34**, 253–259

Garland, T. O. and Patterson, M.W. H. (1967). Six cases of acrylamide poisoning. *Br. Med. J.*, **4**, 134–138

Gold, B. G., Griffin, J. W. and Price, D. L. (1985). Slow axonal transport in acrylamide neuropathy: different abnormalities produced by single-dose and continuous administration. *J. Neurosci.*, **5**, 1755–1768

Gross, J. A., Haas, M. L. and Swift, T. R. (1979). Ethylene oxide neurotoxicity: report of four cases and review of the literature. *Neurology (Minneapolis)*, **29**, 978–985

Gutmann, M. L., Martin, J. D. and Welton, W. (1976). Dapsone motor neuropathy – an axonal disease. *Neurology*, **26**, 514–516

He, F., Lu, B., Zhang, S. *et al.* (1985). Chronic allyl chloride poisoning. An epidemiological, clinical, toxicological and neuropathological study. *G. Ital. Med. Lav.*, **7**, 5

Helander, I. and Partanen, J. (1978). Dapsone-induced distal axonal degeneration of the motor neurons. *Dermatologia*, **156**, 321–324

Heller, C. A. and Friedman, P. A. (1983). Pyridoxine deficiency and peripheral neuropathy associated with long-term phenylzine therapy. *Am. J. Med.*, **75**, 887–888

Hirsch, M. S. and D'Aquila, R. T. (1993). Therapy for human immunodeficiency virus infection. *N. Engl. J. Med.*, **23**, 1686–1695

Johnson, M. K. (1990). Organophosphates and delayed neuropathy – is NTE alive and well? *Toxicol. Appl. Pharmacol.*, **102**, 385–389

Joy, R. J. T., Scalettar, R. and Sodee, D. B. (1960). Optic and peripheral neuritis. Probable effect of prolonged chloramphenicol therapy. *JAMA*, **173**, 1731–1734

Kantarijian, A. D. and Shaheen, A. S. (1963). Methyl bromide poisoning with nervous system manifestations resembling polyneuropathy. *Neurology*, **13**, 1054–1058

Kaplan, J. G. (1980). Neurotoxicity of selected biological toxins. In *Experimental and Clinical Neurotoxicology* (P. S. Spencer and H. H. Schaumburg, eds), pp. 631–648, Baltimore: Williams and Wilkins

Kaplan. J. G., Kessler, J., Pack, D. R. *et al.* (1986). Dursban causes peripheral neuropathy. *Neurology*, **36**, 176

Kaplan, J. G., Kessler, J., Rosenberg, N. *et al.* (1992). Chlorpyrifos (Dursban) causes peripheral neuropathy and cognitive dysfunction. *Neurology*, **42**, 269

Kaplan, J. G., Einzig, A. I. and Schaumburg, H. H. (1993a). Taxol causes permanent large fiber peripheral nerve dysfunction: a lesson for preventative strategies. *J. Neurooncol.*, **16**, 105–107

Kaplan J. G., Kessler, J., Rosenberg, N. *et al.* (1993b). Sensory neuropathy associated with Dursban (chlorpyrifos) exposure. *Neurology*, **43**, 2193–2196

Katrak, S. M., Pollock, M., O'Brien, C. P. *et al.* (1980). Clinical and morphological features of gold neuropathy. *Brain*, **103**, 671–693

Koller, W. C., Gehlmann, L. K., Malkinson, F. D. and Davis, F. A. (1977). Dapsone-induced peripheral neuropathy. *Arch. Neurol.*, **34**, 644–646

Korobkin R., Asbury, A. K., Sumner, A. J. and Nielsen, S. L. (1975). Glue-sniffing neuropathy. *Arch. Neurol.*, **32**, 158–162

Kuncl, R. W., Duncan, G., Watson, D. *et al.* (1987). Colchicine myopathy and neuropathy. *N. Engl. J. Med.*, **316**, 1562–1568

La Rocca, R. V., Meer, J., Gilliatt, R. W. *et al.* (1990). Suramin-induced polyneuropathy. *Neurology*, **40**, 954–960

Layzer, R., Fishman, R. A. and Schafer, J. A. (1978). Neuropathy following abuse of nitrous oxide. *Neurology (Minneapolis)*, **28**, 504–506

Leggat, P. O. (1962). Ethionamide neuropathy. *Tubercle*, **43**, 95–99

LeQuesne, P. M. (1993). Neuropathy due to drugs. In *Peripheral Neuropathy* (P. J. Dyck, P. K. Thomas, J. W. Griffin, *et al.*, eds), pp. 1571–1581, W. B. Saunders Co

LeQuesne, P. M. and McLeod, J. G. (1977). Peripheral neuropathy following a single exposure to arsenic. Clinical course in four patients with electrophysiological and histological studies. *J. Neurol. Sci.*, **32**, 437–451

LeWitt, P. (1980). The neurotoxicity of the rat poison vacor. *N. Engl. J. Med.*, **302**, 73–77

LeWitt, P. A. and Forno, L. S. (1985). Peripheral neuropathy following amitriptyline overdose. *Muscle Nerve*, **8**, 723–724

Lipton, R. B., Apfel, S. F., and Dutcher, J. P. (1989). Taxol produces a predominantely sensory neuropathy. *Neurology*, **39**, 368–373

Lovelace, R. E. and Horwitz, S. J. (1968). Peripheral neuropathy in long-term diphenylhydantoin therapy. *Arch. Neurol.*, **18**, 69–77

Mamoli, B., Wessely, P., Kogelnik, H. D. *et al.* (1979). Electroneurographic investigations of misonidazole polyneuropathy. *Eur. Neurol.*, **18**, 405–414

Martinez, A. C., Perez-Conde, M. C., Ferrer, M. T. *et al.* (1984). Neuromuscular disorders in a new toxic syndrome: electrophysiological study – a preliminary report. *Muscle Nerve*, **7**, 12–22

Martinez-Arizala, A., Sobol, S. M., McCarty, G. E. *et al.* (1983). Amiodarone neuropathy. *Neurology*, **33**, 643–645

Meier, C., Kauer, B., Muller, U. and Ludin, H. P. (1979). Neuromyopathy during chronic amiodarone treatment. A case report. *J. Neurol.*, **220**, 231–239.

Moddel, G., Bilbao, J. M., Payne, D. and Ashby, P. (1978). Disulfiram neuropathy. *Arch. Neurol.*, **35**, 658–660

Mokri, B., Oshnishi, A. and Dyck, P. J. (1981). Disulfiram neuropathy. *Neurology*, **31**, 730–735.

Murai, Y. and Kuroiwa, Y. (1971). Peripheral neuropathy in chlorobiphenyl poisoning. *Neurology (Minneapolis)*, **21**, 1173–1176

Nair, V. S., LeBrun, M. and Kass, I. (1980). Peripheral neuropathy associated with ethambutol. *Chest*, **77**, 98–100

Namba, T., Nolte, C. T., Jackrel, J. and Grob, D. (1971). Poisoning due to organophosphate insecticides. *Am. J. Med.*, **50**, 475–492

Nover, R. (1967). Persistent neuropathy following chronic use of glutethimide. *Clin. Pharmacol. Ther.*, **8**, 283–285

Ochoa, J. (1970). Isoniazid neuropathy in man: quantitative electron microscope study. *Brain*, **93**, 831–850

Ogawa, M. (1971). Electrophysiological and histological studies of experimental chlorobiphenyl poisoning. *Fukuoka Acta Med.*, **62**, 74–77

Ohnishi, A., Inoue, N., Yamamoto, T. *et al.* (1986). Ethylene oxide neuropathy in rats. Exposure to 250 ppm. *J. Neurol. Sci.*, **74**, 215–221

Osuntokun, B. O., Aladetoyindo, A. and Adevja, A. O. G. (1970). Free cyanide levels in tropical or toxic neuropathy. *Lancet*, **2**, 372–373

Parry, G. J. and Bredesen, D. E. (1985). Sensory neuropathy with low dose pyridoxine. *Neurology*, **35**, 1466–1468

Paulsen, I. and Nilsson, L. G. (1985). Distribution of acetylator phenotype in relation to age and sex in Swedish patients. A retrospective study. *Eur. J. Clin. Pharmacol.*, **28**, 311–315

Petersen, C. M., Tsairis, P., Ohnishi, A. *et al.* (1974). Sodium cyanate-induced polyneuropathy in patients with sickle cell disease. *Ann. Intern. Med.*, **81**, 152–158

Pollet, S., Hauw, J. J., Escourolle, R. and Baumann, N. (1977). Peripheral nerve lipid abnormalities in patients on perhexiline meleate. *Lancet*, **1**, 1258

Pomes, A., Frustaci, S., Cattaino, G. *et al.* (1986). Local neurotoxicity of cis-platinum after intra-arterial chemotherapy. *Acta Neurol. Scand.*, **73**, 302–303

Pont, A., Rubino, J. M., Bishop, D. *et al.* (1979). Diabetes mellitus and neuropathy following vacor ingestion in man. *Arch. Intern. Med.*, **139**, 185–187

Prick, J. J. G. (1979). Thallium poisoning. In *Handbook of Clinical Neurology* (P. J. Vinken and G. E. Bruyn, eds), Vol. 36, pp. 239–259, Amsterdam: North Holland Publishing

Ramirez, J. A., Mendell, J. R., Warmolts, J. R. and Griggs, R. C. (1986). Phenytoin neuropathy: structural changes in the sural nerve. *Ann. Neurol.*, **19**, 162–167

Raskin, N. H. and Fishman, R. A. (1965). Pyridoxine-deficiency neuropathy due to hydralazine. *N. Engl. J. Med.*, **273**, 1182–1185

Richardson, R. J. (1992). Interactions of organophosphate compounds with neurotoxic esterase. In *Organophosphates*, (J. E. Chambers and P. E. Levi, eds), pp. 299–323, San Diego: Academic Press

Ricoy, J. R., Cabello, A., Rodriguez, J. *et al.* (1983). Neuropathological studies related to the toxic syndrome related to adulterated rapeseed oil in Spain. *Brain*, **106**, 817–835

Roelofs, R. I., Hrushesky. W., Rogin, J. and Rosenberg, L. (1984). Peripheral sensory neuropathy and cisplatin chemotherapy. *Neurology*, **34**, 934–938

Russell, J. A. and Powles, R. L. (1974). Neuropathy due to cytosine arabinoside. *Br. Med. J.*, **14**, 652–653

Sahenk, Z., Mendell, J. R., Couri, D. and Nachtman, J. (1978). Polyneuropathy from inhalation of nitrous oxide cartridges through a whipped cream dispenser. *Neurology (Minneapolis)*, **28**, 485–487

Sahenk, Z., Brady, S. T. and Mendell, J. R. (1987). Studies on the pathogenesis of vincristine-induced neuropathy. *Muscle Nerve*, **10**, 80–84

Said, G. (1978). Perhexiline neuropathy: a clinicopathological study. *Ann. Neurol.*, **3**, 259–266

Schaumburg, H. H. (1991). Occupational biologic and environmental agents. In *Disorders of Peripheral Nerves* (H. H. Schaumburg, A. R. Berger and P. K. Thomas, eds), pp. 274–302, Philadelphia: F. A. Davis Company

Schaumburg, H. H. and Berger, A. R. (1993). Human toxic neuropathy due to industrial agents. In *Peripheral Neuropathy* (P. J. Dyck, P. K. Thomas, J. W. Griffin *et al.* eds), pp. 1533–1548, Philadelphia: W. B. Saunders

Schaumburg, H. H. and Spencer, P. S. (1979). Clinical and experimental studies of distal axonopathy – a frequent form of brain and nerve damage produced by environmental chemical hazards. *Ann. N. Y. Acad. Sci.*, **329**, 14–28

Schaumburg, H. H., Kaplan, J., Windebank, A. *et al.* (1983). Sensory neuropathy from pyridoxine abuse: a new megavitamin syndrome. *N. Engl. J. Med.*, **309**, 445–448

Senanayake, N. and Karalliedde, L. (1987). Neurotoxic effects of organophosphorus insecticides. An intermediate syndrome. *N. Engl. J. Med.*, **316**, 761–763

Seppalainen, A. M. and Haltia, M. (1980). Carbon disulfide. In *Experimental and Clinical Neurotoxicology* (P. S. Spencer and H. H. Schaumburg, eds), pp. 356–373, Baltimore: Williams and Wilkins

Seppalainen, A. M., Hernberg, S. and Kock, B. (1979). Relationship between blood lead levels and nerve conduction velocities. *Neurotoxicology*, **1**, 313–332

Smith, H. V. and Spalding, J.M.K. (1959). Outbreak of paralysis in Morocco due to ortho-cresyl phosphate poisoning. *Lancet*, **2**, 1019–1021

Spencer, P. S. and Schaumburg, H. H. (1974). A review of acrylamide neurotoxicity. I. Properties, users and human exposure. *Can. J. Neurol. Sci.*, **1**, 143–150

Spencer, P. S., Peterson, E. R., Madrid, R. and Raine, C. S. (1973). Effects of thallium salts on neuronal mitochondria in organotypic cord–ganglia–muscle combination cultures. *J. Cell Biol.*, **58**, 79–95

Sumner, A. J. and Asbury, A. K. (1975). Physiological studies of the dying-back phenomenon. Muscle stretch afferents in acrylamide neuropathy. *Brain*, **98**, 91–100

Taylor, L. P. and Posner, J. B. (1989). Phenobarbital rheumatism in patients with brain tumor. *Ann. Neurol.*, **25**, 92–94

Tellez-Nagel, I., Korthals, J. K., Vlassara, H. V. and Cerami, A. (1977). An ultrastructural study of chronic sodium cyanate-induced neuropathy. *J. Neuropath. Exp. Neurol.*, **36**, 351–363

Thomas, P. K. (1980). The peripheral nervous system as a target for toxic substances. In *Experimental and Clinical Neurotoxicology* (P. S. Spencer and H. H. Schaumburg, eds), pp. 35–47, Baltimore: Williams and Wilkins

Toole, J. F., Gergen, J. A., Hayes, D. M. and Felts, J. H. (1968). Neural effects of nitrofurantoin. *Arch. Neurol.*, **18**, 680–687

Urtasun, R. C., Chapman, J. D., Feldstein, M. L. *et al.* (1978). Peripheral neuropathy related to misonidazole: incidence and pathology. *Br. J. Cancer*, **111**, 271–275

Vanhooren, G., Dehaene, I., Van Zandycke, M. *et al.* (1990). Polyneuropathy in lithium intoxication. *Muscle Nerve*, **13**, 204–208

Walsh, J. (1970). Gold neuropathy. *Neurology*, **20**, 455–458

Watson, D. F. and Griffin, J. W. (1987). Vacor neuropathy: ultrastructural and axonal transport studies. *J. Neuropathol. Exp. Neurol.*, **46**, 96–108

Weller, R. O., Mitchell, J. and Doyle Daves, G. (1980). Buckthorn toxins. In *Experimental and Clinical Neurotoxicology* (P. S. Spencer and H. H. Schaumburg, eds), pp. 336–347, Baltimore: Williams and Wilkins

Whisnant, J. P., Espinosa, R. E., Kierland, R. R. and Lambert, E. H. (1963). Chloroquine neuromyopathy. *Mayo Clin. Proc.*, **38**, 501–513

Windebank, A. J. (1993). Metal neuropathy. In *Peripheral Neuropathy* (P. J. Dyck, P. K. Thomas, J. Griffin, P. Low, *et al.*, eds), pp. 1549–1570, Philadelphia: W. B. Saunders

Windebank, A. J. and Blexrud, M. D. (1989). Residual ethylene oxide in hollow fiber hemodialysis units is neurotoxic in vitro. *Ann. Neurol.*, **26**, 63–68

13
Critical illness polyneuropathy
C. F. Bolton

HISTORICAL REVIEW

Between 1977 and 1981 five unusual patients were observed in the critical care unit who presented as difficulty in weaning from the ventilator and severe weakness in the limbs (Bolton *et al.*, 1983, 1984). Comprehensive electrophysiological and morphological studies established this as a primary distal axonal degeneration of motor and sensory fibres (Bolton *et al.*, 1984). The aetiology was uncertain, but conditions such as Guillain–Barré syndrome, nutritional deficiency neuropathy, neuropathy secondary to collagen vascular disease, toxic neuropathy possibly due to antibiotics or heavy metals, and spinal cord trauma were considered. These possibilities were discounted and it seemed likely that sepsis and multiple organ failure were the chief underlying factors (Bolton and Young, 1986). An immediate reaction to our initial reports was that this was simply a variant of Guillain–Barré syndrome. However, a comparison of 15 patients with critical illness polyneuropathy, and 15 patients with Guillain-Barré syndrome, all studied in our unit during the same time period, indicated that the two types of polyneuropathies were quite distinctive with regard to antecedent or associated illnesses and electrophysiological and morphological features (Bolton *et al.*, 1986). Guillain–Barré syndrome was often preceded by a minor infection or inoculation, and with a latent period of days or weeks before the onset of the polyneuropathy, whereas critical illness polyneuropathy developed during the nidus of the critical illness (Bolton *et al.*, 1986). It was recognized that electrophysiological studies were crucial to identifying this type of polyneuropathy and, hence, they were used with increasing frequency in the Critical Care/Trauma Centre (Bolton, 1987). Thus, by 1983, 19 cases had been collected, were named 'critical illness polyneuropathy' and reported as a complication of sepsis and multiple organ failure (Zochodne *et al.*, 1987). During this time, it became evident that virtually all of these cases had had a septic encephalopathy preceding the development of the polyneuropathy and this as yet poorly recognized entity was to be more clearly defined in prospective investigations by Jackson *et al.* (1985) and Young *et al.* (1990). A prospective study of 43 patients was then conducted (Witt *et al.*, 1991) and determined that the incidence of the polyneuropathy in patients who had sepsis and multiple organ failure was 70%. In addition, antibiotics, neuromuscular blocking agents and nutritional deficiencies could not be proven to be aetiological factors, but features of the sepsis and multiple organ failure syndrome were. It was speculated that disturbances of the microcirculation to peripheral nerves, a phenomenon which seems to accompany all organ systems in the septic syndrome, was a possible pathophysiological mechanism (Zochodne *et al.*, 1987). From the beginning, it was clear that critical illness polyneuropathy was an important cause of difficulty in weaning from the ventilator when pulmonary and cardiac causes had been excluded, since confirmed in studies by Spitzer *et al.* (1989). Finally, electrophysiological and morphological features in some of our cases strongly suggested that sepsis also affected the muscle in the form of scattered muscle fibre necrosis, which was termed the 'myopathy in critical illness' (Zochodne *et al.*, 1986).

It is likely that polyneuropathy has always been a complication of severe sepsis, but before the advent of aggressive treatment with antibiotics, and support of blood pressure and breathing in intensive care units, death usually occurred quickly, before the polyneuropathy was clinically evident. Nonetheless, Osler (1892) mentioned muscle wasting as a complication of prolonged sepsis. In 1961, Mertens described 'coma–polyneuropathies' in patients who had circulatory shock associated with acute intoxication and severe metabolic crises, seemingly due to metabolic and ischaemic lesions of the peripheral nervous system. Erbsloh *et al.* (1989) observed a polyneuropathy following anoxic coma after cardiac arrest, but this may have been due to anterior horn cell ischaemia, which may be a cause of post-cardiac arrest quadriplegia. Erbsloh also described instances of polyneuropathy following the shock associated with haemorrhagic pancreatitis. In 1971, Henderson and colleagues described a peripheral neuropathy in patients with burns. In 1977, Bischoff *et al.* reported 4 patients who developed a severe polyneuropathy who were septic and had been treated with gentamicin. These investigators, on ultrastructural examination of the peripheral nerves, observed lysosomal abnormalities similar to those found in the kidney as a result of gentamicin nephrotoxicity. Thus they speculated that the polyneuropathy was secondary to the gentamicin. In 1983, Roelofs *et al.*, in the United States, reported in abstract form 'prolonged respiratory insufficiency due to an acute motor neuropathy: a new syndrome'. During the years that we were first observing our patients with critical illness polyneuropathy, Couturier and co-workers, in France, were making remarkably similar observations, and reported 11 patients in 1984. Four further cases were reported in 1987 by Barat and colleagues in France. In Holland, Lycklama *et al.* (1987) observed cases of critical illness polyneuropathy and because some patients recovered remarkably quickly, they proposed that there must be significant primary involvement of the muscle fibre membrane.

In 1985, Op de Coul and colleagues, in Holland, first reported 12 patients who had a severe, but reversible, axonal motor neuropathy which appeared due to the use of the competitive neuromuscular blocking agent, pancuronium bromide (Pavulon) to ease artificial ventilation. A number of similar cases have since been reported (Op de Coul *et al.*, 1985, 1991; Gooch *et al.*, 1991; Kupfer *et al.*, 1991; Rossiter *et al.*, 1991; Subramony *et al.*, 1991). Many of these patients also received corticosteroids and, particularly when this combination is used in association with the treatment of acute asthma, a severe myopathy results (Lacomis *et al.*, 1993), first reported by MacFarlene and Rosenthal in 1977. Sher and colleagues, in 1979, reported a patient who had acute pulmonary infection and shock and suffered a severe myopathy characterized by selective loss of myosin filaments. Zochodne *et al.* (1994) described seven patients with an 'acute necrotizing myopathy of intensive care' in which non-depolarizing neuromuscular blocking agents seemed to trigger the myopathy. Many of the patients in these reports were septic, often overlooked as a significant factor by the investigators.

It has now become recognized that neuromuscular conditions associated with sepsis are frequent but often unrecognized complications that occur in critical care units and which lead to difficulty in weaning from the ventilator and delay in recovery. The identification of these conditions has important implications in management, in determining prognosis and in assessing the cost effectiveness of procedures used in critical care units (Bolton *et al.*, 1994).

Finally, the recent adoption of the term 'systemic inflammatory response syndrome' (SIRS) to replace the 'septic syndrome' and greater knowledge of the mechanism of SIRS, allow inclusion of a variety of neuromuscular conditions, not all associated with management in critical care units. This chapter, therefore, will include a discussion of these more broadly defined conditions.

SEPSIS, THE SYSTEMIC INFLAMMATORY RESPONSE SYNDROME AND NERVOUS SYSTEM COMPLICATIONS

It was observed that patients with this polyneuropathy suffered from sepsis and multiple organ failure, or critical illness, a term commonly applied by intensivists to this group of patients. Hence, the condition was termed 'critical illness polyneuropathy' (Zochodne *et al.*, 1987). Critical illness is particularly common in intensive or critical care units, with incidences varying from 20 to 50% (Tran *et al.*, 1990). It is a major cause of morbidity and has a mortality rate of at least 50%.

A major problem has been confusion over definitions (Sibbald *et al.*, 1991). A meeting of the American College of Chest Physicians and The Society of Critical Care Medicine led to some agreement being reached (American College of Chest Physicians, 1992). There was a consensus that the term, 'systemic inflammatory response syndrome' (SIRS) should now be applied to a severe clinical insult that arose, not only as the result of infection but also as a result of non-infective processes such as trauma, burns and pancreatitis. The chief clinical features of this syndrome are two or more of: temperature $> 38°C$ or $< 36°C$; heart rate > 90 beats/min; respiratory rate > 20 breaths/min or $PaCO_2 < 32$ Torr (< 4.3 kPa); and white blood cell count (WBC) $> 12\,000$ cells/mm^3, or < 4000 cells/mm^3 or $> 10\%$ immature (band) forms. SIRS may be accompanied by hypotension (blood pressure < 90 mmHg or a reduction of > 40 mmHg from baseline in the absence of other causes for hypotension).

The concept of SIRS is important, since it suggests an explanation for certain nervous system conditions which have been ill-defined (Figure 13.1). Critical illness polyneuropathy, according to our view, has been a complication of SIRS (sepsis) in which there is multiple organ failure. However, SIRS may be associated with other neuromuscular conditions in the critical care unit (Table 13.1) (Figure 13.1). Moreover, critical illness polyneuropathy can clearly occur in patients who do not have infection but other critical conditions, such as severe trauma or burns, and its variants may occur outside the critical care unit.

We have not, nor to our knowledge have others, studied patients systematically in the earliest stages of sepsis to determine if the peripheral nerves are affected at that time. This would involve serial studies of the same patient beginning at the time of admission to the critical care unit. We are strongly suspicious that peripheral nerve dysfunction does occur at this time. Regression analysis of 43 patients in our pro-

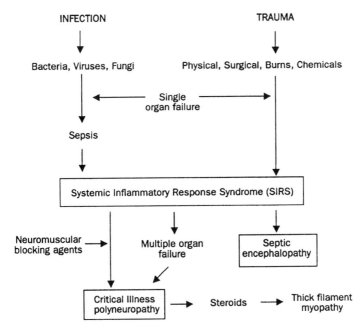

Figure 13.1 The various factors associated with the development of the systemic inflammatory response syndrome (SIRS) and its nervous system complications, septic encephalopathy and not only critical illness polyneuropathy but other neuromuscular complications.

spective study indicated that peripheral nerve function was at the lower limit of normal on admission to the critical care unit, and it progressively deteriorated thereafter (Witt *et al.*, 1991). The central nervous system (CNS) is clearly affected in the earliest stages of sepsis by septic encephalopathy, as shown in prospective studies by Young *et al.* (1990). Once the sepsis and multiple organ failure are treated successfully, these neurological complications progressively improve.

The pathophysiology of SIRS is currently under intensive investigation. The insulting agent, infection, trauma, etc., activate humoral and cellular mechanisms that initiate a series of events which ultimately lead to a severe disturbance of the microcirculation to various organs (Figure 13.2). The result is inadequate organ perfusion and multiple organ failure. Our clinical, electrophysiological and morphological investigations of the central and peripheral nervous systems in sepsis are consistent with these mechanisms affecting the microcirculation to brain and peripheral nerve.

CRITICAL ILLNESS POLYNEUROPATHY: A COMPLICATION OF SEPSIS AND MULTIPLE ORGAN FAILURE

Clinical and electrophysiological features

After the development of SIRS, the earliest nervous system manifestation is septic encephalopathy. Within hours of the appearance of a positive blood culture, careful

Table 13.1 Neuromuscular conditions in the critical care unit associated with the systemic inflammatory response syndrome (sepsis)

Conditions	Incidence	Clinical features	Electromyography	Creatine phosphokinase	Muscle biopsy
Polyneuropathy					
Critical illness polyneuropathy	Common	Flaccid limbs, respiratory weakness	Axonal degeneration of motor and sensory fibres	Near normal	Denervation atrophy
Motor neuropathy	Common with neuromuscular blocking agents	Flaccid limbs, respiratory weakness	Axonal degeneration of motor fibres	Near normal	Denervation atrophy
Neuromuscular transmission defect					
Transient neuromuscular blockage	Common with neuromuscular blocking agents	Flaccid limbs, respiratory weakness	Abnormal repetitive nerve stimulation studies	Normal	Normal
Myopathy					
Thick filament myopathy	Common with steroids, neuromuscular blocking agents and asthma	Flaccid limbs, respiratory weakness	Abnormal spontaneous activity	Elevated	Central loss of thick filaments
Disuse (cachectic myopathy)	Common(?)	Muscle wasting	Normal	Normal	Normal or type 2 fibre atrophy
Necrotizing myopathy of intensive care	Rare	Flaccid weakness, myoglobinuria	Abnormal spontaneous activity in muscle	Markedly elevated	Panfascicular muscle fibre necrosis

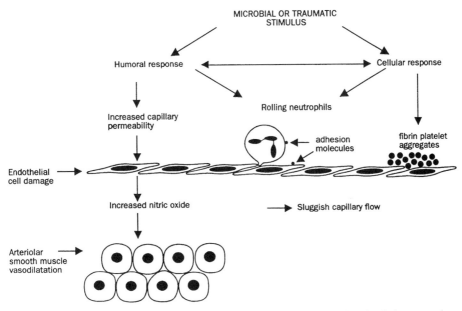

Figure 13.2 Schematic, theoretical presentation of disturbances in the microcirculation to various organs, including brain, peripheral nerve and muscle, in the systemic inflammatory response syndrome (sepsis). The result is impaired perfusion due to excessive vasodilatation through overproduction of nitric oxide, and aggregation of cellular elements through activation of adhesion molecules. Increaed capillary permeability causes oedema and the potential for entry of toxic substances.

testing reveals impaired attention, concentration, orientation and writing (Young *et al.*, 1990). If SIRS continues, the patient gradually slips into deep coma, usually without the development of focal signs, seizures, myoclonus or asterixis. The electroencephalogram (EEG) is a sensitive indicator of the presence and severity of septic encephalopathy. Computed tomography (CT) head scans and cerebrospinal fluid (CSF) examinations are usually unremarkable. Sedative or narcotic medication frequently used in the critical care unit is often a confounding factor, but the presence of significant elevation of blood levels of these drugs and the presence of excessive beta activity on the EEG may be helpful in diagnosis (Young *et al.*, 1992).

If the sepsis, and at this point multiple organ failure, can be brought under control, the encephalopathy usually improves rapidly but, at this time, it will be noticed that there is difficulty in weaning from the ventilator. Studies in our unit indicate that the commonest neuromuscular cause for this, after cardiac and pulmonary causes have been excluded, is critical illness polyneuropathy (Zochodne *et al.*, 1987; Maher *et al.*, 1993). However, clinical signs of neuropathy, including depressed tendon reflexes, are absent in only half of these patients. Hence, electrophysiological studies are necessary to firmly establish the diagnosis. The clinical presence of the polyneuropathy can be suspected when, on deep painful stimulation of the distal extremities, it will be noted that limb movements seem clearly weak despite strong grimacing of facial musculature. It is often quite safe to discontinue intermittent mandatory ventilation, providing that adequate amounts of pressure support are given through the ventilator with each inspiration. Then, on attempts at voluntary respiration, if there is a neuromuscular cause for the respiratory insufficiency, it will be noted that respiratory movements are rapid and weak and there is a progressive rise in the blood CO_2 level.

The earliest electrophysiological sign is a depression of compound muscle action potential amplitudes without any significant change in latency. This occurs within 1 week of axonal damage. Fibrillation potentials and positive sharp waves may not appear in muscle until 3 weeks. Motor unit potentials, if they can be activated by the patient (and may not be, due to sedation or septic encephalopathy) will often appear normal or somewhat low in amplitude and polyphasic, suggesting an associated primary involvement of muscle by sepsis. These electrophysiological changes could also be due to a primary myopathy. Hence, it is important to demonstrate depression of sensory compound action potential amplitudes before a firm electrophysiological diagnosis of polyneuropathy can be made. This is often difficult, since the normal range of compound sensory action potential amplitudes is quite large. Thus it is important to perform serial studies and a fall of sensory compound action potential amplitude if sepsis persists, or a rise if sepsis has been cured and recovery is occurring, provides more positive evidence of polyneuropathy.

Repetitive nerve stimulation studies to demonstrate a defect in neuromuscular transmission should also be performed. We have shown that this does not occur in sepsis but will be present if neuromuscular blocking agents have been used. Their effects may persist beyond several hours, a number of days if the patient is in renal or liver failure (Segredo *et al.*, 1992). It is also important to perform phrenic nerve conduction studies and needle electromyography of the chest wall and diaphragm to establish that the difficulty in weaning from the ventilator is, in fact, due to critical illness polyneuropathy (Bolton, 1993a).

Knowledge of the presence of critical illness polyneuropathy aids management on the ventilator and, in particular, indicates that the patient has a neuromuscular problem, which may prolong care in the critical care unit. If it is a mild polyneuropathy, recovery could be expected to occur within a matter of weeks, but if it is severe it may take months. In severe cases recovery may not occur. In patients who are recovering, physiotherapy and rehabilitation tailored to polyneuropathy should be instituted. Because of limb weakness, assistance will be required in eating and also with later attempts at sitting and walking.

Uncomfortable sensations, pain or paraesthesias, are not features of critical illness polyneuropathy. Their presence suggests a polyneuropathy secondary to the use of the antiobiotic, metronidazole, which characteristically affects sensory fibres (Witt *et al.*, 1991).

Since sepsis and multiple organ failure occur in children as well as adults in critical care units, instances of critical illness polyneuropathy might be anticipated in children. Sheth and Pryse-Philips (1994) have provided the first description, in four children. Dimachkie *et al.* (1994) have reported a further child, and we have just observed our first child.

Morphological features

Biopsy of peripheral nerve and muscle and comprehensive study of both the central and peripheral nervous systems in eight patients who died (Zochodne *et al.*, 1987) pointed to the presence of a primary axonal degeneration of peripheral nerve motor and sensory fibres, particularly distally. There was no evidence of inflammation.

Muscle showed scattered atrophic fibres in acute denervation, and grouped atrophy in chronic denervation. There were the occasional necrotic muscle fibres, suggesting an associated primary myopathy. The only CNS manifestation was central chromatolysis of anterior horn cells and loss of dorsal root ganglion cells, secondary to the polyneuropathy. To date, there have been no changes that appear distinctive for critical illness polyneuropathy.

Differential diagnosis

The differential diagnosis of critical illness polyneuropathy involves firstly patients who have been admitted to a critical care unit for a variety of severe, primary illnesses or injury and then, after a period of a few days or weeks, as they appear to be recovering, there is difficulty in weaning from the ventilator and possible weakness of the limbs (although neurological signs may be normal or equivocal in half the patients). A variety of lung or cardiac disorders will have been eliminated as a cause of difficulty in weaning from the ventilator. An underlying neuromuscular condition can be suspected if, on attempted weaning, attempted voluntary respirations are rapid and weak and accompanied by a rising blood CO_2 level.

Several tests may be necessary to solve this problem. Conditions of the high cervical spinal cord, peripheral nerve, neuromuscular junction and muscle should be systematically considered: thus, magnetic resonance image (MRI) scanning of the cervical spinal cord, a variety of electrophysiological tests, including testing of the respiratory system by phrenic nerve conduction studies and needle electromyography of the diaphragm, measurements of creatine kinase and biopsy of muscle, rarely nerve. Anaesthetists recommend testing for a defect in neuromuscular transmission by applying four maximal stimuli to a peripheral nerve (the train of four) and simply visualizing or palpating the muscular response. This is probably too inaccurate and neuromuscular transmission should be tested by repetitive nerve stimulation and recording the compound muscle action potential according to standard techniques.

In most instances, it is possible to exclude conditions such as acute infective or neoplastic spinal cord compression, Guillain–Barré syndrome, myasthenia gravis and muscular dystrophy, since their clinical features are usually obvious before endotracheal intubation and placement on a ventilator. However, occasionally, the conditions develop so rapidly that a diagnosis is not possible. Motor neuron disease, in particular, may present for the first time with primary neuromuscular respiratory failure, requiring intubation and ventilation. The diagnosis must then be established by testing while the patient is in the critical care unit.

A second type of differential diagnosis involves patients who have developed their neuromuscular problem after admission to the critical care unit as a complication of primary illness or injury, outside the nervous system. Most of these patients will be suffering from SIRS (Figure 13.1). Moreover, in the last few years, the use of competitive neuromuscular blocking agents (Klessig *et al.*, 1992), at times in conjunction with high-dose steroids in cases of severe asthma, has produced distinctive neuromuscular conditions, seemingly complications of the use of these agents, but usually in the setting of SIRS. These should probably be regarded as variants of critical illness polyneuropathy.

VARIANTS OF CRITICAL ILLNESS POLYNEUROPATHY ENCOUNTERED IN THE CRITICAL CARE UNIT (Table 13.1)

Acute motor neuropathy associated with competitive neuromuscular blocking agents

In this condition (Op de Coul *et al.*, 1985; Gooch *et al.*, 1991; Kupfer *et al.*, 1991; Rossiter *et al.*, 1991; Subramony *et al.*, 1991), the patient will have been in the critical care unit for several days, or possibly even weeks, and competitive neuromuscular blocking agents, such as pancuronium bromide, or the shorter-acting vecuronium, will have been given to ease mechanical ventilation. Atracurium appears to be relatively free of neuromuscular side effects. These neuromuscular blocking agents will have been used for longer than 48 hours, occasionally for days or weeks. On attempted weaning from the ventilator, it is noted that, in addition to severe respiratory neuromuscular paralysis, there is paralysis of all four limbs. Plasma creatine kinase activity is mildly or moderately elevated. Electrophysiological testing may or may not reveal a defect in neuromuscular transmission. If present, it will be demonstrated on slower rates of stimulation, to be expected in a postsynaptic defect. There is evidence of a severe primary axonal degeneration, predominantly of motor fibres, on nerve conduction and needle electromyographic studies. Muscle biopsy shows varying degrees of denervation atrophy and muscle necrosis. It is believed that SIRS is an important underlying factor in most, if not all, of these patients. Thus, if the various systemic complications can be treated successfully, the neuromuscular condition, itself, improves spontaneously and good recovery may occur, sometimes quite rapidly.

Transient neuromuscular blockade

The competitive neuromuscular blocking agents, notably vecuronium, are cleared by the liver and kidney. Hence in the presence of failure of these organs, the effect of the neuromuscular blocking agent may be quite prolonged after it has been discontinued, for up to a number of days (Segredo *et al.*, 1992). In our experience, repetitive stimulation studies will correctly identify the defect in neuromuscular transmission if the effect is only going to be transient. However, by the time of testing, many of these patients will already have developed an underlying critical illness polyneuropathy and, here, recovery will not occur within a short period but may be prolonged for several weeks, or even months in severe cases.

Myopathy

Thick filament myopathy

A distinctive syndrome (Danon and Carpenter, 1991; Douglass *et al.*, 1992; Hirano *et al.*, 1992; Lacomis *et al.*, 1993) occurs in children or adults in the setting of sudden, severe asthma. Endotracheal intubation and placement on a ventilator is necessary. High-dose steroids to treat the asthma and neuromuscular blocking agents to ease ventilation are given, often for a number of days. Again, on attempted weaning from the ventilator, it will be noted that the patient has severe neuromuscular respiratory insufficiency and severe weakness in all four limbs. In one patient, complete ophthalmoplegia was present, in addition to weakness of limb and respiratory muscles (Sitwell *et al.*, 1991). Plasma creatine kinase levels are often considerably elevated. Repetitive stimulation studies do not usually reveal a defect in neuromuscular transmission. Nerve conduction studies reveal normal sensory conduction but a low-amplitude compound muscle action potential in the presence of normal latencies. Needle electromyography usually gives the finding of a primary myopathy; that is, motor unit potentials tend to be low-amplitude, short-duration and polyphasic. Muscle biopsy shows a loss of structure centrally in muscle fibres which, under the electron microscope has been shown to be due to destruction of the thick myosin filaments (Danon and Carpenter, 1991).

Recovery occurs quite rapidly. The clinical and electrophysiological features are usually so distinctive in this syndrome that open muscle biopsy is often not necessary, a particularly worthwhile consideration in children because of the disfiguring scar.

Many now recommend that neuromuscular blocking agents should be used to ease ventilation only when there are clear-cut indications, in as low a dosage, and for as short a period as possible.

Disuse (cachectic) myopathy

Cachectic myopathy or disuse atrophy, catabolic myopathy (Clowes *et al.*, 1983) or diaphragmatic fatigue (Roussos and Macklem, 1982) are often cited as complications of critical illness. However, all three are ill-defined in clinical terms. Motor and sensory nerve conduction studies, needle electromyography of muscle and plasma creatine kinase levels are all normal. Muscle biopsy may be normal or show type 2 muscle fibre atrophy.

Acute necrotizing myopathy of intensive care

Rarer, but more well-defined, is 'acute necrotizing myopathy of intensive care.' It may be precipitated by a wide variety of infective, chemical and other insults, basically involving the differential diagnosis of acute myoglobinuria (Penn, 1986). It would be expected to occur with increased frequency in critical care units, in which there is a high incidence of trauma, the use of various medications, etc. Thus Ramsay *et al.*, (1993) and Zochodne *et al.*, (1994) reported 11 cases in the critical care unit in which there was severe weakness with high levels of creatine kinase and often myoglobinuria. Electromyography was consistent with a severe myopathy, and muscle biopsy showed severe necrosis. Often, rapid and sponteneous recovery occurs, but in more severe cases, notably those reported by Ramsay and colleagues, the prognosis was not as good.

Mild elevations of creatine kinase have been observed and on muscle biopsy scattered necrosis of muscle fibres, in some critically ill patients, suggesting primary involvement of muscle in critical illness, as well as denervation atrophy. This may be due to a reduction in bioenergetic reserves as measured by ^{31}P NMR spectroscopy, since two of our patients had very low ratios of phosphocreatine to inorganic phosphate, more than would be expected from denervation of muscle alone (Bolton *et al.*, 1994). These abnormalities returned towards normal as the patients recovered from the critical illness and from the polyneuropathy. Nonetheless, biopsy performed in

11 of our patients in the critical care unit, because of uncertainties about the nature of the neuromuscular condition, were all dominated by denervation atrophy, presumably secondary to a critical illness polyneuropathy (Pringle *et al.*, 1992).

THE PATHOPHYSIOLOGY OF THE NEUROMUSCULAR COMPLICATIONS OF SIRS (SEPSIS)

The initial stimulus may be either infective or traumatic. Both humoral and cellular processes are activated (Figure 13.2). These interact with resulting release of mediators of SIRS: cytokines, arachidonic acid, oxygen free radicals and proteases. The chief deleterious effect is disturbances of the microcirculation throughout the body. Here, adhesion molecules are formed (Glauser *et al.*, 1991) which cause the phenomenon of 'rolling neutrophils'. Fibrin–platelet aggregates are also formed. These cellular elements impede microcirculatory flow. The mediators also cause increased capillary permeability and endothelial cell damage. There is excessive release of nitric oxide from damaged endothelial cells. Nitric oxide is now known to be the endovascular relaxing factor (Palmer *et al.*, 1987). As a result, there is relaxation of arteriolar smooth muscles and vasodilatation. This further enhances poor flow and resulting stasis in capillaries. Thus various essential nutrients and substrates are prevented from reaching the end organ. For example, despite adequate oxygenation through endotracheal intubation and ventilation, there is a severe oxygen deficit at the level of the microcirculation. The severe dysfunction of both the central and peripheral nervous systems that occurs in sepsis could therefore be anticipated.

Retrospective (Zochodne *et al.*, 1987) and prospective (Witt *et al.*, 1991) studies have failed to incriminate a variety of potential causes for critical illness polyneuropathy, including types of primary illness or injury, Guillain–Barré syndrome, medications including aminoglycoside antibiotics and neuromuscular blocking agents and specific nutritional deficiencies. Thus it seemed likely that sepsis was the cause (Zochodne *et al.*, 1987; Witt *et al.*, 1991). The severity of the polyneuropathy can be quantified from electrophysiological data (Witt *et al.*, 1991). It tends to be more severe the longer each patient is in the critical care unit. Sepsis and multiple organ failure also tend to increase in frequency and severity under similar conditions. Increasing blood glucose and decreasing serum albumin concentrations correlate with decreasing peripheral nerve function (Witt *et al.*, 1991). Both biochemical changes are well-recognized manifestations of the sepsis and multiple organ failure syndrome.

As has been noted, the microcirculation of various organs is disturbed in sepsis (Figure 13.3). Blood vessels supplying peripheral nerves lack autoregulation (Low *et al.*, 1987), rendering them particularly susceptible to such disturbances. Moreover, cytokines that are secreted in sepsis have histamine-like properties which may increase microvascular permeability. The resulting endoneurial oedema could induce hypoxia by increase in intercapillary distance and other mechanisms. This could result in severe energy deficits and induce primary axonal degeneration, most likely distally, if highly energy-dependent systems involving axonal transport of structural proteins are involved. The predominantly distal involvement may explain why the recovery phase in some patients may be surprisingly short, conforming to the short length of nerve through which axonal regeneration takes place. It is also possible that cytokines, themselves, may have a direct toxic effect on peripheral nerve. To our knowledge, such has not been demonstrated, either in humans or experimental

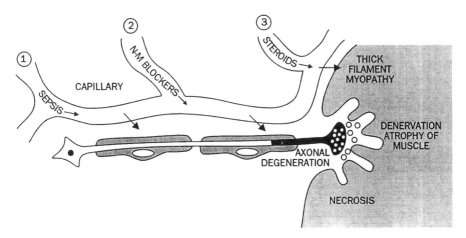

Figure 13.3 Schematic illustration of theoretical mechanisms of neuromuscular syndromes associated with sepsis. Sepsis induces release of cytokines which cause increased capillary permeability. 1. This, and other microvascular mechanisms, may induce critical illness polyneuropathy, with distal axonal degeneration of nerve and denervation atrophy of muscle. 2. Neuromuscular (N-M) blocking agents traverse the hyperpermeable capillary membrane and have direct toxic effect on nerve, to increase denervation of muscle. 3. Steroids gain access to muscle by this mechanism and, in the presence of denervation due to 1 and 2, induce a thick filament myopathy. (Reproduced from Bolton (1993b), with permission.)

animals. However, tumour necrosis factor decreases the resting transmembrane potential of skeletal muscle fibres *in vitro* (Tracey *et al.* 1986). It also induces muscle proteolysis in animals (Fong, 1989). However, we (G. P. Rice, C. F. Bolton and N. J. Witt, 1989, unpublished data) investigated seven patients who were in the critical care unit for between 2 to 67 days; five of these patients had critical illness polyneuropathy. No patient showed elevated levels of tumour necrosis factor. However, it is known that these levels rise only transiently over a matter of a few hours with each episode of sepsis. Thus only well-designed prospective studies with frequent clinical and electrophysiological testing and measurements of tumour necrosis factor, would determine the true role of this and other cytokines in the genesis of the polyneuropathy.

Disturbances of the microcirculation to nerve and muscle may also explain the effects of neuromuscular blocking agents and steroids. Through increased capillary permeability induced by the sepsis, neuromuscular blocking agents, notably vecuronium or its metabolite, 3-desacetyl-vecuronium (Segredo *et al.*, 1992), could have a direct toxic effect on peripheral nerve axons. These neuromuscular blocking agents may also cause functional denervation through their prolonged neuromuscular blocking action (Wernig *et al.*, 1980). The result would be denervation atrophy of muscle and a relatively pure motor neuropathy.

Concern has always been expressed that antibiotics, particularly aminoglycosides with their known neural toxicity, might cause critical illness polyneuropathy. They might gain access to peripheral nerve as a result of capillary permeability. However, there has been no statistical proof that antibiotics cause peripheral nerve dysfunction in sepsis (Witt *et al.*, 1991). Nonetheless, this possibility should be explored in experimental animals.

This schema (Figure 13.3) also explains the acute myopathy which develops when asthmatic patients are treated with neuromuscular blocking agents and steroids. It is suspected that many of these patients suffer from the systemic inflammatory response syndrome since infection is often a precipitating event in acute, severe asthma. Thus critical illness polyneuropathy, in its very early stages, and then the additive effect of neuromuscular blocking agents, would produce acute denervation of muscle. Novel experiments by Karpati *et al.* (1972) have shown in the experimental animal that if the muscle is first denervated by nerve transection and then steriods are given, a thick filament myopathy similar to that seen in humans can be induced. Thus, in the human condition, critical illness polyneuropathy and the additional effects of neuromuscular blocking agents would be the necessary mechanisms of the initiating neuropathy before steroids could produce the typical myopathy changes.

This mechanism may also explain further myopathies reported in critical care unit patients. A rapidly evolving myopathy, reported recently by Al-Lozi *et al.* (1994), was characterized by deficiency of thick filaments throughout the muscle fibres, not just centrally. The extensive necrosis of muscle fibres in the syndrome of acute, severe muscle necrosis in intensive care unit patients, reported by Ramsay *et al.* (1993) and Zochodne *et al.* (1994) may simply represent a further stage of this process.

VARIANTS OF CRITICAL ILLNESS POLYNEUROPATHY SEEN OUTSIDE THE CRITICAL CARE UNIT

Up to this point, critical illness polyneuropathy and the differential diagnosis of this condition has been considered in the setting of the critical care unit and the underlying factors of the systemic inflammatory response syndrome (sepsis) and multiple organ failure. However, taking a broader view, it should be considered in other clinical situations, including those outside the critical care unit. Here, trauma or infection may combine with single organ failure to produce SIRS and then critical illness polyneuropathy (Figure 13.1).

Patients in end-stage renal disease may develop a particularly severe and rapidly-developing axonal, predominantly motor, polyneuropathy should they experience trauma or sepsis (Bolton and Young, 1990). Recurring attacks of sepsis were particularly common during the early years of chronic haemodialysis, when Scribner shunts were used. It is possible that the lessening incidence of this severe type of polyneuropathy coincided with the switch to Cimino–Brescia fistulas in which recurring attacks of sepsis were less frequent. This, rather than changes in dialysis techniques, may be the major reason for the decline in the incidence of severe uraemic neuropathy.

Chronic liver disease induces a mild, predominantly demyelinating motor and sensory polyneuropathy (Asbury, 1993). Severe sepsis might be expected to induce a critical illness polyneuropathy in this setting. The authors have had one such case, briefly reported here (M. J. Strong, D. Munoz and C. F. Bolton, unpublished data).

Case report: critical illness polyneuropathy due to sepsis and severe liver disease

The patient was aged 50 years and had suffered from alcohol-induced cirrhosis of the liver. However, he had stopped drinking alcoholic beverages 8 years previously. He was admitted to hospital for possible liver transplantation when it was noticed that he had developed peritonitis secondary to a shunt infection. The shunt was removed but the offending organism was never cultured. He was treated with gentamicin and cloxacillin, with good results, over a period of 2 weeks. The gentamicin blood levels were never in the toxic range and he was never shown to have impairment of hearing or of renal function. Ten days after the onset of the sepsis, it was noticed he was unsteady when walking and had numbness in his hands which extended proximally to the elbows. Less severe numbness was present distally in the lower limbs. There was no evidence of postural hypotension or fluctuation in blood pressure.

On examination, he was emaciated but was alert and cheerful and had never shown signs of encephalopathy. There was mild hand tremor and asterixis. There was mild weakness distally in all four limbs. The tendon reflexes were absent. Vibration sense was markedly impaired in all four limbs. Position sense was lost to the wrists but was only mildly impaired in the toes. Two-point discrimination was absent over the palms and soles of the feet. There was a mild distal loss to pinprick below the mid-forearms and upper calves. He had moderately severe ataxia in the upper limbs, worse with the eyes closed. This ataxia was milder on heel–shin testing in the lower limbs. His gait was moderately ataxic.

CSF examination was normal. Electrophysiological studies revealed only mild prolongation of latencies but reduction in compound muscle and sensory nerve action potentials. Needle electromyography showed some fibrillation potentials and positive sharp waves in muscles in the upper and lower limbs. The findings were consistent with an axonal motor and sensory polyneuropathy.

The right superficial and deep peroneal nerves and adjacent muscle were biopsied. The nerves showed evidence of a primary axonal degeneration of motor and sensory fibres without inflammation (Figure 13.4). There were many acutely degenerating, large myelinated fibres. Schwann cells were swollen and contained lipid and myelin debris. There were signs of axonal regeneration, axonal sprouts and thinly myelinated fibres. Electron microscopy showed that unmyelinated nerve fibres were also affected.

The muscle biopsy showed denervation atrophy, manifested by atrophic fibres with nuclear clusters, small, dark, angulated fibres and type grouping, with predominance of type I fibres. There were no signs of vasculitis or inflammation.

A variety of tests was performed to exclude commonly recognized causes for polyneuropathy, such as deficiency of vitamin B_{12}, folate and vitamin E. All were normal.

It was concluded the patient had critical illness polyneuropathy. It stabilized in hospital. A liver transplantation was attempted but he died postoperatively.

Other variants of critical illness polyneuropathy

Gorson and Ropper (1993) have described five patients who developed critical illness polyneuropathy as an unusually early complication of severe respiratory insufficiency, later requiring ventilator support. Four of the five had multiple organ failure

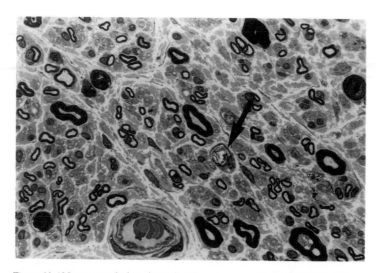

Figure 13.4 Nerve morphology in patient (see case report) who had critical illness polyneuropathy associated with liver failure and sepsis. Plastic-embedded, toluidine blue-stained section of superficial peroneal nerve, showing numerous fibres undergoing Wallerian degeneration (one labelled with an arrow). Decreased fibre density and clusters of regenerated fibres are seen. No inflammatory infiltrates are present (magnification × 1000).

and received steroids and polyneuropathy blocking agents; two recovered substantially from the polyneuropathy.

Post-transplantation

Patients in the postoperative state following organ transplantation, because of immunosuppression, have a tendency to recurring infections. Hence, critical illness polyneuropathy might be expected to occur in this setting. However, there appear to have been no such reports in the scientific literature. Amato *et al.* (1993) reported four patients who developed a severe, generalized polyneuropathy as a presumed complication of graft-versus-host disease. There was electrophysiological evidence of more demyelination than has been observed in critical illness polyneuropathy, and the authors speculated that this was a different form of polyneuropathy. The polyneuropathy improved after treatment with immunosuppression, or with the resolution of the graft-versus-host disease or the tissue rejection.

Burns

Severe burns are an important traumatic cause of the systemic inflammatory response syndrome. In a landmark study by Koepke and colleagues (Henderson *et al.*, 1971) at the University of Michigan Burn Unit, clinical and electrophysiological studies showed that a polyneuropathy was present in 15% of the patients. They anticipated present theories by speculating underlying metabolic or toxic causes.

The incidence in further studies varied from 3 to 50% (Helm *et al.*, 1977; Marquez *et al.*, 1993). Marquez *et al.* (1993) believed that the polyneuropathy in their patients consisted chiefly of a mononeuritis multiplex. However, most of the patients suffered from either sepsis or renal failure and it is likely these were important underlying factors. In two well-described patients, de Saint-Victor and colleagues in France (1994) emphasized that patients with severe burns have a typical critical illness polyneuropathy which is simply a manifestation of the systemic inflammatory response syndrome.

Demoic acid

Teitelbaum *et al.* (1990) reported a polyneuropathy as a toxic effect of the ingestion of demoic acid through eating mussels. Leijten and De Weerd (1990) have questioned whether sepsis and multiple organ failure was the main mechanism for the polyneuropathy. I agree with this, and speculate that the severe chemical insult induced a systemic inflammatory response syndrome, with complicating septic encephalopathy and critical illness polyneuropathy.

HIV-1 infection

A variety of types of polyneuropathy may be associated with HIV-1 infection (Lange, 1994). Because of immunosuppression, these patients are susceptible to recurring infections. However, the axonal polyneuropathy that occurs is predominatly sensory in its manifestation. It seems unlikely, therefore, that critical illness polyneuropathy is a complication of AIDS.

Guillain–Barré syndrome

Finally, patients who have severe Guillain–Barré syndrome, are in critical care units and on ventilators, may have sepsis and multiple organ failure secondary to the invasive procedures of endotracheal intubation and intravascular lines. Thus a worsening in their peripheral neuropathy may be attributed to an exacerbation of the Guillain–Barré syndrome. But if electrophysiological studies show this worsening to be entirely due to axonal degeneration, in my view it is more likely to be due to critical illness polyneuropathy. Thus instead of further attempts at immunosuppression, management of sepsis should be the prime consideration.

ACKNOWLEDGEMENTS

I am grateful to Betsy Toth for secretarial assistance, to Dr George Rice for measuring levels of tumour necrosis factor, to Dr David Munoz for supplying the pathological slide for Figure 13.4, and to my colleagues in Clinical Neurological Sciences and Critical Care Medicine.

REFERENCES

Al-Lozi, M. T., Pestronk, A., Yee, W. C. *et al.* (1994). Rapidly evolving myopathy with myosin-deficient muscle fibres. *Ann. Neurol.*, **35**, 273–279

Amato, A. A., Barohn, R. J., Sahenk, Z. *et al.* (1993). Polyneuropathy complicating bone marrow and solid organ transplantation. *Neurology*, **43**, 1513–1518

American College of Chest Physicians/Society of Critical Care Medicine Consensus Conference: definitions for sepsis and organ failure and guidelines for the use of innovative therapies in sepsis. (1992). *Crit. Care Med.*, **20**(6), 864–874

Asbury, A. K. (1993). Neuropathies with renal failure, hepatic disorders, chronic respiratory insufficiency, and critical illness. In *Peripheral Neuropathy* (P. J. Dyck and P. K. Thomas, eds), pp. 1251–1265, W. B. Saunders Co

Barat, M., Brochet, P., Bital, C. *et al.* (1987). Polyneuropathies au cours de sejours prolonges en reanimation. *Rev. Neurol. (Paris)*, **143**, 823–831

Bischoff, A., Meier, C. and Roth, F. (1977). Gentamicin-neurotoxizität (Polyneuropathie-enkephalopathie). *Schweiz. Med. Wochenschr.*, **107**(1), 3–8

Bolton, C. F. (1987). Electrophysiologic studies of critically ill patients. *Muscle Nerve*, **10**, 129–135

Bolton, C. F. (1993a). Clinical neurophysiology of the respiratory system. A.A.E.M. Minimonograph #40. *Muscle Nerve*, **16**, 809–818

Bolton, C. F. (1993b). Neuromuscular complications of sepsis. *Intensive Care Med.*, **19**, 558–563

Bolton, C. F. and Young, G. B. (1986). Sepsis and septic shock: central and peripheral nervous systems. In *New Horizons: Perspectives on Sepsis and Septic Shock* (W. J. Sibbald and C. L. Sprung, eds), pp. 157–171, Society of Critical Care Medicine

Bolton, C. F. and Young, G. B. (1990). *Neurological Complications of Renal Disease*, p. 79, Butterworth

Bolton, C. F., Brown, J. D. and Sibbald, W. J. (1983). The electrophysiologic investigation of respiratory paralysis in critically ill patients. *Neurology (Cleveland)*, **33**, 186

Bolton, C. F., Gilbert, J. J., Hahn, A. F. and Sibbald, W. J. (1984). Polyneuropathy in critically ill patients. *J. Neurol. Neurosurg. Psychiatry*, **47**, 1223–1231

Bolton, C. F., Laverty, D. A., Brown, J. D. *et al.* (1986). Critically ill polyneuropathy: electrophysiological studies and differentiation from Guillain–Barré syndrome. *J. Neurol. Neurosurg. Psychiatry*, **49**, 563–573

Bolton, C. F., Young, G. B. and Zochodne, D. W. (1994). Neurological changes during severe sepsis. In *Current Topics in Intensive Care*, **1**, 180–217

Clowes, G. H. A., George B. C. and Villee, C. A. (1983). Muscle proteolysis induced by a circulating peptide in patients with sepsis or trauma. *N. Engl. J. Med.*, **308**, 545–552

Couturier, J. C., Robert, D. and Monier, P. (1984). Polynévrites compliquant des sejours prolongés en réanimation: a propos de 11 cas d'étiologie encore inconnue. *Lyon Méd.*, **252**, 247–249

Danon, M. J. and Carpenter, S. (1991). Myopathy and thick filament (myosin) loss following prolonged paralysis with vecuronium during steroid treatment. *Muscle Nerve*, **14**, 1131–1139

de Saint-Victor, J. F., Durand, G., Le Gulluche, Y. and Hoffmann, J. J. (1994). Neuropathies du syndrome de sepsis avec defaillance multiviscerale chez les brules: 2 cas avec revue de la litterature. *Rev. Neurol. (Paris)*, **150**, 149–154

Dimachkie, M., Austin, S. G., Slopis, J. M. and Vriesendorp, F. J. (1994). Critical illness polyneuropathy in childhood. *J. Child Neurol.*, **9**, 207

Douglass, J. A., Tuxen, D. V., Horne, M. *et al.* (1992). Myopathy in severe asthma. *Am. Rev. Respir. Dis.*, **146**, 517–519

Erbsloh, F. and Abel, M. (1989). Deficiency neuropathies. In *Handbook of Clinical Neurology* (J. Vinken and G. W. Bruyn, eds), Chapter 23, North Holland

Fong, Y. (1989). Cachectin/TNF or II-1a induces cachexia with redistribution of body proteins. *Am. J. Physiol.*, **256**, 659–665

Glauser, M. P., Zanetti, G., Baumgartner, J-D. *et al.* (1991). Septic shock: pathogenesis. *Lancet*, **338**, 732–736

Gooch, J. L., Suchyta, M. R. and Balbierz, J. M. (1991). Prolonged paralysis after treatment with neuromuscular junction blocking agents. *Crit. Care Med.*, **19**, 1125–1131

Gorson, K. C. and Ropper, A. H. (1993). Acute respiratory failure neuropathy: a variant of critical illness polyneuropathy. *Crit. Care Med.*, **21**, 267–271

Helm, P. A., Johnson, E. R. and Carlton, A. M. (1977). Peripheral neurological problems in the acute burn patient. *Burns*, **3**, 123–125

Henderson, B., Koepke, G. H. and Feller, I. (1971). Peripheral polyneuropathy among patients with burns. *Arch. Phys. Med. Rehabil.*, **52**, 149–151

Hirano, M., Ott, B. R. and Raps, E. C. (1992). Acute quadriplegic myopathy: complication of treatment with steroids, nondepolarizing blocking agents, or both. *Neurology*, **42**, 2082–2087

Jackson, A. C., Gilbert, J. J., Young, G. B. and Bolton, C. F. (1985). The encephalopathy of sepsis. *Can. J. Neurol. Sci.*, **12**, 303–307

Karpati, G., Carpenter, S. and Eisen, A. A. (1972). Experimental core-like lesions and nemaline rods: a correlative morphological and physiological study. *Arch. Neurol.*, **27**, 247–266

Klessig, H. T., Geiger, H. J., Murray, M. J. and Coursin, D. B. (1992). A national survey on the practice patterns of anesthesiologist intensivists in the use of muscle relaxants. *Crit. Care Med.*, **20**, 1341–1345

Kupfer, Y., Namba, T., Kaldawi, E. *et al.* (1991). Prolonged weakness after long-term infusion of vecuronium bromide. *Ann. Intern. Med.*, **117**, 484–486

Lacomis, D., Smith, T. W. and Chad, D. A. (1993). Acute myopathy and neuropathy in status asthmaticus: case report and literature review. *Muscle Nerve*, **16**, 84–90

Lange, D. J. (1994). Neuromuscular diseases associated with HIV-1 infection. *Muscle Nerve*, **17**, 16–30

Leijten, F.S. S. and de Weerd, A. W. (1990). Letter to the Editor. *N. Engl. J. Med.*, **323**, 1631

Low, P. A., Tuck, R. R. and Takeuchi, M. (1987). Nerve microenvironment in diabetic neuropathy. In *Diabetic Neuropathy* (P. J. Dyck, P. K. Thomas, A.K.Asbury, *et al.*, eds), pp. 268–277, W. B. Saunders

Lycklama, J., Nijeholt, A. and Troost, J. (1987). Critical illness polyneuropathy. In *Handbook of Clinical Neurology* (W. B. Matthews, ed), pp. 129–135. Elsevier Science Publishers BV

MacFarlene, I. A. and Rosenthal, F. D. (1977). Severe myopathy after status asthmaticus. *Lancet*, **11**, 615

Maher, J., Rutledge, F., Remtulla, H. *et al.* (1993). Neurophysiological assessment of failure to wean from a ventilator. *Can. J. Neurol. Sci.*, **20** (suppl. 2), S28

Marquez, S., Turley, J. J. E. and Peters, W. J. (1993). Neuropathy in burn patients. *Brain*, **116**, 471–483

Mertens, H. G. (1961). Die disseminierte Neuropathie nach Koma. *Nervenarzt*, **32**, 71–79

Op de Coul, A. A. W., Lambregts, P. C. L. A., Koeman, J. *et al.* (1985). Neuromuscular complications in patients given Pavulon (pancuronium bromide) during artifical ventilation. *Clin. Neurol. Neurosurg.*, **87**, 17–22

Op de Coul, A. A. W., Verheul, G. A. M., Leyten, A. C. M. *et al.* (1991). Critical illness polyneuromyopathy after artificial respiration. *Clin. Neurol. Neurosurg.*, **93**, 27–33

Osler, W. (1892). *The Principles and Practice of Medicine*, pp. 114–118. D. Appleton

Palmer, R. M. J., Ferrige, A. G. and Moncada, S. (1987). Nitric oxide release accounts for the biological activity of endothelium-derived relaxing factor. *Nature*, **327**, 524–526

Penn, A. S. (1986). Myoglobinuria. In *Myology*, Vol. 2 (A. G. Engel and B. Q. Baker, eds), pp. 1792–1793, McGraw-Hill

Pringle, C. E., Bolton, C. F., Ramsay, D. A. *et al.* (1992). Muscle biopsy in critical illness: electrophysiological and morphological correlations. *Can. J. Neurol. Sci.*, **19**, 297

Ramsay, D. A., Zochodne, D. W., Robertson, D. M. *et al.* (1993). A syndrome of acute severe muscle necrosis in intensive care unit patients. *J. Neuropath. Exper. Neurol.*, **52**, 387–398

Roelofs, R. I., Cerra, F., Bielka, N. *et al.* (1983). Prolonged respiratory insufficiency due to acute motor neuropathy: a new syndrome. *Neurology*, **33**, 240

Rossiter, A., Souney, P. F., McGowan, S. *et al.* (1991). Pancuronium-induced prolonged neuromuscular blockade. *Crit. Care Med.*, **19**, 1583–1587

Roussos, C. and Macklem, P. T. (1982). The respiratory muscles. *N. Engl. J. Med.*, **307**, 786–797

Segredo, V., Caldwell, J. E., Matthay, M. A. *et al.* (1992). Persistent paralysis in critically ill patients after long-term administration of vecuronium. *N. Engl. J. Med.*, **327**, 524–528

Sher, J. H., Shafiq, S. A. and Schutta, H. S. (1979). Acute myopathy with selective lysis of myosin filaments. *Neurology*, **29**, 100–106

Sheth, R. D. and Pryse-Philips, W. E. M. (1994). Post-ventilatory quadriplegia: critical illness polyneuropathy in childhood. *Neurology*, **44**, A169

Sibbald, W. J., McCormack, D., Marshall, J. *et al.* (1991). Sepsis – clarity of existing terminology – or more confusion? *Crit. Care Med.*, **19**, 996–998

Sitwell, L. D., Weinshenker, B. G., Monpetit, V. and Reid, D. (1991). Complete ophthalmoplegia as a complication of acute corticosteroid- and pancuronium-associated myopathy. *Neurology*, **41**, 921–922

Spitzer, A. R., Maher, L., Awerbuch, G. *et al.* (1989). Neuromuscular causes of prolonged ventilator dependence. *Muscle Nerve*, **12**, 775

Subramony, S. H., Carpenter, D. E., Raju, S. *et al.* (1991). Myopathy and prolonged neuromuscular blockade after lung transplant. *Crit. Care Med.*, **19**, 1580–1582

Teitelbaum, J. S., Zatorre, R. J., Carpenter, S. *et al.* (1990). Neurologic sequelae of domoic acid intoxication due to the ingestion of contaminated mussels. *N. Engl. J. Med.*, **322**, 1781–1787

Tracey, K. J., Lowry, S. F., Beutler, B. *et al.* (1986). Cachectin/tumour necrosis factor mediates human muscle denervation: topical 31-P NMR spectroscopy studies. *Magn. Reson. Med.*, **7**, 373–383

Tran, D. D., Groeneveld, A. A. J. B., van der Meulen, J. *et al.* (1990). Age, chronic disease, sepsis, organ system failure, and mortality in a medical intensive care unit. *Crit. Care Med.*, **18**, 474–479

Wernig, A., Pecot-Dechavassine, M. and Stover, H. (1980). Sprouting and regression of the nerve at the frog neuromuscular junction in normal conditions and after prolonged paralysis with curare. *J. Neurocytol.*, **9**, 277–303

Witt, N. J., Zochodne, D. W., Bolton, C. F. *et al.* (1991). Peripheral nerve function in sepsis and multiple organ failure. *Chest*, **99**, 176–184

Young, G. B., Bolton, C. F., Austin, T. W. *et al.* (1990). The encephalopathy associated with septic illness. *Clin. Invest. Med.*, **13**, 297–304

Young, G. B., Bolton, C. F., Austin, T. W. *et al.* (1992). The electroencephalogram in sepsis-associated encephalopathy. *J. Clin. Neurophysiol.*, **9**, 145–152

Zochodne, D. W., Bolton, C. F., Thompson, R. T. *et al.* (1986). Myopathy in critical illness. *Muscle Nerve*, **9**, 652

Zochodne, D. W., Bolton, C. F., Wells, G. A. *et al.* (1987). Critical illness polyneuropathy: a complication of sepsis and multiple organ failure. *Brain*, **110**, 819–842

Zochodne, D. W., Ramsay, D. A., Saly, V. *et al.* (1994). Acute necrotizing myopathy of intensive care: electrophysiological studies. *Muscle Nerve*, **17**, 285–292

14
Biopsy of peripheral nerve tissue

P. K. Thomas

INTRODUCTION

Until about 25 years ago nerve biopsy was infrequently employed as a diagnostic procedure, its use largely being confined to the diagnosis of leprosy, vasculitis and inherited storage disorders. With the introduction of electron microscopy, the reintroduction of teased fibre studies, and the use of morphometric assessment (Thomas, 1971) and, later, the availability of immunohistochemical and immunocytochemical techniques, nerve biopsy became considerably more informative. It is now widely employed. Nevertheless, it is an invasive procedure with a significant complication rate. Its indications therefore need to be precisely defined. Apart from biopsy of cutaneous sensory nerves, peripheral nerve tissue can be sampled from other sites, ranging from the dorsal root ganglia to terminal nerve plexuses in the skin and mucous membranes. This chapter surveys the range of procedures that are now available and assesses the clinical utility of biopsy of peripheral nerve tissues.

TYPE OF BIOPSY

Dorsal root ganglia and spinal roots

Biopsy of dorsal root ganglia is rarely merited but has been undertaken in patients with dorsal root ganglionitis associated with Sjögren syndrome (Griffin et al., 1990). As a research procedure it has been performed in patients with Friedreich's ataxia (Lamarche et al., 1982; Small et al., 1993). It may be merited in cases of progressive sensory ganglionitis with inflammatory changes in the cerebrospinal fluid (CSF) if a diagnosis cannot be achieved by other means. A mid-thoracic ganglion with adjacent spinal root is obtained under general anaesthesia through a midline incision over the spine and dissection to the junction of the facet and transverse process on one side. A partial facetectomy allows exposure of the ganglion. In patients with Friedreich's ataxia the T4 ganglion was obtained at the time of a corrective operation for kyphoscoliosis (Small et al., 1993). Because of dermatomal overlap there is no sensory loss following removal of a single mid-thoracic ganglion and postoperative pain or dysaesthesias have not been encountered.

Brachial plexus

Open surgical biopsy from the brachial plexus may be necessary for diagnostic purposes. This is most likely to arise when there is difficulty in distinguishing between postradiation damage and malignant infiltration, usually in patients with a previous history of carcinoma of the breast. Computed tomography (CT) or magnetic resonance (MR) imaging may yield equivocal findings (Cascino *et al.*, 1983). Exposure of the brachial plexus may be sufficient to reveal malignant tissue that can be sampled, but as the carcinoma can spread intrafascicularly it may be necessary to remove a thickened fascicle (Thomas and Holdorff, 1993). Diagnostic difficulty may also arise in distinguishing between malignant invasion and focal hypertrophic inflammatory neuropathy (Cusimano *et al.*, 1988) which may require fascicular biopsy for clarification.

Cutaneous sensory nerves

Some neuropathies have a proximal distribution and in these sampling of a proximal nerve may be informative. In hypertrophic neuropathies with nerve enlargement, the great auricular nerve, which often stands out prominently in the neck, has been chosen at times (Thévenard and Berdet, 1958). Such neuropathies are usually diffuse and however tempting this nerve may appear, it is generally more justifiable to select a distal nerve. Proximal sensory nerves in the upper arm are not readily accessible, but if a somewhat more distal sensory nerve is acceptable, the anterior branch of the medial cutaneous nerve of the forearm is available and can be exposed on the medial aspect of the upper arm before it crosses anterior to the medial epicondyle of the humerus. It supplies the medial border of the forearm. The lateral antebrachial cutaneous nerve, which is the sensory branch of the musculocutaneous nerve and supplies the lateral aspect of the forearm, has also been used (Dyck *et al.*, 1984). It can be biopsied in the proximal forearm. Normative morphometric data are not available for these nerves.

In the lower limb, the intermediate cutaneous nerve of the thigh can be sampled. It is readily found superficial to the deep fascia over the rectus femoris muscle through an incision in the midline of the thigh halfway between the groin and the knee. It was recently used by Said *et al.* (1994) in the investigation of patients with diabetic proximal lower-limb neuropathy.

As most polyneuropathies have a distally accentuated distribution, biopsy of a distal cutaneous sensory nerve is usually appropriate. In the lower limbs the sural nerve at a retromalleolar site is most often selected as a large body of normative data is available (e.g. Jacobs and Love, 1985). The superficial peroneal (musculocutaneous) nerve is also favoured in some centres as a muscle biopsy can be taken from peroneus brevis at the same time (Gherardi *et al.*, 1986). The saphenous nerve at the ankle can be biopsied just proximal to the medial malleolus. In multifocal neuropathies in which the medial aspect of the lower leg is affected to a greater extent, this nerve may be selected. Biopsy of the saphenous nerve has also been undertaken proximally in the thigh where it passes through the femoral trigone (Dyck *et al.*, 1984). The terminal sensory branch of the deep peroneal nerve was chosen for biopsy in some early studies (Greenfield and Carmichael, 1935; Aring *et al.*, 1941) but the high variability found in normal subjects by Swallow (1966) makes this nerve less suitable for morphometric evaluation.

In the upper limb, the radial nerve at the wrist is most commonly chosen, although leprologists tend to favour the second dorsal digital branch to the medial side of the thumb. In patients with multifocal neuropathies in which the ulnar territory is predominantly involved the dorsal branch of this nerve as it winds around the medial side of the wrist is useful.

The size of the biopsy that is required will depend upon the suspected pathology. In a disorder such as a hereditary or toxic neuropathy that will affect the peripheral nerves diffusely, a restricted fascicular biopsy is likely to be informative. If a patchy process is suspected, such as vasculitis, amyloidosis, leprosy or chronic inflammatory demyelinating polyneuropathy (CIDP), a larger portion is merited, either subtotal (i.e. removing the major width of the nerve but leaving one or two fascicles in continuity) or total.

Mixed and motor nerves

Biopsy of motor nerves is rarely undertaken but may be necessary in purely motor inflammatory neuropathies. A fascicular biopsy from the deep peroneal nerve just distal to the neck of the fibula can be obtained but carries the risk of increasing the severity of muscle weakness. Alternatively, nerves to muscles, weakness of which would produce little detectable functional deficit, can be chosen. The nerves to anconeus, palmaris longus and peroneus brevis have been used in this way. Stevens *et al.* (1973) described a technique for simultaneous biopsy from the superficial peroneal nerve and the distal deep peroneal nerve.

Fascicular biopsy from a major nerve trunk such as the ulnar, median, radial, tibial or peroneal nerves may be necessary in patients with a focal neuropathy affecting one of these nerves and in whom focal enlargement of the nerve has been demonstrated by MR imaging. Distinction between a nerve tumour and focal hypertrophic inflammatory neuropathy (Mitsumoto *et al.*, 1990) or focal hypertrophic neurofibrosis (Simpson and Fowler, 1966) is not always possible clinically and electrophysiologically. Biopsy may prevent sacrifice of the whole nerve if the pathology is shown to be benign. Focal amyloid deposition (amyloidoma) is a further possibility in such cases (Birch, 1993).

Terminal regions

Motor point biopsy with intravital methylene blue staining was introduced in the 1950s (Coërs and Woolf, 1959) and although this revealed interesting findings, it did not prove clinically useful. Muscle biopsy to examine motor end plate morphology has been informative in research studies on disorders of neuromuscular transmission (Engel and Santa, 1971).

Cutaneous innervation can be studied in skin biopsies and the ganglion cells of the myenteric plexus in rectal biopsies. In the past this was helpful in the diagnosis of neuronal storage disorders. It is now less frequently required as leucocyte enzyme estimation is available for the investigation of GM1 and GM2 gangliosidosis and for the sphingolipidoses. Skin biopsy is still valuable in the diagnosis of neuronal ceroid lipofuscinosis (Carpenter *et al.*, 1977) and GM2 gangliosidosis related to activator protein deficiency.

Although attempts have been made in the past to study cutaneous innervation in skin biopsies, this has been handicapped by problems in identifying the finer ramifications of the cutaneous nerve plexuses. Johnson and Doll (1984), using electron microscopy, demonstrated thickening of the perineurial basal laminae in small skin nerve fascicles in diabetic neuropathy.

It had generally been believed that cutaneous receptors were situated in the dermis or in the deepest part of the epidermis. The ability to reveal fine nerve fibres by the immunohistochemical demonstration of reactivity to protein gene product (PGP) 9.5 and the use of confocal microscopy showed that the dermis contains a profuse network of fine nerve fibres that penetrate the epidermis to reach the surface of the skin (Kennedy and Wendelschafer-Crabb, 1993). The presence of nerve fibres in the epidermis was confirmed by electron microscopy. Kennedy and Wendelschafer-Crabb (1994) found that in comparison with the PGP 9.5-reactive fibres, those reacting for calcitonin gene-related peptide (CGRP) were less numerous, with fewer again reactive for substance P. In normal skin there were dense networks of nerve fibres around the sweat ducts. Biopsies from patients with diabetic neuropathy either showed a paucity of such fibres or there was hyperinnervation with multiple short branches. Also employing PGP 9.5 immunoreactivity, McArthur *et al.*, (1994) showed reduced cutaneous innervation in sensory neuropathies and in denervated skin after nerve biopsy. Cutaneous innervation can be quantified by these techniques which are likely to be useful in the future in the diagnosis of neuropathies and in monitoring therapy.

Combined nerve and muscle biopsy

In some disorders both peripheral nerve and muscle may be affected and a higher diagnostic yield is obtained by combined nerve and muscle biopsy. This applies in particular to vasculitis but it may be appropriate in a number of other conditions such as sarcoidosis and mitochondrial disorders. Combined nerve and muscle biopsy can be achieved through a single incision for the superficial peroneal nerve and peroneus brevis, the sural nerve in the calf and gastrocnemius and the intermediate cutaneous nerve of the thigh and rectus femoris.

INDICATIONS FOR BIOPSY

Confirmation of neuropathy

The clinical features, in combination with nerve conduction studies, are usually sufficient to establish a diagnosis of neuropathy, although difficulties can arise in some circumstances. This is most likely to be encountered in selective small-fibre neuropathies where nerve conduction studies, which assess large-fibre function, may be normal. Such patients may show elevated thermal sensory thresholds but this does not establish peripheral nerve disease. Even in patients with sensory neuropathies that have affected large fibres, because of the wide range of sensory nerve action potential amplitude in normal subjects, an individual with neuropathy may lose a substantial number of nerve fibres and still retain a sensory action potential with an amplitude that falls within the normal range. Nerve biopsy in patients in both these categories may be crucial in demonstrating the presence of neuropathy by morphometric analysis to assess nerve fibre density and involvement of small myelinated and unmyelinated axons and to look for evidence of active nerve fibre degeneration. In most other circumstances it is inadvisable to undertake biopsy unless the nerve action potential is demonstrably abnormal.

Diagnosis of cause of neuropathy

The usual indication for nerve biopsy is in an attempt to establish the cause of the disorder in an undiagnosed neuropathy. In general terms, biopsy is most useful in suspected inflammatory disorders such as leprosy, vasculitis and CIDP and in amyloid neuropathy. It is helpful in the recognition of acquired and inherited disorders of myelination in which there are distinctive changes, in some axonopathies such as those producing giant axonal neuropathy, and in a variety of storage disorders. The salient pathological changes in these conditions are discussed below.

In most chronic axonopathies, diagnostic changes are not seen. Nevertheless, in an undiagnosed chronic progressive neuropathy, with significant disability, a 'last resort' nerve biposy is justifiable. Gratifying surprises do happen!

Biopsy for research purposes

With informed consent, nerve biopsy may be undertaken as part of a research study. As an example, the spectacular advances that have taken place in recent years in the molecular genetics of the hereditary motor and sensory neuropathies (see Chapter 6) depended upon the prior establishment of genetic heterogeneity and the identification of different genetic entities. In this, nerve biopsy played a vital role in combination with clinical, genetic and electrophysiological studies. For the future, nerve biopsy is likely to play an important role in working out the way in which a particular gene defect leads to the observed structural changes in nerve. It is also likely to continue to be valuable in elucidating the immunological mechanisms involved in acute and chronic inflammatory demyelinating polyneuropathy. Studies on dorsal root ganglia may well be helpful in elucidating disease mechanisms in the spinocerebellar degenerations that include degeneration of the primary sensory neurons.

In recent years, serial nerve biopsies have come to be used in the evaluation of treatment for diabetic neuropathy (Sima *et al.*, 1988). Structural changes in nerve have been used as a surrogate for clinical assessment on the basis that changes in nerve fibre density in sensory nerves have been shown to be correlated with changes in sensation. The main variables employed have been nerve fibre density and the amount of remyelination and regenerative activity. A substantial number of questions still require to be answered before this type of assessment can convincingly be used to evaluate treatment effects. In the first place it needs to be shown that regenerating axon sprouts achieve functional connections at the periphery. Moreover, diabetic polyneuropathy involves a distal 'dying-back' axonopathy (Said *et al.*, 1983). It is not yet established whether the centrally directed axons entering the central nervous system (CNS) are similarly affected, that is, whether diabetic neuropathy is a central–peripheral distal axonopathy (Spencer and Schaumburg, 1976). If so, regeneration in the peripheral nervous system would be of no advantage.

Assessment of the extent of regeneration is not simple. Counts of the numbers of regenerative clusters of myelinated axons give an inadequate estimate as to the amount of regeneration unless regenerative clusters that have not yet myelinated and regenerating unmyelinated axons are also taken into account. This can only be done by electron microscopy which presents considerable difficulties. Assessment of regeneration in teased fibres can only be achieved effectively for fibres of larger diameter (see below) which will exclude a high proportion of regenerating fibres. These will be of small calibre. Remyelination can be recognized in teased fibre preparations, but a greater number of remyelinating fibres in the second biopsy will indicate that a greater amount of demyelination has taken place in the period that has intervened since the first biopsy. The same could also be argued for axonal regeneration.

BIOPSY TECHNIQUE AND SPECIMEN PROCESSING

Nerve biopsy is only a minor surgical procedure but should be undertaken with particular care to avoid damage to the specimen from crushing, stretching or drying. It is preferably performed by the same person on a regular basis. The laboratory technician who will process the specimen should be present in the operating department to receive it. Processing should only be performed by a committed laboratory as it differs considerably from that afforded to routine surgical specimens. Routine procedures may be satisfactory for the diagnosis of inflammatory disorders such as leprosy or vasculitis but not for most other conditions.

The techniques employed have now been relatively well standardized between laboratories. In brief, the specimen is carefully divided with a sharp blade into three or more portions after trimming off the divided ends which will have been damaged during surgical removal. Two portions are fixed in a buffered paraformaldehyde/glutaraldehyde solution and subdivided. Following postosmication and dehydration, subdivided segments are in epoxy resin for semithin sectioning for observations by light microscopy and ultrathin sections for electron microscopy. One segment is processed into epoxy resin without accelerator and kept refrigerated until required for teasing. A third unfixed portion is frozen in liquid nitrogen and stored at −70°C for frozen sections for histochemistry and immunocytochemistry. Paraffin sections are still used in some laboratories.

The range of procedures employed for a given biopsy will depend upon the clinical problem. Semithin transverse sections of epoxy resin-embedded material are routine. Laboratories have preferences for the staining technique utilized. Toluidine blue is frequently adopted, but a combination of thionin and acridine orange (Sievers, 1971) or methylene blue, azure II and basic fuchsin (Humphrey and Pittman, 1974) gives better differentiation between tissue components. If morphometric studies on myelinated nerve fibres are required, these are undertaken on semithin transverse sections employing a semi-automatic image analysis system. Morphometry of unmyelinated axons requires electron miscroscopy. Teased fibre analysis is laborious and unless a laboratory is particularly well staffed it is often reserved for selected cases. Electron microscopy is probably desirable in most cases. Immunocytochemistry to identify lymphocyte subsets or immunohistochemistry to recognize immunoglobulin deposition or to characterize amyloid deposits is performed when required.

INFORMATION OBTAINED BY NERVE BIOPSY

What follows is an abbreviated account of the range of information that may be derived by the examination of nerve bioposies so that the clinical usefulness of the procedure can be appreciated. Detailed accounts of peripheral nerve pathology can be found elsewhere (Vital and Vallat, 1987; Bouche and Vallat, 1992; Thomas *et al.*, 1992; Dyck *et al.*, 1993).

Axonal changes

Axonal loss

Active degeneration of myelinated nerve fibres of Wallerian type can be recognized in semithin sections by the presence of myelin debris, usually within Schwann cells or macrophages. If very acute, myelin ovoids containing degenerate axoplasm will be seen. Active axonal degeneration is also detectable in teased fibre preparations as linear rows of myelin droplets in degenerating fibres. Completed axonal degeneration is revealed by electron microscopy as groups of proliferated Schwann cells within the persisting basal lamina of the fibre, the so-called bands of Büngner. Active degeneration of unmyelinated axons is more difficult to recognize and to distinguish from poor fixation but loss of unmyelinated axons is indicated by the presence of stacks of flattened Schwann cell processes.

Fibre loss can be assessed by total counts of myelinated and unmyelinated axons if a total nerve biopsy has been performed. This involves counting randomly selected areas and obtaining total counts from estimates of fascicular area. If a fascicular biopsy has been performed, fibre density is estimated. This can be made difficult by the presence of endoneurial oedema. Also, representative values can only be obtained from fascicles of medium or large size; small fascicles tend to have abnormally low densities (O'Sullivan and Swallow, 1968). Fibre loss may be relatively uniform between fascicles but can affect individual fascicles selectively or parts of fascicles. Patchy fibre loss is most often seen in ischaemic neuropathies and leprosy and can be a feature in CIDP.

Axonal loss may involve myelinated fibres of all diameters and also unmyelinated axons, or it may be selective. This is demonstrated from histograms of fibre size distribution. Fibre (and axon) diameter should be obtained by measurements of perimeter, converting this to the diameter of an equivalent circle. Estimates based on measurements of cross-sectional area introduce errors in fibres that are laterally compressed. Fibres sectioned in the paranodal region or through Schwann call nuclei should be excluded. A number of broad patterns of fibre loss are recognizable. Predominant loss of the large alpha myelinated fibres is seen in conditions such as Friedreich's ataxia (Dyck *et al.*, 1971b; McLeod, 1971) and uraemic neuropathy (Thomas *et al.*, 1971). Care has to be taken in accepting selective large-fibre loss as this pattern can be produced spuriously in a neuropathy in which there has been loss of fibres of all sizes but in which large numbers of small regenerating fibres are present. In 'small-fibre neuropathies', as may be seen in amyloidosis (Dyck and Lambert, 1969), dominantly inherited sensory neuropathy (Dyck *et al.*, 1971b), Fabry's disease (Kocen and Thomas, 1970; Ohnishi and Dyck, 1974) and Tangier disease (Kocen *et al.*, 1973), there is a predominant loss of the small myelinated A delta fibres and of unmyelinated axons. Other patterns of loss are also encountered.

These various patterns can be diagnostically helpful, particularly in the categorization of the hereditary sensory neuropathies (see Thomas, 1993a).

Axonal pathology

Axonal atrophy is a feature of some neuropathies and its recognition is considered later. Giant axonal change (Figures 14.1 and 14.2) consists of focal enlargement by collections or irregularly orientated neurofilaments and it is seen in inherited giant axonal neuropathy (Asbury *et al.*, 1972a; Donaghy *et al.*, 1988) and as a conse-

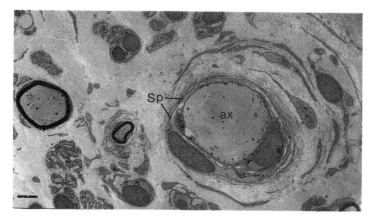

Figure 14.1 Hereditary giant axonal neuropathy. Electron micrograph of transverse section through sural nerve showing greatly enlarged axon (ax) containing neurofilaments surrounded by circumferentially orientated Schwann cell processes (Sp). Bar = 5μm.

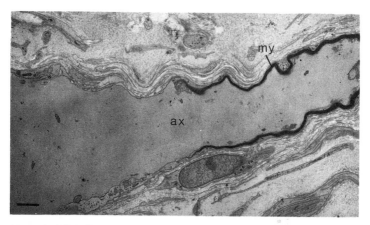

Figure 14.2 Hereditary giant axonal neuropathy. Electron micrograph of longitudinal section through sural nerve. A greatly enlarged axon (ax) containing neurofilaments is ensheathed by a thin myelin layer (my) to the right of the figure but is completely demyelinated where it expands in the left side of the figure. Bar = 5μm.

quence of solvent abuse (Korobkin *et al.*, 1975). Intervening regions of the axon are often atrophic and contain microtubules without neurofilaments. Specific abnormal intra-axonal inclusions are encountered infrequently but are occasionally seen in some lysosomal storage disorders. Glycogenosomes may be found non-specifically but are particularly frequent in adult polyglucosan body disease. 'Dystrophic' axons containing abnormal accumulations of mitochondria and secondary lysosomes are a non-specific feature.

Axonal regeneration

Evidence of early regeneration is occasionally seen in the presence of growth cones. The main hallmark of regeneration of myelinated axons is the occurrence of clusters of myelinated and unmyelinated axons associated with Schwann cells, initially within the confines of the basal lamina that had surrounded the degenerated fibre. Regeneration can also be recognized in teased fibre preparations by the presence of fibres with uniformly short internodes in relation to the diameter of the fibre. This becomes difficult in small-calibre fibres which are then hard to distinguish from normal small fibres as the range of internode lengths for a given diameter is wide. Regeneration of unmyelinated axons is recognized on electron microscopy where they are seen as groups of small axons surrounded but not enveloped by Schwann cell processes.

Disturbances of myelination: Schwann cell pathology

Demyelination

Loss of myelin with preservation of axonal continuity can be the result of pathology affecting the myelin directly or Schwann cell (primary demyelination) or it may be secondary to disturbances in axons (secondary demyelination). Primary demyelination can be recognized in teased fibre preparations and in sectioned nerve, both by light and electron microscopy. It may result from direct mechanical damage as in compression neuropathy (Ochoa, 1980), but this is rarely the occasion for nerve biopsy. A few toxic neuropathies are demyelinating, such as those due to perhexilene (Said, 1978) and amiodarone (Meier *et al.*, 1979). Active demyelination is rarely seen in paraproteinaemic neuropathy or in the hereditary demyelinating neuropathies because of their chronicity, although it may be encountered in the latter during childhood. It is most often observed in the Guillain–Barré syndrome and CIDP when it is the result of active stripping of myelin by macrophages (Prineas, 1972). Intramyelinic oedema can be observed during demyelination (Waddy *et al.*, 1989). Secondary demyelination is related both to axonal atrophy which occurs, for example, in uraemic neuropathy (Dyck *et al.*, 1971a) or around expanded axons in giant axonal neuropathy (Figure 14.2). Secondary demyelination tends to be clustered along the length of individual fibres whereas primary demyelination affects internodes randomly. Teased fibre preparations are required to assess this.

Remyelination

Remyelination is most easily recognized in teased fibres. It can take the form of restricted areas of thin myelin following paranodal demyelination or short intercalated internodes often with thin myelin. Remyelination of whole internodal segments that had been demyelinated results in a series of consecutive short internodes, again often with thin myelin, between internodes of normal length and myelin thickness. Once mature myelin has formed, remyelination is recognized as abnormal variability in internodal length along individual fibres.

The relationship between myelin thickness and axon diameter can be examined by plotting one against the other graphically. A measure of relative myelin thickness is given by the 'g' ratio (axon diameter/total fibre diameter). If the 'g' ratio is plotted against axon diameter, two clouds will be observed, one with smaller axons and a higher 'g' ratio (i.e. thinner myelin), the other with axons of larger size but relatively thicker myelin sheaths and a lower 'g' ratio (Friede and Beuche, 1985a; Jacobs and Love, 1985). Remyelinated and regenerated fibres both possess relatively thin myelin sheaths in proportion to axon diameter. This is related to their shorter internodal length (Friede and Beuche, 1985b). In some disorders, such as type III hereditary motor and sensory neuropathy (HMSN III), Schwann cells never produce myelin of normal thickness (Dyck *et al.*, 1971c; Guzzetta *et al.*, 1982), the myelin sheath remaining thin (hypomyelination).

Demyelination leads to Schwann cell proliferation. Following remyelination Schwann cells that have failed to remyelinate the axon persist and if remyelination is recurrent they accumulate as a concentric array of laminae with intervening layers of collagen. This constitutes hypertrophic or 'onion bulb' neuropathy (Figure 14.3).

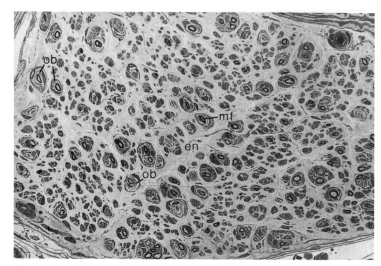

Figure 14.3 Transverse semithin section through sural nerve from a patient with an IgM paraproteinaemic neuropathy showing depletion of the myelinated nerve fibre (mf) population and increased quantities of endoneurial collagen (en). Scattered onion bulbs (ob) are present containing single or multiple myelinated nerve fibres. The presence of multiple fibres within the onion bulbs indicates regenerative sprouting after axonal degeneration. Araldite embedding, thionin and acridine orange stain (magnification × 400).

Probably unmyelinated axons have to become associated with these supernumerary Schwann cells for them to persist.

Dysmyelination

Abnormal myelination is encountered in a variety of neuropathies. One type is the occurrence of focal areas of thickened myelin referred to as tomacula and, although non-specific, they are a particular feature of hereditary neuropathy with liability to pressure palsies (HNPP). They are most easily identified in teased fibre preparations and are the result of redundant folds of myelin that are incorporated, often asymmetrically, within the myelin sheath (Behse *et al.*, 1972; Madrid and Bradley, 1975). A spectacular form of dysmyelination is observed in a rare autosomal recessive form of HMSN characterized by multiple outpouchings of myelin along the internodes (Ohnishi *et al.*, 1989; Gabreëls-Festen *et al.*, 1990). A further example of dysmyelination is the occurrence of abnormally wide spacing of the myelin because of separation at the intermediate dense line (see King and Thomas, 1984). It is virtually pathognomonic of IgM paraproteinaemic neuropathy (Figures 14.4 and 14.5). It has to be distinguished from failure of compaction of myelin when the major dense line is separated by Schwann cell cytoplasm. It is non-specific change, being seen in many demyelinating processes although particularly evident adaxonally in HNPP.

Schwann cell inclusions

Characteristic inclusions are seen in Schwann cells in a variety of inherited neuropathies including metachromatic and Krabbe leukodystrophy, adrenoleukodystrophy and type A Niemann–Pick disease (see Thomas, 1993b). In the past nerve biopsy was helpful in diagnosing these disorders but this is now possible less invasively from leucocyte and serum enzyme studies. Droplets of neutral lipid and deposits of cholesterol esters are observed in Schwann cells in Tangier disease (Kocen *et al.*, 1973; Dyck *et al.*, 1978).

Schwann cells, particularly those associated with unmyelinated and small myelinated axons are colonized by *Mycobacterium leprae* in pluribacillary leprosy. Currently the most satisfactory way of recognizing these is by electron microscopy (Figure 14.6) rather than by acid fast staining of tissue sections. Ultrastructurally, they have a dense core surrounded by a clear halo.

Connective tissue changes

Endoneurial oedema, collagenization and Schwann cell basal laminal changes

Endoneurial oedema is a feature in a variety of neuropathies, being most obtrusive in the presence of extensive acute axonal degeneration and in CIDP (Waddy *et al.*, 1989) when it is most evident subperineurially. Increased endoneurial collagen production is a non-specific consequence of nerve fibre loss. It also occurs if oedema is persistent. In paucibacillary (tuberculoid) leprosy, in which tissue destruction is

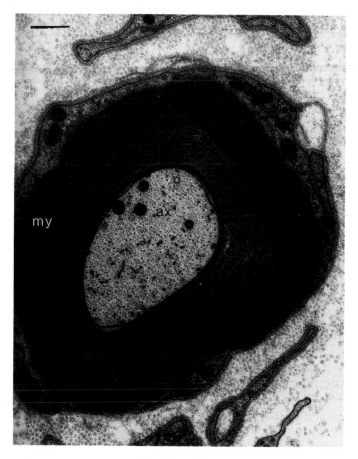

Figure 14.4 Electron micrograph of transverse section through myelinated axon (ax) from a patient with an IgM paraproteinaemic neuropathy. The surrounding myelin displays alternating zones of compact (dark regions) and widely-spaced (light regions) myelin (my). Bar = 0.5μm.

pronounced, in the later stages of the disease the nerve trunks may be virtually replaced by fibrosis, few neural elements being detectable.

When axonal degeneration of Wallerian type occurs, with removal of the myelin and axonal debris, as already stated the basal lamina that had ensheathed the fibre normally collapses and assumes a crenated appearance in transverse section. Schwann cell proliferation occurs within the basal laminal tube preparatory to axonal regeneration. In diabetic neuropathy the basal laminal tube frequently fails to collapse and retains a circular profile. It is also abnormally persistent when regeneration takes place, encircling regenerating clusters of axons (King *et al.*, 1989). This is virtually the only pathognomonic structural appearance for diabetic neuropathy. It is likely that non-enzymatic glycation leads to abnormal cross-linking of proteins in the basal lamina so that it becomes more rigid and also less susceptible to digestion by proteolysis.

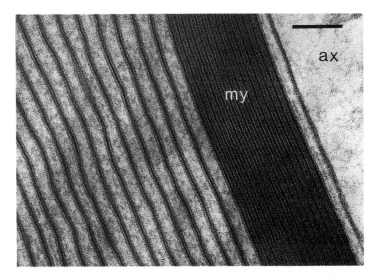

Figure 14.5 Electron micrograph through myelin from a patient with an IgM paraproteinaemic neuropathy. The myelin (my) to the right of the figure has a normal periodicity whereas that to the left shows abnormally wide spacing because of expansion of the space between the major dense lines. ax, axon. Bar = 0.1μm.

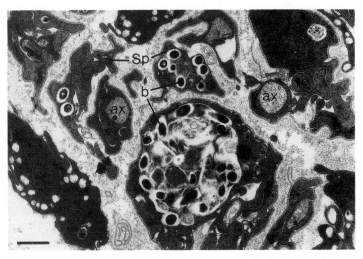

Figure 14.6 Pluribacillary leprosy. Electron micrograph from a sural nerve biopsy. b, multiple *M. leprae* profiles; Sp, Schwann cell processes; ax, unmyelinated axons. Bar = 1μm.

Cellular infiltration

Collections of inflammatory cells may be detected in the endoneurium or in the neighbourhood of epineurial vessels in CIDP (Thomas *et al.*, 1969; Dyck *et al.*, 1975) although in many cases in which this disease seems clinically likely they are not detected. This could reflect sampling difficulty or differences in type of pathology. Such inflammatory cells are most readily demonstrable immunocytochemically when a mixed population of CD4 and CD8 T lymphocytes is usually observed, the CD4 cells predominating.

Infiltration with inflammatory cells is conspicuous in leprosy, affecting the endoneurium, perineurium and epineurium. Highly vacuolated 'foamy' macrophages containing numerous *M. leprae* are characteristic of pluribacillary or lepromatous leprosy and 'epithelioid' macrophages with very rare bacilli of paucibacillary or tuberculoid leprosy.

Granulomata with giant cells may be encountered in sarcoid neuropathy (Nemni *et al.*, 1981; Vital *et al.*, 1982) although this is an uncommon finding. Peripheral nerves may be infiltrated by carcinoma, leukaemic cells or lymphoma (see McLeod 1993a,b), sometimes restricted to the intrafascicular compartment and extending subperineurially. This is more often encountered in spinal roots and the limb girdle plexuses than in biopsies of peripheral nerve trunks

Amyloid infiltration

Both in primary or AL amyloidosis and in the inherited amyloid neuropathies, deposits of amyloid are observed either in relation to the endoneurial and epineurial microvessels or as endoneurial deposits. These have a characteristic appearance in semithin sections, consisting of amorphous masses with irregular margins. They give a positive reaction with Congo red staining and show apple-green birefringence when viewed with polarization optics. It may be possible to identify the nature of the amyloid immunohistochemically, AL amyloid giving a positive reaction with antibodies for kappa or lambda immunoglobulin light chains. Transthyretin-derived amyloid usually gives a positive reaction with appropriate monoclonal antibodies (see Reilly and King, 1993) although false negative results can be obtained.

Perineurium

The lamellated perineurium that surrounds the fascicles may show distinctive changes. The perineurium is often thickened non-specifically in a variety of neuropathies and thickening of the basal laminae of the perineurial cells, although occurring with ageing, is a particular feature of diabetic neuropathy (Johnson *et al.*, 1986). Calcified foci between the lamellae are especially common in diabetes (King *et al.*, 1988). Inflammatory changes restricted to the perineurium are seen in sensory perineuritis (Asbury *et al.*, 1972b) and may occur in vasculitis in which perineurial necrosis is sometimes seen. They also occurred in Spanish oil syndrome (Ricoy *et al.*, 1983). Lamellar inclusions within perineurial cells are a feature of Fabry's disease (Kocen and Thomas, 1970) and xanthomatous deposits may be encountered in primary biliary cirrhosis (Thomas and Walker, 1965).

An unusual disorder to which reference has already been made is focal hypertrophic neurofibrosis in which the nerve trunk is broken up into multiple minifascicles, each surrounded by a perineurial ensheathment (Bilbao *et al.*, 1984; Cusimano *et al.*, 1988). The origin of this appearance is uncertain.

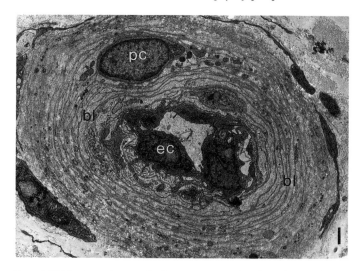

Figure 14.7 Electron micrograph of a transverse section through an endoneur-ial capillary from a patient with diabetic polyneuropathy. The endothelial cells (ec) are surrounded by a wide zone composed of reduplicated basal lamina (bl) containing displaced pericytes (pc). Bar = 1μm. (Reproduced from Bradley *et al.* (1990), with permission.)

Blood vessels

The basal lamina surrounding the endothelial cells of the endoneurial microvessels may become reduplicated in a variety of neuropathies and this also occurs with ageing. It is particularly conspicuous in diabetic neuropathy (Figure 14.7) when it is seen as an amorphous zone surrounding the vessels in semithin sections. It gives a positive reaction to the periodic acid–Schiff (PAS) stain. Proliferation of the endothelial cells of endoneurial capillaries occurs in diabetic and other neuropathies. These cells may be seen to contain lamellar material in Fabry's disease (Ohnishi and Dyck, 1974).

In vasculitis from whatever cause, the walls of the epineurial arterioles are infil-trated with inflammatory cells that extend into the surrounding connective tissues. Vascular leakage may be shown by the histochemical demonstration of fibrin around the vessels.

COMPLICATIONS

Nerve biopsy is invasive and has a significant complication rate. Minor wound infections may occur. For lower-limb biopsies their frequency is probably reduced by keeping the patient in bed for 24 hours after the biopsy. Local thrombophlebitis is occasionally encountered. Although it has been claimed that the extent of sensory loss does not differ between fascicular and total sural nerve biopsies (Pollock *et al.*, 1983) this has not been personal experience or that of others (Stevens and Dyck, 1983). With a restricted fascicular biopsy, it is often not possible to detect any loss. Minor tingling paraesthesias over the lateral side of the heel and along the lateral border of the foot are not infrequent but usually subside after a few months. From a large personal series, painful neuromata or persistent pain have been rare.

The frequency of residual symptoms after sural nerve biopsy was evaluated by questionnaire by Dyck *et al.* (1984). In patients with neuropathy about 60% had no symptoms after 1 year, 30% had mild persisting symptoms which later cleared and 10% had troublesome paraesthesias or pain, although it was considered that some of the symptoms could have been due to the neuropathy and not to the biopsy. Normal subjects having biopsies for control purposes experienced few residual symptoms. In control patients evaluated 5 years after either fascicular or whole sural nerve biopsies by Pollock *et al.* (1983), none had pain, paraesthesias, analgesia or anaesthesia. Contact dysaesthesia to tactile stimulation was a residual symptom in some. Nerve conduction studies suggested that regeneration had taken place whether the patients had had fascicular or total biopsies.

A higher complication rate has been reported in other series. In a survey reported by Poburski *et al.* (1985) on 24 patients who had had total sural nerve biopsies, 14 had persisting discomfort (pain or paraesthesias) in the sural nerve territory. In five the symptoms were rated as severe. However, this study was limited in that it was undertaken on only 29% of the total number of patients biopsied during the 4-year study period, being restricted to those who responded to an invitation to attend for examination. In another survey (Solders, 1988), based on a postal questionnaire sent to 60 patients who had had fascicular sural nerve biopsies out of whom 54 replied, persisting discomfort was reported by six (11%), in three of whom it was graded as severe. Neundörfer *et al.* (1990) were able to examine 56 out of 80 patients who had had a total sural nerve biopsy 6 months to 3 years before. Sensory deficits were reported preoperatively by 30 (53%), paraesthesias and dysaesthesias by 18 (32%) and pain by 16 (28%). At an average time of 21 months postoperatively, persistent sensory loss was found in 52 patients (93%), persistent paraesthesias and dysaesthesias in 17 (30%) and persistent pain in 14 (25%).

Perry and Bril (1994) have recently compared the complication rate from whole nerve and fascicular sural nerve biopsies between 41 patients with diabetic neuropathy and 40 patients with other neuropathies. Of the diabetic patients 22 had a repeat biposy on the same side by extending the incision proximally and three an additional contralateral biopsy. The diabetic patients were followed for a mean of 6.8 years and the non-diabetic for 5.6 years. Mild long-term pain was reported by 18.9% of patients overall with no difference between the two groups. Mild persistent sensory symptoms insufficient to interfere with daily activities were reported significantly more often in the diabetic (63.6%) as compared with the non-diabetic patients. Wound infections and severe pain were uncommon and were not more frequent in the diabetic subjects.

CONCLUSIONS

Peripheral nerve biopsy is now an established and valuable investigative procedure, but as it may give rise to significant residual symptoms it should only be undertaken after careful consideration of the indications and with the informed consent of the patient. Unless it is being undertaken for conditions such as vasculitis or leprosy where routine processing will suffice, nerve biopsies should only be processed and evaluated in a laboratory with particular expertise.

Neundörfer *et al.* (1990) assessed the diagnostic yield in a series of 56 sural nerve biopsies. Of these, in 15 (27%) a diagnosis was reached by the biopsy alone; in 21 (37%) non-specific findings were obtained that nevertheless contributed diagnostically valuable information. In the remaining two cases (4%) the diagnosis remained obscure despite the biopsy. In another series of 53 cases (Argov *et al.*, 1989), sural nerve biopsy contributed to the diagnosis in 20 (38%).

Nerve biopsy is not the only means of sampling peripheral nerve tissue. Thus the introduction of newer technques is likely to make the examination of the innervation of the skin increasingly informative, particularly for research purposes. The same is likely to be true for motor point muscle biopsy. The range of techniques available for the examination of peripheral nerve tissues will undoubtedly continue to expand. This chapter has been confined to the examination of peripheral nerve tissue morphologically. Chemical analysis has also been undertaken, again mainly for research purposes.

REFERENCES

Argov, Z., Steiner I. and Soffer, D. (1989). The yield of sural nerve biopsy in the evaluation of peripheral neuropathies. *Acta Neurol. Scand.*, **79**, 243–245

Aring, C. D., Dean, W. B., Roseman, E. *et al.* (1941). The peripheral nerves in cases of nutritional deficiency. *Arch. Neurol.*, **45**, 772–787

Asbury, A. K., Gale, M. K., Cox, S. C. *et al.* (1972a). Giant axonal neuropathy. A unique case with segmental neurofilamentous masses. *Acta Neuropathol. (Berlin)*, **20**, 237–247

Asbury, A. K., Picard, E. H. and Baringer, J. R. (1972b). Sensory perineuritis. *Arch. Neurol.*, **26**, 302–312

Behse, F., Buchthal, F., Carlsen, F. and Knappeis, G. (1972). Hereditary neuropathy with liability to pressure palsies. Electrophysiological and histopathological aspects. *Brain*, **95**, 777–794

Bilboa, J. M., Khoury, N. J. S, Hudson, A. R. and Briggs, S. J. (1984). Perineurioma (localized hypertrophic neuropathy). *Arch. Pathol. Lab. Med.*, **108**, 557–562

Birch, R. (1963). Peripheral nerve tumors. In *Peripheral Neuropathy*, 3rd edn (P. J. Dyck, P. K. Thomas, J. W. Griffin, P. A. Low, and J. F. Poduslo, eds), pp. 1623–1640, Philadelphia: W. B. Saunders

Bouche, P. and Vallat, J-M. (1992). *Neuropathies Periphériques: Polyneuropathies et Mononeuropathies Multiples.* Paris: Doin

Bradley, J., Thomas, P. K., King, R. H. M. *et al.* (1990). Morphometry of endoneurial capillaries in diabetic sensory and autonomic neuropathy. *Diabetologia*, **33**, 611–618

Carpenter, S., Karpati, G., Andermann, F. *et al.* (1977). The ultrastructural characteristics of the abnormal cytosomes in Batten–Kufs disease. *Brain*, **100**, 137–156

Cascino, T. L., Kori, S., Krol, G. and Foley, K. M. (1983). CT of the brachial plexus in patients with cancer. *Neurology*, **33**, 1553–1557

Coërs, C. and Woolf, A. L. (1959). *The Innervation of Muscle.* Oxford: Blackwell Scientific

Cusimano, M. D., Bilboa, J. M. and Cohen, S. M. (1988). Hypertrophic brachial plexus neuritis: a pathological study of two cases. *Ann. Neurol.*, **24**, 615–622

Donaghy, M., King, R. H. M., Thomas, P. K. and Workman, J. M. (1988). Abnormalities of the axonal cytoskeleton in giant axonal neuropathy. *J. Neurocytol.*, **17**, 197–208

Dyck, P. J. and Lambert, E. H. (1969). Dissociated sensation in amyloidosis. *Arch. Neurol.*, **18**, 619–625

Dyck P. J., Johnson, W. J., Lambert, E. H. and O'Brien, P. C. (1971a). Segmental demyelination secondary to axonal degeneration in uremic neuropathy. *Mayo Clin. Proc.*, **36**, 400–431

Dyck, P. J., Lambert, E. H. and Nichols, P. C. (1971b). Quantitative measurement of sensation related to compound action potential and number and sizes of myelinated and unmyelinated fibers of sural nerve in health, Friedreich's ataxia, hereditary sensory neuropathy, and tabes dorsalis. In *Handbook of Electroencephalography and Clinical Neurophysiology*, Vol. 9 (W. A. Cobb, ed.), pp. 83–118, Amsterdam: Elsevier Publishing Co

Dyck, P. J., Lambert, E. H., Sanders, K. and O'Brien, P. C. (1971c). Severe hypomyelination and marked abnormality of conduction in Dejerine–Sottas hypertrophic neuropathy: myelin thickness and compound action potential of sural nerve in vitro. *Mayo Clin. Proc.*, **46**, 432–436

Dyck, P. J., Lais, A. C., Ohta, M. *et al.* (1975). Chronic inflammatory polyradiculoneuropathy. *Mayo Clin. Proc.*, **50**, 621–637

Dyck, P. J., Ellefson, R. D., Yao, J. K. and Herbert, P. N. (1978). Adult onset Tangier disease: I. Morphometric and pathological studies suggesting delayed degradation of neutral lipids after fiber degeneration. *J. Neuropathol. Exp. Neurol.*, **37**, 119–137

Dyck, P. J., Karnes, J., Lais, A. *et al.* (1984). Pathological alterations of the peripheral nervous system of humans. In *Peripheral Neuropathy*, 2nd edn (P. J. Dyck, P. K. Thomas, E. H. Lambert and R. Bunge, eds), pp. 760–870, Philadelphia: W. B. Saunders

Dyck, P. J., Giannini, C. and Lais, A. (1993). Pathologic alterations in nerves. In *Peripheral Neuropathy*, 3rd edn (P. J. Dyck, P. K. Thomas, J. W. Griffin, P. A. Low and J. F. Poduslo, eds), pp. 514–595, Philadelphia: W. B. Saunders

Engel, A. G. and Santa, T. (1971). Histometric analysis of the ultrastructure of the neuromuscular junction in myasthenia gravis and in the myasthenic syndrome. *Ann. N.Y. Acad. Sci.*, **183**, 46–52

Friede, R. L. and Beuche, W. (1985a). Combined scatter diagrams of sheath thickness and fibre calibre in human sural nerves: changes with age and neuropathy. *J. Neurol. Neurosurg. Psychiatry*, **48**, 749–756

Friede, R. L. and Beuche, W. (1985b). A new approach towards analyzing peripheral nerve fibre populations. I. Variance in sheath thickness corresponds to different geometric proportions of the internodes. *J. Neuropathol. Exp. Neurol.*, **44**, 60–72

Gabreëls-Festen, A. A. W. M., Joosten, E. M. G., Gabreëls, F. J. M. *et al.* (1990). Congenital demyelinating motor and sensory neuropathy and focally folded myelin sheaths. *Brain*, **113**, 1629–1643

Gherardi, R., Benaid, J. P., Mussini, J. M. and Hauw, J. J. (1986). Etude morphométrique de la biopsie du nerf musculo-cutané: résultats normaux. *Arch. Anat. Cytol. Pathol.*, **34**, 261–267

Greenfield, J. G. and Carmichael, E. A. (1935). The peripheral nerves in cases of subacute combined degeneration of the cord. *Brain*, **58**, 483–491

Griffin, J. W., Cornblath, D. R., Alexander, E. *et al.*, (1990). Ataxic sensory neuropathy and dorsal root ganglionitis associated with Sjögren's syndrome. *Ann. Neurol.*, **27**, 304–315

Guzzetta, F., Ferrière, G. and Lyon, G. (1982). Congenital hypomyelination polyneuropathy: pathological findings compared with polyneuropathies starting in late life. *Brain*, **105**, 395–416

Humphrey, C. D. and Pittman, F. E. (1974). A simple methylene blue – azure II – basic fuchsin stain for epoxy-embedded tissue sections. *Stain Technol.*, **49**, 9–12

Jacobs, J. M. and Love, S. (1985). Qualitative and quantitative morphology of human sural nerve at different ages. *Brain*, **108**, 897–924

Johnson, P. C. and Doll, S. C. (1984). Dermal nerves in human diabetic subjects. *Diabetes*, **33**, 244–250

Johnson, P. C., Brendel, K. and Meezan, E. (1986). Human diabetic perineurial basement membrane thickening. *Lab. Invest.*, **44**, 265–270

Kennedy, W. R. and Wendelschafer-Crabb, G. (1993). The innervation of the human epidermis. *J. Neurol. Sci.*, **115**, 184–190

Kennedy, W. R. and Wendelschafer-Crabb, G. (1994). Quantification of nerve in skin biopsies from control and diabetic subjects. *Neurology*, **44** (suppl 2), A275

King, R. H. M. and Thomas, P. K. (1989). The occurrence and significance of myelin with unusually large periodicity. *Acta Neuropathol. (Berlin)*, **63**, 319–329

King, R. H. M., Llewelyn, J. G., Thomas, P. K. *et al.* (1988). Perineurial calcification. *Neuropathol. Exp. Neurol.*, **14**, 105–123

King, R. H. M., Llewelyn, J. G., Thomas, P. K. *et al.* (1989). Diabetic neuropathy: abnormalities of Schwann cell and perineurial basal laminae. Implications for diabetic vasculopathy. *Neuropathol. Appl. Neurobiol.*, **15**, 339–355

Kocen, R. S. and Thomas, P. K. (1970). Peripheral nerve involvement in Fabry's disease. *Arch. Neurol. (Chicago)*, **22**, 81–88

Kocen, R. S., King, R. H. M., Thomas, P. K. and Haas, L. F. (1973). Nerve biopsy findings in two cases of Tangier disease. *Acta Neuropathol. (Berlin)*, **26**, 317–327

Korobkin, R., Asbury, A. K., Sumner, A. J. and Nielsen, S. L. (1975). Glue-sniffing neuropathy. *Arch. Neurol.*, **32**, 158–162

Lamarche, J., Luneau, C. and Lemieux, B. (1982). Ultrastructural observations on spinal ganglion in Friedreich's ataxia: a preliminary report. *Can. J. Neurol. Sci.*, **9**, 137–139

Madrid, R. and Bradley, W. G. (1975). The pathology of neuropathies with focal thickening of the myelin sheath (tomaculous neuropathy): studies on the formation of the abnormal myelin sheath. *J. Neurol. Sci.*, **25**, 415–418

McArthur, J. C., Hsieh, S.-T., McCarthy, B. *et al.* (1994). Quantitation of intra-epidermal nerves in sensory neuropathies and after nerve transection using punch skin biopsies. *Neurology*, **44** (suppl 2), A275

McLeod, J. G. (1971). An electrophysiological and pathological study of peripheral nerves in Freidreich's ataxia. *J. Neurol. Sci.*, **12**, 333–349

McLeod, J. G. (1993a). Paraneoplastic neuropathies. In *Peripheral Neuropathy*, 3rd edn (P. J. Dyck, P. K. Thomas, J. W. Griffin, P. A. Low, and J. F. Poduslo, eds), pp. 1583–1590, Philadelphia: W. B. Saunders

McLeod, J. G. (1993b). Peripheral neuropathy associated with lymphomas, leukemias, and polycythemia vera. In *Peripheral Neuropathy*, 3rd edn, (P. J. Dyck, P. K. Thomas, J. W. Griffin, P. A. Low and J. F. Poduslo, eds), pp. 1591–1598, Philadelphia: W. B. Saunders

Meier, C., Kauer, B., Müller, U. and Ludin, H. P. (1979). Neuromyopathy during chronic amiodarone treatment. A case report. *J. Neurol.*, **220**, 231–239

Mitsumoto, H., Levin, K. H., Wilbourn, A. J. and Chou, S. M. (1990). Hypertrophic mononeuritis clinically presenting with painful legs and moving toes. *Muscle Nerve*, **13**, 215–221

Nemni, R., Galassi, G., Cohen, M. *et al.* (1981). Symmetric sarcoid polyneuropathy: analysis of a sural nerve biopsy. *Neurology*, **31**, 1217–1223

Neundörfer, B., Grahmann, F., Engelgardt, A. and Harte, J. (1990). Postoperative effects and value of sural nerve biopsies: a retrospective study. *Eur. Neurol.*, **30**, 350–352

Ochoa, J. (1980). Nerve fiber pathology in acute and chronic compression. In *Management of Peripheral Nerves Problems* (G. E. Omer and M. Spinner, eds), pp. 487–501, Philadelphia: W. B. Saunders

Ohnishi, A. and Dyck, P. J. (1974). Loss of small peripheral sensory neurons in Fabry's disease. *Arch. Neurol.*, **31**, 120–127

Ohnishi A., Murai, Y., Ikeda, M. *et al.* (1989). Autosomal recessive motor and sensory neuropathy with excessive myelin outfolding. *Muscle Nerve*, **12**, 568–575

O'Sullivan, D. J. and Swallow, M. (1968). The fibre size and content of the radial and sural nerves. *J. Neurol. Neurosurg. Psychiatry*, **31**, 464–470

Perry, J. R. and Bril, V. (1994). Complications of sural nerve biopsy in diabetic versus non-diabetic patients. *Can. J. Neurol. Sci.*, **21**, 34–37

Poburski, R., Malin, J.-P. and Starck, E. (1985). Sequelae of sural nerve biopsies. *Clin. Neurol. Neurosurg.*, **87**, 193–198

Pollock, M., Nukuda, H., Taylor, P. *et al.* (1983). Comparison between fascicular and whole sural nerve biopsy. *Ann. Neurol.*, **13**, 65–68

Prineas, J. W. (1972). Acute idiopathic polyneuritis. An electron microscope study. *Lab. Invest.*, **26**, 133–147

Reilly, M. M. and King, R. H. M. (1993). Familial amyloid polyneuropathy. *Brain Pathol.*, **3**, 165–176

Ricoy, J. R., Cabello, A., Rodriguez, J. and Téllez, I. (1983). Neuropathological studies on the toxic syndrome related to adulterated rapeseed oil in Spain. *Brain*, **106**, 817–835

Said, G. (1978). Perhexilene neuropathy: a clinicopathological study. *Ann. Neurol.*, **3**, 259–266

Said, G., Slama, G. and Selva, J. (1983). Progressive centripetal degeneration of axons in small fibre diabetic neuropathy. *Brain*, **106**, 791–807

Said, G., Gulon-Goeau, C., Lacroix, C. and Moulonguet, A. (1994). Nerve biopsy findings in different patterns of proximal diabetic neuropathy. *Ann. Neurol.*, **35**, 559–569

Sievers, J. (1971). Basic two-dye stains for epoxy-embedded 0.3–1μm sections. *Stain Technol.*, **46**, 195–199

Sima, A. A. F., Bril, V., Nathaniel, V., McLewen, T. A. J. *et al.* (1988). Regeneration and repair of myelinated fibers in sural nerve biopsy specimens from patients with diabetic neuropathy treated with sorbinil. *N. Eng. J. Med.*, **319**, 548–555

Simpson, D. A. and Fowler, M. (1966). Two cases of localized hypertrophic neurofibrosis. *J. Neurol. Neurosurg. Psychiatry*, **29**, 80–93

Small, J. R., Thomas, P. K. and Schapira, A. H. V. (1993). Dorsal root ganglion proteins in Friedreich's ataxia. *Neurosci. Lett.*, **163**, 182–184

Solders, G. (1988). Discomfort after sural nerve fascicular biopsy. *Acta Neurol. Scand.*, **77**, 503–504

Spencer, P. S. and Schaumburg, H. H. (1976). Central-peripheral distal axonopathy – the pathology of dying-back polyneuropathies. *Prog. Neuropathol.*, **3**, 253–295

Stevens, J. C. and Dyck, P. J. (1983). Sensory loss from whole sural nerve biopsy. *Ann. Neurol.*, **14**, 493–494

Stevens, J. C., Lofgren E. P. and Dyck, P. J. (1973). Histometric evaluation of branches of peroneal nerve: technique for combined biopsy of muscle nerve and cutaneous nerve. *Brain Res.*, **52**, 37–45

Swallow, M. (1966). Fibre size and content of the anterior tibial nerve of the foot. *J. Neurol. Neurosurg. Psychiatry*, **29**, 205–213

Thévenard, A. and Berdet, H. (1958). Remarques sur l'hypertrophie des nerfs péripheriques: intérét de l'exploration clinique du plexus cervical superficial en particulier de sans branche auriculaire et son examen histologique après biopsie. *Presse Méd.*, **66**, 529–541

Thomas, P. K. (1971). The quantitation of nerve biopsy findings. *J. Neurol. Sci.*, **11**, 285–295

Thomas, P. K. (1993a). Hereditary sensory neuropathies. *Brain Pathol.*, **3**, 157–163

Thomas P. K. (1993b). Other inherited neuropathies. In *Peripheral Neuropathy*, 3rd edn, (P. J. Dyck, P. K. Thomas, J. W. Griffin, P. A. Low and J. F. Poduslo, eds), pp. 1194–1218, Philadelphia: W. B. Saunders

Thomas, P. K. and Walker, J. G. (1965). Xanthomatous neuropathy in primary biliary cirrhosis. *Brain*, **88**, 1079–1088

Thomas, P. K., Lascelles, R. G., Hallpike, J. F. and Hewer, R. L. (1969). Recurrent and chronic relapsing Guillain–Barré polyneuritis. *Brain*, **92**, 589–606

Thomas, P. K., Hollinrake, K., Lascelles, R. G. *et al.* (1971). The polyneuropathy of chronic renal failure. *Brain*, **94**, 761–780

Thomas, P. K., Landon, D. N. and King, R. H. M. (1992). Diseases of the peripheral nerves. In *Greenfield's Neuropathology*, 5th edn (J. H. Adams and L. W. Duchen, eds), pp. 1116–1245, London: Edward Arnold

Thomas, P. K. and Holdorff, F. (1993). Neuropathy due to physical agents. In *Peripheral Neuropathy*, 3rd edn (P. J. Dyck, P. K. Thomas, J. W. Griffin, P. A. Low and J. F. Poduslo, eds), pp. 990–1013, Philadelphia: W. B. Saunders

Vital, C. and Vallat, J.-M. (1987). *Ultrastructural Study of the Human Diseased Peripheral Nerve*, 2nd edn. New York: Elsevier

Vital, C., Aubertin, J. M., Ragnault, J. M. *et al.* (1982). Sarcoidosis of the peripheral nerve: a histological and ultrastructural study of two cases. *Acta Neuropathol. (Berlin)*, **58**, 111-114

Waddy, H. M., Misra, V. P., King, R. H. M. *et al.* (1989). Focal cranial nerve involvement in chronic inflammatory demyelinating polyneuropathy: clinical and MRI evidence of peripheral and central lesions. *J. Neurol.*, **236**, 400–410

Index